Sexual Grooming

AF180415

Georgia M. Winters • Elizabeth L. Jeglic

Sexual Grooming

Integrating Research, Practice, Prevention, and Policy

Springer

Georgia M. Winters
School of Psychology and Counseling
Fairleigh Dickinson University
Teaneck, NJ, USA

Elizabeth L. Jeglic
Department of Psychology
John Jay College of Criminal Justice
New York, NY, USA

ISBN 978-3-031-07224-6 ISBN 978-3-031-07222-2 (eBook)
https://doi.org/10.1007/978-3-031-07222-2

© The Editor(s) (if applicable) and The Author(s), under exclusive license to Springer Nature Switzerland AG 2022
This work is subject to copyright. All rights are solely and exclusively licensed by the Publisher, whether the whole or part of the material is concerned, specifically the rights of translation, reprinting, reuse of illustrations, recitation, broadcasting, reproduction on microfilms or in any other physical way, and transmission or information storage and retrieval, electronic adaptation, computer software, or by similar or dissimilar methodology now known or hereafter developed.
The use of general descriptive names, registered names, trademarks, service marks, etc. in this publication does not imply, even in the absence of a specific statement, that such names are exempt from the relevant protective laws and regulations and therefore free for general use.
The publisher, the authors and the editors are safe to assume that the advice and information in this book are believed to be true and accurate at the date of publication. Neither the publisher nor the authors or the editors give a warranty, expressed or implied, with respect to the material contained herein or for any errors or omissions that may have been made. The publisher remains neutral with regard to jurisdictional claims in published maps and institutional affiliations.

This Springer imprint is published by the registered company Springer Nature Switzerland AG
The registered company address is: Gewerbestrasse 11, 6330 Cham, Switzerland

This book is dedicated to the survivors, families, and communities who have been impacted by child sexual abuse who motivate us to find ways in which we intervene before the abuse occurs, and provide support to those who have been affected by abuse; to our families, whose unwavering support have allowed us to devote our careers to sexual violence prevention; to our mentors, colleagues, and students who have provided guidance and assistance every step of the way; and to the researchers, professionals, and organizations who are dedicated to understanding, investigating, prosecuting, treating, and preventing child sexual abuse.

Acknowledgment

A special thank you to doctoral student Caitlin Krause, our editorial assistant, for the many hours she has dedicated to making this book a reality; this book would not be possible without her motivation and commitment to producing literature that can help others understand and prevent sexual violence.

Contents

About the Authors

Georgia M. Winters is an Assistant Professor in the School of Psychology and Counseling at Fairleigh Dickinson University (FDU) and serves as the director of the forensic psychology master's program at FDU. She received her Ph.D. in clinical psychology from John Jay College of Criminal Justice and the City University of New York, The Graduate Center. Dr. Winters has been conducting research related to sexual offending and the prevention of sexual violence for over a decade, and she is one of the foremost experts in sexual grooming along with Dr. Elizabeth Jeglic. She is the director of a research lab at FDU targeting prevention of sexual violence. Dr. Winters has published over 40 peer-reviewed publications and book chapters. Moreover, she has conducted clinical evaluations and treatment with individuals who have committed or been victimized by sexual violence during her predoctoral internship at University of Massachusetts Medical School and postdoctoral training at the Institute of Law, Psychiatry and Public Policy at the University of Virginia.

Elizabeth L. Jeglic is Professor of Psychology at John Jay College of Criminal Justice in New York. She received her doctorate in clinical psychology from Binghamton University. Dr. Jeglic conducts research on sexual violence prevention and evidence-based public policy and along with Dr. Georgia Winters is one of the foremost experts on sexual grooming. She has published over 140 peer-reviewed articles and book chapters. Dr. Jeglic is the co-author/editor of five books: *Handbook of Youth Suicide Prevention* (Springer, 2022); *Handbook of Issues in Criminal Justice Reform in the United States* (Springer, 2021); *New Frontiers in Offender Treatment: The Translation of Evidence Based Practices to Correctional Settings* (Springer, 2018); *Sexual Offending: Evidence Based Legislation and Prevention* (Springer 2016), and *Protecting your Child from Sexual Abuse: What You Need to Know to Keep your Kids Safe* (Skyhorse, 2018). She is the former Associate Editor of the journal *Sexual Abuse* and is on the editorial board of *Sexual Abuse* and *Psychology, Public Policy and Law*. Along with Dr. Cynthia Calkins, she is co-director of the Sex Offender Research Lab (SORL). She was awarded the Fay Honey Knopp Award from the New York State Association for the Treatment of Sexual Abusers for her contributions to the prevention of sexual violence.

Chapter 1
Introduction

In the United States (US), the estimated lifetime prevalence for child sexual abuse (CSA) is 26.6% for girls and 5.1% for boys (Finkelhor et al., 2014). It is believed that as many as half of these CSA cases involved elements of pre-offense behaviors utilized by the individual to facilitate the sexual abuse, a process known as "sexual grooming" (Canter et al., 1998; Groth & Birnbaum, 1978; Winters & Jeglic, 2021). While the exact definition of the term varies (see Chap. 3), sexual grooming is typically used to describe the behaviors or tactics a person may use in preparation for committing a sex crime against a minor (e.g., Craven et al., 2006; McAlinden, 2013; van Dam, 2001). These behaviors are used to manipulate the potential victim and those around them in order to more easily enact the sexual abuse. Of note, in this book we will be using the terms "child sexual grooming" and "sexual grooming" interchangeably to refer to the tactics an individual may use in preparation for sexual abuse of the minor.

The aims of sexual grooming are to ultimately prevent detection from others and disclosure from the victim, as well as to facilitate future abuse of the minor. As such, it is difficult to establish true prevalence rates of these behaviors. Nonetheless, several empirical studies have sought to provide some evidence as to the frequency of which these tactics are used in cases of CSA. Groth and Birnbaum (1978) categorized 175 adults with CSA offenses based on the methods they used to lure their victims into the sexual abuse. Results suggested that in 30% of cases, the individual used "seduction" and "enticement" strategies (e.g., bribes, rewards, use of authority) to facilitate the sexual abuse. Canter et al. (1998) coded 97 police records of CSA cases and found that 45% involved intimate (i.e., grooming) behaviors, as defined by the authors as desensitization, affection, reassurance, the promise of gifts, kissing, and oral sex performed by the individual on the victim. Of note, these studies were published more than two decades ago and thus likely reflect an underestimate of the number of CSA cases that involve sexual grooming. The understanding and operationalization of grooming-like behaviors in these studies may not fully encapsulate the current conceptualization of the construct, as the current literature

© The Author(s), under exclusive license to Springer Nature Switzerland AG 2022

G. M. Winters, E. L. Jeglic, *Sexual Grooming*,
https://doi.org/10.1007/978-3-031-07222-2_1

on sexual grooming includes far more potential behaviors than were examined in these studies (Winters et al., 2020). Moreover, these numbers likely underrepresent the prevalence given that they only capture sexual grooming rates in reported cases of CSA, meaning cases that were *not* reported to law enforcement were not included in these estimates. Indeed, a recent pilot study of a newly developed self-report measure of sexual grooming (*Sexual Grooming Scale – Victim Version*) by Winters and Jeglic (2021) found that 99% of a sample of 100 adult victims of CSA self-reported having experienced at least one sexual grooming behavior during the offense process, with an average of 15 out of 42 possible behaviors being reported by the victims. However, this study included a relatively small sample size consisting of adult undergraduate students who endorsed experiencing CSA; therefore, the results may not be fully representative of victims' experiences of sexual grooming. In sum, while the exact prevalence rates are largely undetermined, sexual grooming has nevertheless become a construct that has become synonymous with the process of CSA (McAlinden, 2013; Thornton, 2003).

Broadly speaking, as outlined in Fig. 1.1, sexual grooming can be conceptualized in five overarching stages that describe the tactics used throughout the process which is based on the content-validated Sexual Grooming Model (SGM; see Chap. 2; Winters et al., 2020). First, the adult seeks to identify a potential victim based on psychological, emotional, and environmental vulnerabilities. Second, the individual will attempt to gain access to the victim and then isolate him/her from others. Third, in the trust development phase, the individual seeking to commit the sexual offense deceptively creates an emotional attachment with the potential victim and those around the child. Fourth, the child is gradually exposed to sexual content and physical contact over time in order to desensitize him/her to sexualized acts before the impending abuse. Fifth, after the initial sexual abuse incident, the adult may seek to maintain the sexual grooming of the child to prevent them from disclosing the abuse and/or to continue ongoing sexual abuse of the victim.

These overarching steps involved in the grooming process may be used by an adult to lure the child victim into sexual abuse. However, it is important to note that sexual grooming is a complex and nuanced process that varies widely in terms of the behaviors used and the time spent grooming the child. While the adult may progress sequentially through the stages outlined above, it is likely that many would simultaneously use tactics from multiple stages (e.g., continue to use trust development techniques intertwined with sexual desensitization tactics), vacillate between the stages (e.g., select a new victim if they have difficulty gaining access to their selected target), or skip certain stages if not applicable in their situation (e.g., a family member living with the child has a preselected victim whom they have access to). The stages and/or specific behaviors used in the process may also differ depending on the characteristics of the adult and minor. For example, it has been suggested that males and females who commit CSA may employ different types of sexual grooming behaviors (Love & Fremouw, 2009; see Chap. 9). Additionally, the adult may use age-specific tactics with the minor they are sexually grooming, such as providing an adolescent with alcohol or drugs and pornography (Christiansen & Blake, 1990). Contextual (e.g., the relationship between the adult and victim; the

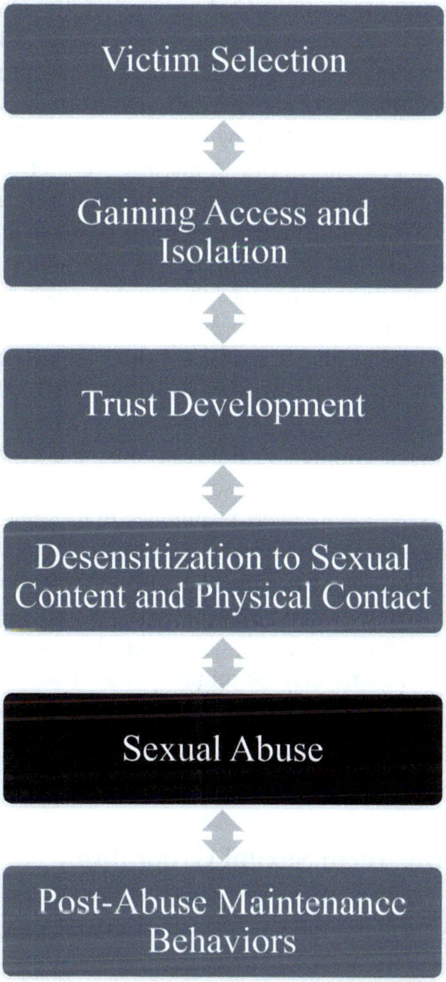

Fig. 1.1 Stages of sexual grooming

setting in which the sexual grooming is occurring) and cultural factors (e.g., socio-economic status, religious and cultural beliefs, and practices) may further influence the sexual grooming process. Regarding the context, sexual grooming differs depending on whether these behaviors occur in-person versus online (see Chap. 5; Davidson, & Gottschalk, 2011). The relationship between the adult and minor can also have an impact on which sexual grooming behaviors are employed; though strangers may use sexual grooming tactics, there may be more extensive sexual grooming involved in cases where the perpetrator is a relative or acquaintance (McAlinden, 2006). Lastly, as sexual grooming is designed to increase the likelihood the individual goes unnoticed, the "effectiveness" of the strategies and fear of disclosure will drive the types of behaviors used, and the timing for when the sexual abuse will occur (Conte et al., 1989; Elliott et al., 1995).

While the adult aiming to commit CSA may generally adhere to the five overarching stages, it is clear that there are nonetheless many variations and permutations of behaviors and tactics employed in the sexual grooming process, and thus one case of sexual grooming can look very different from the next. In turn, this can result in difficulty identifying some of the more nuanced and subtle tactics. Sexual grooming is difficult to recognize prior to the discovery or disclosure of CSA, as many of these behaviors are similar to normal adult/child interactions but with underlying deviant sexual motivations. Empirical research has shown there is a hindsight bias related to sexual grooming, in that individuals tend to overestimate the likelihood they would have recognized these behaviors before learning that sexual abuse indeed occurred (Winters & Jeglic, 2016). Moreover, there is further evidence to suggest that people have a difficult time identifying sexual grooming behaviors as potentially predatory (Winters & Jeglic, 2017), although they may be more likely to deem behaviors related to isolation (e.g., taking select children to get ice cream, accompanying children to the restroom) and desensitization to touch (e.g., having children sit on their lap, horse playing with children, hugging) as inappropriate compared to the more covert techniques (e.g., selecting vulnerable children, trust development tactics; Winters & Jeglic, 2016). Not only are these behaviors not easily recognized by others, but also the likelihood of the victim disclosing the abuse may be reduced when sexual grooming behaviors are present (Terry, 2008; van Dam, 2001). Then, even if concern is raised by the victim or those around the child, these reports may be minimized as it would be unlikely for law enforcement to be able to intervene if sexual abuse has not yet taken place (Salter, 1995).

1.1 History of the Term Sexual Grooming

Historically, dating back to the 1800s, the term "grooming" was used in reference to preparing or mentoring an individual for a specific career, or process of beatifying oneself or animals (British Broadcasting Corporation [BBC], 2008). Yet today, this term is now commonly associated with sexual offenses committed against a minor (Thornton, 2003). It is unknown at what exact point of time the term sexual grooming became part of the lexicon of CSA (McAlinden, 2013). Burgess and Hartman (2017) proposed the term originated from Ken Lanning in the Federal Bureau of Investigation Academy's Behavioral Science Unit in the 1970s. Lanning (2010) described that historically the term "seduction" was used to describe the behavior of adults who engaged in sexual grooming, which he argues may be the more appropriate term given that it is more easily understood and common in vernacular. Others have suggested that the term was first associated with CSA in a 1985 Chicago Tribune article that noted, "These 'friendly molesters' become acquainted with their targeted victim, gaining their trust while secretly grooming the child as a sexual partner" (BBC, 2008).

Regardless of the exact origin, sexual grooming has since been deemed "a ubiquitous feature of the sexual abuse of children" (Thornton, 2003, p. 144). Other terms used to describe sexual grooming include "entrapment," "engagement," "subjection," "coercive control," or "enticement" (Bennett & O'Donohue, 2014; Conte, 2018; Gallagher, 1998; Howitt, 1995; Kierkegaard, 2008; Salter, 1995). The term has been used as a noun (i.e., "sexual groomer," "sexual grooming"), verb (i.e., "sexually groom a victim"), and adjective (i.e., "the sexually groomed victim"; Burgess & Hartman, 2017). It has been suggested that the evolution of the term over time has improved both victims' and the public's understanding of the complex reactions victims may have to their sexual abuse (Burgess & Hartman, 2017), and it may explain why a person may not disclose the abuse. This information has been helpful for both clinical contexts (e.g., understanding the victim's experiences), as well as the criminal justice system (e.g., law enforcement profiling cases of CSA).

In the 1990s, the concept of sexual grooming became increasingly used in the mainstream media. With the surge of the Internet, there was concern about individuals who target potential victims and sexually groom them through online chatrooms (BBC, 2008). Subsequently, empirical research and theoretical literature on the subject of in-person and online grooming began to proliferate in the 2000s (Craven et al., 2006; McAlinden, 2007). Throughout the past two decades, the use of the term sexual grooming has become increasingly popular in cultures across the world (Burgess & Hartman, 2017), in large part due to several high-profile cases in the US and other countries. These well-known cases of CSA often contain evidence showing the individual who committed the abuse went undiscovered for years (decades, in some cases), despite numerous "red flags" in the individual's behaviors toward children. It was hypothesized that the elusiveness in these high-profile cases was due to these manipulative, pre-offense behaviors, which ultimately led to the term sexual grooming becoming a part of common vernacular.

1.2 Public Recognition of Sexual Grooming

1.2.1 The Case of Jerry Sandusky

One of the most prominent cases that put the concept of grooming on the global map was that of Jerry Sandusky. Sandusky was a Pennsylvania State University (Penn State) assistant football coach from 1969 to 1999. In 2011, the nation was stunned by accusations of numerous counts of CSA committed against at least eight male victims during a 15-year period spanning from 1994 to 2009. Sandusky was convicted of 45 CSA-related counts for these crimes and sentenced to 30–60 years in prison (see CNN, 2020 for a detailed description of the counts). Through the publicization of this case, the term sexual grooming moved to the forefront of society, as it soon became clear that Sandusky had utilized sexual grooming behaviors to help avoid detection and disclosure from his victims for over a decade. To further

Victim Selection

- At-risk youth (e.g., troubled, needy)
- In need of a "father figure"
- Lacked supervision

Gaining Access and Isolation

- Involvement in youth-serving organization (e.g., Second Mile, foster care)
- Activities alone with the child (e.g., driving children; workouts in the athletic facility)
- Overnight outings

Trust Development

- Presenting as likable (e.g., "nice guy"; "pillar of the community")
- Giving them attention/affection
- Relating to the child on their level (e.g., playing in the pool; telling jokes)
- Giving gifts (e.g., trips to games, money, games)

Desensitization to Sexual Content and Physical Touch

- Watching child undressing
- Exposing naked body
- Seemingly innocent touch (e.g., kissing and hugging; "horse playing")
- Increasing sexual touching over time (e.g., escalating to showering with the boys)

Post-Abuse Maintenance Behaviors

- Threatened to harm the victim and his family if they alerted anyone to the abuse
- Affection (e.g., telling the boys he loves them)

Fig. 1.2 Sexual grooming behaviors in the Jerry Sandusky case

elucidate this case, the sexual grooming behaviors documented in this incident are summarized in Fig. 1.2 and described in-depth in text.

1.2.1.1 Selecting a Vulnerable Victim

Sandusky targeted at-risk youth who were perceived as needy or troubled and/or came from difficult family situations. In 1977, Sandusky founded a nonprofit organization, The Second Mile, which provided millions of dollars in support to as many as 100,000 underprivileged youth annually (ESPN, 2011; Gladwell, 2012). Most of his victims were at-risk children he met through The Second Mile organization, typically those without a father figure and who were 8–12 years of age (O'Neill, 2012). Court records further outlined the vulnerabilities of his victims, including that three resided in public housing, three were in foster homes, and one resided in a trailer with his single mother (O'Neill, 2012). In a *New York Times* article, it was noted that Sandusky screened potential victims to select those who lacked supervision; he asked the young boys if they wanted to stay after school, and those who were not able to stay without parental permission were "screened out" by Sandusky. Moreover, Sandusky even adopted one boy whom he previously sexually abused (Moody, 2015). The boy had been using illicit substances and alcohol and was sent to a juvenile detention center. Sandusky then adopted the boy who moved into his family home, where he continued to abuse the child.

1.2.1.2 Gaining Access and Isolation

As noted above, Sandusky used his roles within youth-serving organizations to gain access to his victims. He utilized his position at Penn State and The Second Mile organization to have contact with children, including at special events and youth football camps. He even continued to be actively engaged in these organizations following his retirement from Penn State. In a Penn State report, they acknowledged that Penn State "empowered Sandusky to attract potential victims by allowing him to have unrestricted and unsupervised access to the University's facilities and affiliation with the University's prominent football program. Indeed, the continued access provided Sandusky with the very currency that enabled him to attract his victims" (Dutton, 2012).

Regarding isolation, once Sandusky had access to a potential victim, he would create situations in which he could be alone with the child without other adults. As examples, he would offer to drive the child home or bring the child for individual workouts at the Penn State athletic facilities. Penn State acknowledges in their internal report that Sandusky had sexually assaulted a number of his victims on Penn State's campus locations. Additionally, Sandusky utilized overnight stays and outings to get time alone with the victims, including having young boys stay in his basement bedroom or bringing the victims to a hotel room.

1.2.1.3 Trust Development

First and foremost, Sandusky was highly respected in the community due to his involvement with the Penn State football team and his charitable work. He was well liked by most due to his "goofiness" (Gladwell, 2012). He even received a presidential award from President George H. W. Bush for the charitable work he did through The Second Mile. Sandusky showed the boys attention and affection; he was noted to kiss one of his victims on his head and say "I love you" and write "love letters" to another victim. One victim described viewing Sandusky as a "father figure" (O'Neill, 2012). Sandusky made efforts to relate to his victims through childlike activities, such as shuffleboard, video games, playing in the pool, and telling jokes (Moody, 2015). Sandusky took the boys on fun outings, such as Penn State football games, picnics, tailgate parties, and meals at restaurants. He would also provide the victims with gifts and rewards, such as money, athletic apparel, games, clothing, and electronics (O'Neill, 2012).

1.2.1.4 Desensitization to Sexual Content and Physical Contact

Evidence showed that Sandusky desensitized his victims to sexual content and physical contact gradually over time. He engaged in seemingly innocent touch, such as frequently "horse playing" with the children or placing his hand on their knees during car rides (Gladwell, 2012). Sandusky reportedly kissed the boys atop their heads and blew "raspberries" on their stomachs. He would also hug, tickle, and cuddle with his victims (Danahy, 2011; Gladwell, 2012; Moody, 2015); Sandusky even sometimes called himself "the Tickle Monster". Sandusky would then increase the intensity of the sexual contact over time. CNN (2012) reported that he would grope the boys down their shorts in the swimming pool, give "naked bear hugs," and start soap fights in the shower of the locker room. Records indicate that in one instance in 1998, Sandusky invited an 11-year-old boy from The Second Mile to the athletic facility at Penn State. He drove the boy to the facility where they worked out on exercise machines and wrestled together. This eventually led to one of the most infamous sexual grooming tactics used by Sandusky, which involved him showering naked with his victims at the athletic facility following workouts. In this particular case, he "wrapped his hands around the boy's chest" and "lifted the boy to 'get the soap out of' the boy's hair" in the shower.

1.2.1.5 Post-abuse Maintenance

Sandusky was known to engage in post-abuse maintenance behaviors in an effort to prevent the victims from disclosing. One victim described during his testimony that Sandusky threatened him, stating that he would remain in foster care and not see his family if he told anyone about the abuse (O'Neill, 2012). Moreover, Sandusky was known to continue abusing the boys over time with ongoing gifts ("perks" as one victim put it) and told the boys he loved them.

In sum, the Penn State Sandusky scandal drew the attention of the public globally. With clear evidence of sexual grooming, many were left wondering how this pervasive abuse was not recognized sooner. One particularly interesting circumstance of this case was that concerns *had* been raised about Sandusky's behavior with young boys one decade before he was formally charged. In 1998, the Penn State police, alongside the Pennsylvania Department of Public Welfare, investigated a reported incident committed by Sandusky (CNN, 2020; Gladwell, 2012). A mother of an 11-year-old boy raised concerns that Sandusky showered with her son. Sandusky was subsequently interviewed by a psychologist, Alycia Chambers, who concluded this was "likely pedophile's pattern of building trust and gradual introduction of physical touch, within a context of a 'loving,' 'special' relationship (Gladwell, 2012)." However, a caseworker assigned to the incident, Jerry Laura, reported that he disagreed with the psychologist's assessment, noting these behaviors were in the "gray" area related to "boundary issues." An evaluation of the boy was conducted by a counselor, John Seasock, who indicated, "There seems to be no incident which could be termed as sexual abuse, nor did there appear to be any sequential pattern of logic and behavior which is usually consistent with adults who have difficulty with sexual abuse of children." Seasock stated he did not see evidence of sexual grooming and rather Sandusky should be informed about how to "stay out of such gray area situations in the future." Ultimately, Sandusky admitted to showering with the boy but denied any further wrongdoing and assured the behavior would not happen again. The district attorney determined no formal criminal charges should be filed and advised the Penn State police chief to close the case. The discrepancy between trained professionals and the failure to detect Sandusky's abusive behavior resulting in over a decade more of sexual abuse clearly demonstrates the difficulty of recognizing and preventing these potentially predatory behaviors.

1.2.2 *Sexual Grooming Cases in the Spotlight*

Sadly, the Sandusky case is not an anomaly as reports of sexual abuse in the media are a daily occurrence. One of the more recent high-profile cases involving grooming was that of Larry Nassar, the former US Gymnastics national team doctor (Hauser & Zraick, 2019). Following a 2016 investigation by the *Indianapolis Star*, there were hundreds of female victims who accused Nassar of sexually abusing them over the course of three decades (Evans et al., 2018). Nassar used the guise of medical practice to commit inappropriate sexual contact against young gymnasts. Like Sandusky, Nassar was a valued member of the community, who was respected and liked by many; he was deemed the National Contributor of the Year from the US Elite Coaches Association and noted to be a "highly respected, visible, eager osteopathic physician." Victim testimony revealed that Nassar created situations in which he was alone with potential victims (e.g., inviting a young girl to his home for an alleged medical study). He would provide victims with candy, gifts, and emotional support (Lapook, 2018) and send private messages via email and texting (Evans et al., 2018). Eventually, he would increase touching over time, mainly under the guise of medical practice, such as massaging private areas and conducting invasive pelvic examinations that were not medically necessary (Evans et al., 2018).

On a larger scale, there have been numerous sexual abuse scandals among global and national organizations that have involved sexual grooming. For the past two decades, there have been documented cases of sexual grooming involving CSA in the Catholic Church in both media and empirical research. Research conducted on a large sample of CSA cases in the Catholic Church found that these premeditated behaviors (i.e., sexual grooming) were not uncommon in that setting (Terry &

Tallon, 2004; Winters et al., 2022). Another study found that priests convicted of CSA had used tactics such as providing alcohol, cigarettes, or drugs to the victim, going on overnight stays and trips, establishing trusting relationships with the victim's family, showing favoritism, physical playing, gift giving, and misusing the respect and authority of their position (see Chap. 8; Spraitz & Bowen, 2018). Similarly, the Boy Scouts of America is currently facing nearly 100,000 claims of sexual abuse said to have been committed by scoutmasters and volunteers. It was reported that 81% of these cases involved grooming techniques (Abused in Scouting, 2020).

Not only has there been an increase in attention to in-person grooming, but also the notion of adults sexually grooming children online has drawn considerable attention. In 2004, a new Dateline NBC television show, To Catch a Predator, featured host Chris Hansen confronting individuals attempting to meet minors they conversed with on the Internet. These so-called "sting" operations were in partnership with a volunteer organization, Perverted Justice, which trained adults to pose as child decoys in chatrooms. This show, along with individual cases in the media, has highlighted the potential dangers of children in online forums. More recently, with children having increased access to social media and online gaming, there has been a rise in children being targeted through these online platforms (BBC, 2019).

Ultimately, all these cases of online and in-person sexual grooming that have flooded the media in recent years have led to the public becoming more aware of the role of sexual grooming in CSA. It is hard for many to understand how adults who commit sexual abuse can go undetected for so long and how these sexual grooming behaviors are not recognized sooner. In order to better prevent CSA before it occurs or to stop ongoing abuse, it is paramount that these potentially observable and identifiable pre-offense behaviors be better understood. Clearly, there remains a great need to better examine these elusive pre-offense behaviors in an effort to prevent CSA.

1.3 Conclusion

There has been increased attention to the concept of sexual grooming in recent decades, yet there remains much to be explored about this construct. To date, there have been notable advances in the empirical literature of online grooming due to the increased use of the Internet by minors; however, in-person grooming has somewhat fallen to the wayside. A significant portion of the in-person sexual grooming literature has included theoretical reviews (e.g., Bennett & O'Donohue, 2014; Craven et al., 2006), and of the few empirical studies that have been conducted, many are outdated and may not reflect the current conceptualization of the term (e.g., Berliner & Conte, 1990; Conte et al., 1989; Elliott et al., 1995). Despite the importance of the subject, sexual grooming remains an understudied phenomenon, and there remains confusion in the field as to the true definition and conceptualization of the term. To this end, in this book we aim to provide an in-depth examination of the current understanding and research regarding sexual grooming.

Below, we provide an overview of the remaining content of this book:

> The book will begin in Chap. 2 with a review of existing models that have been developed to describe the sexual grooming process, including a more detailed description of the SGM (Winters et al., 2020). Chapter 3 will review previously proposed definitions and culminate in the proposal of our new operational definition based upon the SGM. In Chap. 4, we will focus on the developing research examining the impact that sexual grooming may have on its victims at the individual, family, and community levels. The advent of the Internet has given those aiming to commit sexual offenses against children access to large numbers of victims on online platforms (e.g., gaming, social media, chatrooms); therefore, Chap. 5 will review what is known about online sexual grooming, including a discussion regarding how it differs from in-person grooming. Chapters 6, 7 and 8 will investigate what is known about self (i.e., as personal grooming or self-grooming in order to justify, deny, or minimize the harm caused by their abuse), familial and community (i.e., strategies that perpetrators use to groom a child's family and community so that they may gain access victims and prevent detection or disclosure), and institutional grooming (i.e., individuals who commit non-familial CSA working in child-serving organizations, such as Boy Scouts of America, educators, coaches, etc.). For Chaps. 9, 10, 11 and 12, we focus on sexual grooming for specific populations, including females who commit CSA, juveniles who commit CSA, and sexual grooming of adult victims. Chapter 13 is a clinically focused chapter that will provide an overview of assessment tools, including the newly developed *Sexual Grooming Scale–Victim Version* (Winters & Jeglic, 2021), and strategies for treatment of victims of CSA and those who have been convicted of sexual abuse involving sexual grooming. Chapter 14 will use the Centers for Disease Control and Prevention (CDC)'s socioecological model to highlight sexual grooming efforts to prevent grooming at the individual, relational, community, and societal level. Chapters 15 and 16 address the role that sexual grooming plays in law enforcement and the courts, as well as the importance of national and international legislation designed to punish those who engage in sexual grooming. Lastly, the book will conclude with Chap. 17, which will summarize the most important conclusions about the current state of the sexual grooming field, as well as propose future directions for the research and prevention of sexual grooming.

This book is a research-oriented book addressing the problem of sexual grooming in cases of CSA. We believe having a comprehensive review of sexual grooming is important for various areas of practice, including research, primary prevention, clinical work, law enforcement, and policy. Improved empirical research on sexual grooming can further our understanding of the construct, which can provide evidence-based data for what the process entails and how to intervene and treat these individuals. Knowledge of sexual grooming can help children, caregivers, and those working closely with children (e.g., teachers, doctors, coaches) recognize potentially concerning behaviors of adults toward children before the abuse occurs. Clinicians can utilize this information when assessing or treating victims of CSA, as well as those adults who used sexual grooming in their offense process. Criminal justice agencies may improve their investigation and prosecution of CSA cases with aspects of sexual grooming. Lastly, policies and legislation regarding sexual grooming can be improved based on a solid understanding of what this process may entail. All of these important domains would benefit from a comprehensive examination of the construct of sexual grooming, and thus, we hope the information will be of use to numerous audiences including scholars, academics, students, mental health providers, and organizations that address sexual violence prevention.

References

Abused in Scouting. (2020, March 13). *BSA scouting abuse statistics: Looking at the facts. Abused in Scouting.* https://abusedinscouting.com/bsa-scouting-abuse-statistics-looking-at-thefacts/#:~:text=The%20average%20age%20of%20a,BSA%20was%20twelve%20years%20old.&text=96%25%20of%20the%20abuse%20was,techniques%20and%20situations%20were%20involved

Bennett, N., & O'Donohue, W. (2014). The construct of grooming in child sexual abuse: Conceptual and measurement issues. *Journal of Child Sexual Abuse: Research, Treatment, & Program Innovations for Victims, Survivors, & Offenders, 23*(8), 957–976. https://doi.org/10.1080/10538712.2014.960632

Berliner, L., & Conte, J. R. (1990). The process of victimization: The victims' perspective. *Child Abuse & Neglect, 14*(1), 29–40. https://doi.org/10.1016/0145-2134(90)90078-8

British Broadcasting Corporation. (2008, December 1). When did 'grooming' become a dirty word. *BBC.* http://news.bbc.co.uk/2/hi/uk_news/magazine/7758292.stm

British Broadcasting Corporation [BBC]. (2019, March 1). *Instagram biggest for child grooming online – NSPCC finds.* https://www.bbc.com/news/uk-47410520

Burgess, A. W., & Hartman, C. R. (2017). On the origin of grooming. *Journal of Interpersonal Violence, 33*(1), 17–23. https://doi.org/10.1177/0886260517742048f

Canter, D., Hughes, D., & Kirby, S. (1998). Paedophilia: Pathology, criminality, or both? The development of a multivariate model of offence behaviour in child sexual abuse. *Journal of Forensic Psychiatry, 9*(3), 532–555. https://doi.org/10.1080/09585189808405372

Christiansen, J. R., & Blake, R. H. (1990). The grooming process in father – Daughter incest. In A. L. Horton, B. L. Johnson, L. M. Roundey, & D. Williams (Eds.), *The incest perpetrator: A family member no one wants to treat* (pp. 88–98). Sage Publications.

CNN. (2012, June 17). 'The Sandusky 8' describe seduction, molestation and betrayal. *CNN.* https://www.cnn.com/2012/06/17/justice/sandusky-trial-first-week-wrap/index.html

CNN. (2020, July 1). Penn State scandal fast facts. *CNN.* https://www.cnn.com/2013/10/28/us/penn-state-scandal-fast-facts/index.html

Conte, J. R. (2018). Words matter: Introduction to a commentary on grooming. *Journal of Interpersonal Violence, 33*(1), 3–4. https://doi.org/10.1177/0886260517742039

Conte, J. R., Wolf, S., & Smith, T. (1989). What sexual offenders tell us about prevention strategies. *Child Abuse & Neglect, 13*(2), 293–301. https://doi.org/10.1016/0145-2134(89)90016-1

Craven, S., Brown, S., & Gilchrist, E. (2006). Sexual grooming of children: Review of literature and theoretical considerations. *Journal of Sexual Aggression, 12*(3), 287–299. https://doi.org/10.1080/13552600601069414

Danahy, A. (2011, December 8). Sandusky victims describe grooming, abuses. *Centre Daily Times*. https://www.centredaily.com/news/local/education/penn-state/jerry-sandusky/article42807291.html

Davidson, J., & Gottschalk, P. (2011). Characteristics of the Internet for criminal child sexual abuse by online groomers. *Criminal Justice Studies: A Critical Journal of Crime, Law & Society, 24*(1), 23–36. https://doi.org/10.1080/1478601X.2011.544188

Dutton, N. (2012, July 12). Key passages from Penn State internal review report. *CNN*. https://www.wtvr.com/2012/07/12/key-passages-from-penn-state-internal-review-report

Elliott, M., Browne, K., & Kilcoyne, J. (1995). Child sexual abuse prevention: What offenders tell us. *Child Abuse & Neglect, 19*(5), 579–594. https://doi.org/10.1016/0145-2134(95)00017-3

ESPN. (2011, November 14). President of the second mind resigns. *ESPN*. https://www.espn.com/college-football/story/_/id/7233159/penn-state-nittany-lions-scandal-president-second-mile-resigns

Evans, T., Guillen, J., Kaufman, G., Kwiatdowski, M., Mencarini, M., & Alesa, M. (2018, March 8). How Larry Nassar abused hundreds of gymnasts and eluded justice for decades. *Indy Star*. https://www.indystar.com/story/news/2018/03/08/larry-nassar-sexually-abused-gymnasts-michigan-state-university-usa-gymnastics/339051002/

Finkelhor, D., Shattuck, A., Turner, H. A., & Hamby, S. L. (2014). The lifetime prevalence of child sexual abuse and sexual assault assessed in late adolescence. *Journal of Adolescent Health, 55*(3), 329–333. https://doi.org/10.1016/j.jadohealth.2013.12.026

Gallagher, B. (1998). *Grappling with smoke: Investigating and managing organised abuse – A good practice guide*. NSPCC.

Gladwell, M. (2012, September 17). In plain view: How child molesters get away with it. *The New Yorker*. https://www.newyorker.com/magazine/2012/09/24/in plain-view

Groth, A. N., & Birnbaum, H. J. (1978). Adult sexual orientation and attraction to underage persons. *Archives Of Sexual Behavior, 7*(3), 175–181. https://doi.org/10.1007/BF01542377

Hauser, C., & Zraick, K. (2019, July 30). Larry Nassar sexual abuse scandal: Dozens of officials have been ousted or charged. *The New York Times*. https://www.nytimes.com/2018/10/22/sports/larry-nassar-case-scandal.html

Howitt, D. (1995). *Paedophiles and sexual offences against children*. Wiley.

Kierkegaard, S. (2008). Cybering, online grooming and ageplay. *Computer Law & Security Review, 24*(1), 41–55. https://doi.org/10.1016/j.clsr.2007.11.004

Lanning, K. V. (2010). *Child molesters: A behavioral analysis* (5th ed.). National Center for Missing & Exploited Children.

Lapook, J. (2018). *Aly Raisman speaks out about sexual abuse*. 60 Minutes Sports. https://www.cbsnews.com/news/aly-raisman-60-minutes-us-olympic-gold-medal-gymnast-iam-a-victim-of-sexual-abuse/

Love, J. J., & Fremouw, W. (2009). Female sex offenders: A controlled comparison of offender and victim/crime characteristics. *Journal of Family Violence, 24*(6), 367–376. https://doi.org/10.1007/s10896-009-9236-5

McAlinden, A. M. (2006). Setting 'em up': Personal, familial and institutional grooming in the sexual abuse of children. *Social & Legal Studies, 15*(3), 339–362. https://doi.org/10.1177/0964663906066613

McAlinden, A. M. (2007). *The shaming of sexual offenders: Risk, retribution and reintegration*. Hart.

McAlinden, A. M. (2013). *'Grooming' and the sexual abuse of children*. https://blog.oup.com/2013/01/grooming-child-abuse/

Moody, J. (2015, March 18). *Jerry Sandusky groomed him before abuse, victim tells criminal justice conference*. Kearney Hub. https://kearneyhub.com/news/local/jerry-sandusky-groomed-him-before-abuse-victim-tells-criminal-justice-conference/article_4c528fd8-ccf5-11e4-8785-1f6e11dd6a4e.html

O'Neill, A. (2012, October 13). Because of you, I trust no one. *CNN*. https://www.cnn.com/2012/10/10/justice/jerry-sandusky-victim-impact/index.html

Salter, A. C. (1995). *Transforming trauma: A guide to understanding and treating adult survivors of child sexual abuse*. Sage.

Spraitz, J. D., & Bowen, K. N. (2018). Examination of a nascent taxonomy of priest sexual grooming. *Sexual Abuse, 31*(6), 707–728. https://doi.org/10.1177/1079063218809095

Terry, K. J. (2008). Understanding the sexual abuse crisis in the Catholic Church: Challenged with prevention policies. *Victims & Offenders, 3*(1), 31–44. https://doi.org/10.1080/15564880701750482

Terry, K. J., & Tallon, J. (2004). *Child sexual abuse: A review of the literature*. . http://www.bishop-accountability.org/reports/2004_02_27_JohnJay/LitReview/2004_06_Literature_Review_Complete_Optimized.pdf

Thornton, D. (2003). The Machiavellian sex offender. In A. Matravers (Ed.), *Sex offenders in the community: Managing and reducing the risks* (pp. 144–152). Willan.

van Dam, C. (2001). *Identifying child molesters: Preventing child sexual abuse by recognizing the patterns of the offenders*. Haworth Maltreatment and Trauma Press/The Haworth Press.

Winters, G. M., & Jeglic, E. L. (2016). I knew it all along: The sexual grooming behaviors of child molesters and the hindsight bias. *Journal of Child Sexual Abuse: Research, Treatment, & Program Innovations for Victims, Survivors, & Offenders, 25*(1), 20–36. https://doi.org/10.1080/10538712.2015.1108945

Winters, G. M., & Jeglic, E. L. (2017). Stages of sexual grooming: Recognizing potentially predatory behaviors of child molesters. *Deviant Behavior, 38*(6), 724–733. https://doi.org/10.1080/01639625.2016.1197656

Winters, G. M., & Jeglic, E. L. (2021). The Sexual Grooming Scale – Victim Version: The development and pilot testing of a measure to assess the nature and extent of child sexual grooming. *Victims & Offenders, 1-22*, 1–22. https://doi.org/10.1080/15564886.2021.1974994

Winters, G. M., Jeglic, E. L., & Kaylor, L. E. (2020). Validation of the sexual grooming model of child sexual abusers. *Journal of Child Sexual Abuse: Research, Treatment, & Program Innovations for Victims, Survivors, & Offenders*. https://doi.org/10.1080/10538712.2020.1801935

Winters, G. M., Jeglic, E. L., & Terry, K. J. (2022). The prevalence of sexual grooming behaviors in a large sample of clergy. *Sexual Abuse: A Journal of Research and Treatment*. https://doi.org/10.1177/10790632211070803

Chapter 2
Models of Sexual Grooming

Social scientists use models in the development of theories and constructs. Models in this context are defined as general or hypothetical explanations that are used to assess or define a construct (Glanz & Rimer, 1995). Models are deemed to be an integral part of the social sciences as they aide in guiding both theory development as well as research design by developing a framework through which hypotheses are developed and problems are investigated (Miller & Salkind, 2002). Windahl and McQuail (1993) define a model as "a consciously simplified description in graphic form of a piece of reality" that aims to "show the main elements of any structure or process and the relationships between these elements" (p. 2).

Models are developed or generated through two main stages or steps (Chinn & Kramer, 2011). While these steps are not ubiquitous within social science research, they generally adhere to the following pattern. The first stage in developing a model is the construction of conceptual meaning. In other words, what are the various elements or components of the construct that you are trying to explain? In the social sciences, this process typically involves researching the current state of the field (i.e., past research and theory) to identify key factors or variables that overlap and to understand how the various components of the model interact with one another. A good model should be parsimonious and ultimately measurable. In the second step, the model is structured and contextualized within existing frameworks and theory to be useful in practical settings. Further, context can be applied to the model's findings, and assumptions that are made about the model should be specified (Chinn & Kramer, 2011).

Shoemaker et al. (2004) highlight four main uses for models in research:

1. Models can be used to organize data by highlighting the most important parts of a process and how those parts are related.
2. Models can help to make predictions as they describe the relationship between variables, enabling researchers to test hypotheses.

© The Author(s), under exclusive license to Springer Nature Switzerland AG 2022

G. M. Winters, E. L. Jeglic, *Sexual Grooming*,
https://doi.org/10.1007/978-3-031-07222-2_2

3. Models can be used as heuristic tools for communication and education so that more complex constructs can be more easily communicated, visualized, and understood.
4. Models can help to measure a process or construct.

Shoemaker et al. (2004) state that if a model is clear and well developed, then its parts can be measured and the relationships between variables empirically assessed.

The development of a model is particularly salient for the study of sexual grooming, which remains relatively understudied. In order to move the research on sexual grooming forward, we have to be able to understand what exactly we are studying; otherwise, it cannot be measured and assessed. A comprehensive and parsimonious model of sexual grooming would provide a shared understanding of the construct so that researchers could test and evaluate it. To date, most of the research in the field has been descriptive and qualitive in nature, with little consensus as to what behaviors and tactics encompass sexual grooming and, more fundamentally, how the construct is defined. This chapter will provide an overview of the various models that have been proposed to explain child sexual abuse (CSA) generally; then we will review existing models that pertain to in-person child sexual grooming. Next, we will describe the development of the Sexual Grooming Model (SGM), the first validated model of child sexual grooming, and how this model can be used as a foundation for future research in the field. We will conclude the chapter with a review of models of sexual grooming that are unique to a specific context (e.g., online sexual grooming, adult victims) and population (e.g., priests).

2.1 Models of Child Sexual Offending

It is estimated that as many as half of all cases of CSA involve elements of sexual grooming (Canter et al., 1998; Groth & Birnbaum, 1978; Winters & Jeglic, 2021). Therefore, to better understand sexual grooming, it is also important to understand the theories and models of CSA in general. Theories of sexual abuse have generally arisen from two disciplines—criminology and psychology.

2.1.1 Criminological Models

Criminologists have used the *rational choice perspective* to explain criminal behavior. According to this theoretical framework, criminal acts occur because those who engage in crimes are trying to maximize their pleasure while avoiding pain. Those who commit crimes weigh the costs and benefits of engaging in the offending behavior and ultimately make a choice based on their values, the costs of committing the crime, and the likelihood of achieving their desired outcomes (Cornish & Clarke, 1987). These criminal acts are deemed to be goal-directed as opposed to senseless (Clarke & Cornish, 2001). To test the rational choice perspective and its application to CSA, Proulx et al. (1995) conducted a small exploratory study to assess the motivations of ten individuals who committed sex crimes against children. They proposed that before the abuse can occur, an individual must make a series of decisions, including their hunting ground (e.g., the time and place they will be able to gain access to the child), the erotic valence of the child based upon their sexual preference (e.g., the age, gender, and physical characteristics of the child), the child's physical and psychological vulnerability, and the type and quality of the relationship between the perpetrator and the child (Proulx et al., 1995). Their study also showed that the tactics or strategies used to perpetrate the abuse depended upon situational factors. For example, if the child was a stranger and the adult did not have easy access, then coercion may be necessary, and if the adult had to travel a great distance to abuse the child, then they were more likely to use violence in the commission of the abuse (Proulx et al., 1995). While this model can help to explain the decision tree of how an individual selects a child for sexual abuse and hence provide useful information for situational crime prevention (see Leclerc et al., 2009), it does not detail *how* the abuse occurs.

Gottfredson and Hirschi's (1990) *general theory of crime* is one of the earlier theories of criminal behavior, which explains how crime occurs in general. According to their theory, individuals who have lower self-control will commit offenses if opportunities present themselves; however, the ability to commit the crime is also dependent upon situational factors, which can either facilitate or hinder the commission of the crime. While Gottfredson and Hirschi did not directly apply their theory to CSA, the principles they describe have been used as the basis for later theory. A criminological theory that has been used to explain how CSA occurs specifically is the *crime-commission model*. Cornish (1994) proposed that there are "crime scripts" (i.e., step-by-step events involved in the crime process) that are crime-specific and that can provide a framework for the crime-commission process. In 1998, Cornish presented a paper in which he elaborated on these scripts for those who offended against male children in public spaces and those who abused children in residential settings.

While Cornish's work was theoretical in nature, Leclerc et al. (2011) proposed an empirically derived crime-commission script for committing CSA. Using a sample of 221 individuals who were incarcerated for sexually abusing a child or adolescent, Leclerc et al. (2011) administered the *Modus Operandi Questionnaire* (*MOQ*; Kaufman, 1989) and then calculated the proportion of offenders that used each stage of the crime-commission process. This resulted in the development of a "protoscript" of child sexual offenses, which was comprised of a two-phased model with eight steps (see Table 2.1). Phase I—the crime setup phase—describes the process the individual goes through before committing the sexual abuse. Once the stage is set to commit the abuse, the individual moves into Phase II—crime achievement phase—wherein the actual crime takes place (Leclerc et al., 2011). This model of CSA, which was supported in a subsequent study by Beauregard et al. (2012), highlights the sequential decision-making process that individuals with minor victims engage in prior to and then subsequent to the abuse.

Table 2.1 Leclerc et al. (2011, pp. 217–219) crime-commission process stages in child sexual offending

Phase	Step	Step name/strategy	Step description
I: Crime setup phase	1	Setting	Type of setting where offender first encountered the victim (institutional, public, private [home], multiple locations)
	2	Gaining trust strategies	Giving love and attention to victim; spending time with victim, telling them they are special, giving gift and/or privileges
	3	Proceeding to the crime location strategies	Giving gifts and/or privileges to entice them; using threats or physical force to make victim come
	4	Location	Location for the sexual contact (adult's home; outside adult's home; multiple locations)
	5	Isolation	Exploited or created circumstances to be alone with victim for sexual contact (showering/bathing; watching television)
II: Crime achievement phase	6	Gaining cooperation strategies	Desensitize victims to sexual contact (sex talk, saying loving/caring things); giving gifts and/or privileges; using threats or physical force to engage in sexual acts
	7	Outcomes (proximal and terminal)	Amount of time engaging in sexual acts; victim participation; offender sexual behaviors
	8	Avoiding disclosure strategies	Emotional blackmail

While these criminological models speak more generally to CSA as a whole and not specifically to child sexual grooming, it is clear that there is considerable overlap with models specific to sexual grooming as many of the steps/strategies are the same or similar. Most importantly, understanding the modus operandi of those who abuse children was a significant step forward for the prevention of CSA. Many of the grooming-type situations and behaviors were identified in these models, and criminologists were able to apply them to situational crime prevention frameworks—thus highlighting the utility of such models for the prevention of CSA.

2.1.2 Psychological Models

Psychological approaches to understanding CSA have focused primarily on identifying risk factors for prevention and targets for treatment of sexual abuse. Some of the early psychological models, such as Marshall and Barabree's (1990) *integrated theory* and Ward and Siegert's (2002) *pathways model,* explain the etiology of sexual offending behavior but do not describe the process. Finkelhor (1984) was one of the first to describe the process of CSA in his *four preconditions model*, in which he describes CSA as a multifaceted process that combines the individual's needs as well as situational and contextual factors. Finkelhor proposed that four preconditions must be met in order for sexual abuse of a child to occur. The first precondition relates to motivating factors, including (1) sexual arousal to children (pedophilia), (2) feeling more comfortable around children than adults (emotional congruence), and (3) the inability to meet emotional and sexual needs in adult relationships (blockage). The second precondition is overcoming internal inhibitors preventing the abuse by using alcohol, having limited impulse control, having a cognitive impairment, experiencing severe stress, or having distorted beliefs. The third precondition involves factors predisposing an individual to overcome external inhibitors, which can involve extensive planning or situational factors (e.g., lack of parental supervision). Finally, the fourth precondition involves factors predisposing the perpetrator to overcoming the child's resistance, which refers to the tactics the perpetrator uses to gain and maintain sexual access to the child (i.e., sexual grooming behaviors, including giving gifts, desensitizing the child to sexual contact, the use of threats, and emotional dependency). Notably, Ward and Hudson (2001) critiqued the *four preconditions model*, stating that it was overly vague and had overlapping constructs, it did not integrate the latest research and theory on sexual offending, and that there were too many possible pathways to offending, thereby limiting its clinical utility.

Other psychologically based models of child sexual offending include Ward et al.'s (1998) *self regulation model*, which includes three possible pathways to abuse: (1) the failure to control deviant sexual behaviors or urges, (2) the failure to control deviant cognitions and negative affective states, and (3) intact self-control, but deviant goals. Another early theory is Hall and Hirschman's (1992) *quadripartite model of child sexual abuse* in which they describe a four-factor model to explain the onset and maintenance of CSA, which includes (1) physiological sexual arousal, (2) cognitive distortions, (3) affective dyscontrol, and (4) personality problems.

More recently, Seto (2019) proposed the *motivational-facilitation model* (MFM) of sexual offending. The model was influenced by Finkelhor's (1984) *preconditions model* and Gottfredson and Hirschi's (1990) *general theory of crime*. Seto explains that the MFM differs from these previous models in that motivations for the crime are sexually based (motivation factors) and the commission process is facilitated by specific state and trait factors (facilitation factors). While the model is not specific to CSA, it is broad enough that it can be applied to all types of sexual offending behavior.

According to Seto (2019) the motivation factors (i.e., the psychological factors that drive behavior) for sexual abuse include the following:

1. *Paraphilias*: While Seto highlights that not all individuals who commit sex crimes have sexual paraphilias, paraphilic interests and disorders such as pedophilia (sexual interest in prepubescent children), hebephilia (sexual interest in pubescent children), sadism, biastophilia (interest in nonconsenting sex), exhibitionism (sexual interest derived from exposing one's genitals), frotteurism (sexual interest in touching or rubbing against a nonconsenting individual), and

voyeurism (sexual interest in watching others disrobing or engaging in sexual activity) play a role in sexual offending (see Hanson & Bussiere, 1998; Seto 2008, 2013).
2. *High sex drive*: There is evidence suggesting that high sex drive (e.g., excessive sexual preoccupation, high-frequency masturbation, utilization of pornography, and solicitation of sexual partners) that interferes with functioning is associated with sexual offending against children (Klein et al., 2015; Seto et al., 2010)
3. *Intense mating effort*: While this has not been extensively empirically studied, Lalumiere and colleagues (1996, 2005) found that men who have had multiple sexual partners are more likely to be sexually coercive.

Seto (2019) defines the facilitation factors as those factors that overcome state and trait inhibitions that would ordinarily prevent an individual from acting on their motivations. Trait factors include problems with self-regulation and hostile masculinity, while state factors can encompass negative affect (like anger, stress, and depression) and alcohol use. According to the MFM, motivated individuals who have one or more of these facilitation factors would be at an increased risk for offending.

Similar to the criminological theories of sexual abuse, in the MFM situational factors also play an important role since the commission of the abuse cannot transpire if the opportunity to engage in the abuse is blocked. Seto further discusses the person-environment interaction, such that those who are motivated to offend will create situations that increase the likelihood that the abuse can take place. Similar to those outlined in CSA crime-commission scripts, situational factors can include selecting vulnerable victims (which can also include both trait and state vulnerabilities, such as growing up in a single parent home or victim intoxication), the presence (or absence) of guardians, and the time and place of the abuse. The MFM has the advantage that it is a broad theory of offending that can be applied to many types of sexual abuse, including cases of child abuse that involve sexual grooming. However, the model has yet to be extensively tested, and more research is needed to assess its validity.

2.2 Models of Child Sexual Grooming

Holistic models that are specific to child sexual grooming are a relatively new phenomenon. Some of the earliest descriptions of grooming-like behaviors identified various stages, patterns, or tactics used by those who sexually abused children (see Table 2.2). Subsequently, McAlinden (2006) describes one of the first models of child sexual grooming where she presents the concepts of personal grooming (the emotional/psychological grooming the perpetrator does on him/herself), familial grooming (developing a friendship with the child's parent or guardian to gain access to the child and avoid suspicion), and institution grooming (a motivated individual seeks opportunities, generally through employment of volunteer work, in which

Table 2.2 Models of sexual grooming

Source	Stages/descriptions of sexual grooming tactics
Sgroi (1982)	Engagement phase
	Sexual interaction phase
	Secrecy phase
	Disclosure phase
	Suppression phase
Lang and Frenzel (1988)	Gaining cooperation
	Keeping the victim silent
Budin and Johnson (1989)	Gaining access to victim
	Trust
	Keeping the victim silent
Conte et al. (1989)	Gaining access to victim and cooperation
Christiansen and Blake (1990) *Applies to father-daughter grooming*	Trust
	Favoritism
	Alienation
	Secrecy
	Boundary violation
Berliner and Conte (1990)	Sexualization
	Justification
	Cooperation for secrecy
Elliott et al. (1995)	Gaining access to victim
	Trust
	Cooperation
	Keeping the victim silent
Young (1997)	Gaining access to victim
	Trust
	Cooperation
Harms and van Dam (1992) and van Dam (2001)	Identifying vulnerable child
	Engaging child in peer-like environment
	Desensitize child to touch
	Isolate
	Make child feel responsible
Brackenridge (2001) *Applies to grooming in sport*	Targeting a potential victim
	Building trust and friendship
	Developing isolation and control, building loyalty
	Initiation of sexual abuse and securing secrecy
O'Connell (2003) *Applies to online grooming*	Friendship forming
	Relationship forming
	Risk assessment
	Exclusivity
	Sexual

(continued)

Table 2.2 (continued)

Source	Stages/descriptions of sexual grooming tactics
Leclerc et al. (2005)	Gaining trust
	Cooperation
	Keeping the victim silent
Craven et al. (2006)	Gaining access to the child
	Ensuring the child's compliance
	Maintaining secrecy to avoid disclosure
McAlinden (2006)	Befriend a potential victim
	Cultivate a "special friendship"
	Use of "forbidden fruit"
	Desensitization
Olson et al. (2007)	Gaining access
	Cycle of entrapment
	Intervening
	Outcome
Leclerc et al. (2009)	Gaining access to victim
	Gaining victim's trust
	Gaining cooperation in sexual activity
	Maintaining silence following abuse
Lanning (2010)	Identifying a target
	Gaining access to the victim
	Lowering inhibitions
	Gaining and maintaining control

they will have access to children). While not explicitly described as a model of sexual grooming, McAlinden (2006) generally refers to the "stages of the offender's deviant cycle." She describes the general progression through these stages as the following:

1. Selection of a victim: choosing children and families with obvious vulnerability
2. Befriending the potential victim and getting to know their interests so they can gain their confidence and trust
3. Using enticements such as money, candy, or special outings to distance the child from their guardians
4. Crossing boundaries using sexual talk or pornography to entrap the child and potentially elicit feelings of guilt and shame that can prevent disclosure
5. Increasing physical contact, starting with hugs, tickles, or wrestling, which then escalates depending upon the response of the child

Similarly, Craven et al. (2006) pinpointed the identification of the vulnerable child as the first step in sexual grooming. They then highlight environmental and familial grooming strategies, such as seeking employment or volunteer work in child-serving organizations or befriending the family to gain access to the child.

Next, according to Craven and colleagues, the individual proceeds to groom the child both physically by desensitizing them to physical touch and psychologically by isolating them from their guardians and creating dependency. Lastly, they maintain the child's compliance by using bribes, threats, and making the child feel that they are responsible for the abuse. Later, Lanning (2010), a Federal Bureau of Investigation agent, identified the "seduction process" as the pre-offense strategies used by individuals who abuse children in which he details steps similar to those described by McAlinden (2006) and Craven and colleagues (2006). Thus, McAlinden (2006), Craven et al. (2006), and Lanning (2010) were some of the first to articulate a stage-based model or process that was specific to child sexual grooming, leading the way for more detailed and descriptive models to follow.

2.2.1 *Self-Regulation Model of Illicit Grooming*

More recently, Elliott (2017) proposed the *self-regulation model of illicit grooming*. Elliott used what is described as theory knitting approach to create his model. Theory knitting is a method in which multiple theories are integrated to bring together the strengths of each theory along with any new ideas to form a new, unified theory (see Kalmar & Sternberg, 1988). Elliott (2017) attempted to incorporate aspects of previous models of sexual grooming (i.e., O'Connell, 2003; Olson et al., 2007; Webster et al., 2012) with *control theory* and the self-regulation approach of human behavior (see Carver & Scheier, 2001), as well as the *self-regulation model* of sexual offending (see Ward et al., 1998) to develop a more comprehensive and universal model of illicit grooming. Elliott combined research in sexual offending with established theories of human motivation and behavior.

Elliott's model of sexual grooming comprises two phases which he coined potentiality (Phase I) and disclosure (Phase II). In the potentiality phase, Elliott (2017) expands upon the Ward and Beech's (2006) concept of the ecological niche to describe how the individual who engages in sexual grooming creates and maintains an environment that sets the stage for the sexual abuse to occur. To achieve potentiality, Elliott (2017) describes four mechanisms that are employed by the individual to set the stage for abuse:

1. *Rapport*: This pertains to the development of a relationship between the person seeking to commit the abuse and the victim. Elements that are important for initial rapport formation include friendliness, warmth, and positive interactions; all are employed to develop trust.
2. *Incentive*: This mechanism generally applies to the rewards and punishments that are used to engage the victim in the relationship, such as financial incentives (e.g., presents and money), moral incentives (e.g., praise, approval), coercive incentives (e.g., punishment, violence, threats), and natural incentives (e.g., subconscious motives that are universal and innate).

3. *Disinhibition*: This mechanism seeks to lessen the victim's inhibitions and makes them more susceptible to abuse. Elliott (2017) gives examples of the use of drugs and alcohol as part of the abuse process. However, in online sexual abuse this could refer to the to the anonymity, invisibility, and differential norm of online interactions.
4. *Security*: This fourth and final mechanism refers to the strategies used to prevent the abuse from being detected. This could include obscuring one's identity online to physically and psychologically isolate the victim from their support network in order to prevent disclosure.

In the second phase of the model—disclosure—Elliott (2017) describes how the person seeking to commit the abuse then exploits the advantageous conditions created in Phase I to employ behavioral strategies to abuse the victim. This phase only has one mechanism—sensitivity. The goal of this phase is to use strategies similar to those employed in systematic desensitization to gradually desensitize the victim to the abuse. Strategies used include verbal, physical, and psychological tactics aimed at gradually exposing the victim to sexual content. Elliott explains how the model operates on a self-regulatory feedback loop ending in what Elliott terms "goal achievement," which is the commission of sexual abuse.

Elliott's (2017) *self-regulation model of illicit grooming* has numerous strengths over previous models in that it is based upon existing theories of sexual offending behavior and human motivation that have been well researched. Further, it integrates and builds upon the strengths and commonalities of previous models to form an overarching model that is consistent and not domain specific (i.e., it can be applied both to online and in-person grooming). However, Elliott (2017) recognizes that his model requires validation and remains largely theoretical. Further, Winters et al. (2020) highlight that the model is not easily understood or applied, thereby limiting its clinical utility and widespread adoption.

2.2.2 *The Sexual Grooming Model*

To overcome the limitations of earlier models of child sexual grooming, while also building on the commonalities of existing frameworks, we (Winters & Jeglic, 2017; Winters et al., 2020) set forth to develop the first content validated model of sexual grooming. Like Elliott (2017), we used an integrative approach to theory development wherein we reviewed previous models and descriptions of sexual grooming and synthesized the overarching themes and similarities (see Table 2.2 for list of sexual grooming research reviewed).

In 2017, we (Winters & Jeglic) developed the Sexual Grooming Model (hereafter the SGM) of in-person child sexual grooming. Given that one of the significant limitations of prior models was the lack of ability to measure or detect grooming behaviors, we felt that it was imperative that the SGM encompassed measurable and observable behaviors. The capacity to tangibly measure grooming tactics is also paramount to the psychometric analysis of the construct. Further, given the large role that grooming plays in CSA, we wanted a model that was comprehensive yet could be easily understood by multiple stakeholders (e.g., children, adolescents, parents, educators, mental health professionals, law enforcement, legal professionals, and researchers) and that could serve as a tool for the prevention and detection of child abuse involving sexual grooming. The SGM is comprised of five stages described in Winters and Jeglic (2017) and delineated below:

1. *Victim selection*: In this first stage of the grooming process, the individual identifies a potential victim by selecting a minor who is vulnerable, either because of psychological/emotional reasons or because of family circumstances, such as a lack of supervision, family discord, or living in a single-parent home.
2. *Gaining access and isolating the minor*: The next stage involves gaining access to the minor, either through working or volunteering in youth-serving organizations or by gaining the trust of the minor's guardians. Once they have access to the minor, the perpetrator often tries to separate the minor from peers and caretaking adults so that they can begin the grooming process in private. This may involve driving them places alone, taking them on outings or overnight stays, and/or emotionally distancing them from family and friends.
3. *Developing trust with the minor and other adults in the minor's life*: In this stage, the perpetrator works to gain the trust and compliance of the minor and significant adults in their lives (e.g., caretakers, community members). It should be noted that in this part of the process the perpetrator is often also grooming the minor's family, the organizations in which they may be accessing the child, and their community, in order to gain their trust so they can have easy access to the minor without suspicion.
4. *Desensitizing the minor to sexual content and physical contact*: This stage usually happens right before abuse occurs. During this fourth stage, the perpetrator prepares the minor for abuse by desensitizing them to sexual content (such as showing them pornography and nudity) and increasing nonsexual touch.
5. *Maintenance behaviors following the commission of the abuse*: This last and final stage occurs once the abuse has already happened. The purpose of these maintenance behaviors is for the perpetrator to be able to continue the abuse and avoid detection, often by manipulating the minor into feeling guilty or responsible for the abuse or causing them to fear the consequences of disclosure.

Given that previous models of sexual grooming had yet to be empirically validated—the next logical step for the SGM was to begin the validation process. In Winters et al. (2020), we describe the content validation of the model in detail. First, we conducted a thorough review of the child sexual grooming literature and identified 51 articles and books which provided a description of grooming behaviors and strategies employed by in-person child sexual abusers. This resulted in the identification of 77 potential grooming behaviors. Next, we identified the 99 authors of the aforementioned manuscripts and books and found 44 valid e-mail addresses. These 44 experts were then contacted via e-mail and asked to participate in an expert review survey. A total of 18 experts (response rate 40.9%) completed the survey in

Table 2.3 SGM stage ICVs

Stage	CVI
Victim access	0.89
Gaining access and isolating the minor	0.94
Developing trust with the minor and other adults in the minor's life	0.94
Desensitizing the minor to sexual content and physical contact	0.94
Maintenance behaviors following the commission of the abuse	0.89

which they were asked to rate the relevance of each of the five stages of the SGM on a four-point Likert scale. They were then asked to rate the relevance of each of the 77 identified grooming behaviors to the sexual grooming process and finally, to select one or more of the stages of the SGM that the behavior fell under. Using the content validity index (CVI; Lynn, 1986), stages and behaviors that had an CVI great or equal to .78 (range 0–1.0) were included. All the five stages of the SGM exceeded this cutoff (see Table 2.3), and 42 of the 77 behavior items had CVIs ranging from .78 to 1.0 (see Winters et al., 2020). The behaviors and the stage to which they corresponded are presented in Table 2.4.

2.3 Models of Sexual Grooming for Specific Contexts and Populations

As will be discussed later in this book, grooming does not always occur in-person or with children. Further there may be unique characteristics of the situation, the perpetrator, or the organization (as may be the case with priests) that impact the sexual grooming strategies employed. Consequently, researchers have proposed models of sexual grooming that are specifically tailored to online sexual grooming, sexual grooming involving priests, and adult sexual grooming. While we will argue in later chapters that there is significant overlap with the SGM and the models proposed below, there may be strategies or behaviors that are unique to the situation, perpetrator, and/or victim.

2.3.1 Models of Online Sexual Grooming

It has been noted that online sexual grooming (or the grooming of children using the Internet) has many similarities to in-person sexual grooming (Ioannou et al., 2018); however, others argue that online sexual grooming may be qualitatively different than in-person grooming (Carr, 2004). While we will provide an overview of models of online grooming here, online grooming will be more thoroughly discussed in Chap. 5. One of the first models of online sexual grooming was O'Connell's (2003)

Table 2.4 Grooming behaviors identified in the SGM by stage

Stage 1 Victim selection
Minor is compliant/trusting of adults
Minor lacks confidence/low self-esteem
Minor is lonely/isolated
Minor is troubled
Minor is needy
Minor feels unwanted/unloved
Minor is not close to parents/parents are not resources for them
Minor lives with a single mother/needs "father figure"
Minor has a lack of supervision
Stage 2 Gaining access and isolation
Involved in youth-serving organizations (i.e., school, youth groups, scouts, sports)
Manipulates family to gain access to minor
Engages in activities alone with minor/excludes adults
Takes minor for overnight stays/outings
Separates minor from peers and family
Stage 3 Trust development
Appears charming/nice/likable
Has insider status/good reputation/"pillar of the community"
Is affectionate/loving with minor
Gives the minor attention
Exhibits favoritism/"special relationship" with minor
Gives minor compliments
Spends time with minor/communicating often (texting, phone calls, e-mails)
Engages in childlike activities (e.g., stories, games, sports, music)
Gives minor rewards/privileges (e.g., gifts, toys, treats, money, trips)
Provides minor with drugs and/or alcohol
Stage 4 Desensitization to sexual content and physical contact
Asks questions about minor's sexual experience/relationships
Talks about sexual things they themselves had done
Uses inappropriate sexual language/dirty jokes
Teaches minor sexual education
Use of accidental touching/distraction while touching
Watches the minor undressing
Exposes their own naked body to the minor (e.g., changing/showering)
Shows the minor pornography magazines/videos/images
Seemingly innocent/nonsexual contact (e.g., tickling/hugging/sitting on lap)
Desensitizes minor to touch/increasing sexual touching
Stage 5 Post-abuse maintenance behaviors
Tells minor not to tell anyone what happened
Encourages secrets and secret keeping
Tells the minor "I love you," "You're special"

(continued)

Table 2.4 (continued)

Gives the minor rewards or bribes not to tell or tells them—says by not telling the will avoid punishment
Persuade the minor the sexual abuse was acceptable/normal behavior
The provide the minor with misstated moral standards regarding touch
They make the minor feel responsible for the abuse
They threaten the minor with abandonment/rejection/family breaking up if they tell

model of cybersexploitation. The model was developed using a participant observation method in which O'Connell posed as a minor in chatrooms for over 50 hours during a five-year period. Based upon her observations, she proposed a seven-stage model describing the sequential steps of the online sexual grooming process. These included the following:

1. *Friendship*: The individual gains as much information as they can to gain insight into the child's life so that they can form a friendship.
2. *Relationship forming*: In this stage, the individual uses the information they gathered to connect with the child and share similar interests.
3. *Risk assessment*: In this stage, the individual makes sure that they will not be detected by asking for the location of the computer and the whereabouts of guardians.
4. *Exclusivity stage*: The individual will work to establish a sense of exclusivity with the child, such as serving as a nonjudgmental confidante and encouraging the child to develop an emotional dependence.
5. *Sexual stage*: Strategies may include gentle boundary pressing, expressing affection, reducing inhibition by showing the child pornography, and sending/receiving images.
6. *Fantasy reenactment*: The perpetrator will have the child engage in their sexual fantasies either by encouraging them (mutuality) or by using threats and aggression.
7. *Damage limitation*: The final stage wherein the perpetrator ceases communication or continued contact.

Research on this model showed that online grooming was more heterogeneous than what this model described and that not all the stages were observed or followed sequentially (Whittle et al., 2014).

More recently, Kloess et al. (2019) detailed the offense process of online sexual grooming by outlining three main phases: (1) *the approach phase* (either direct, the adult went directly to sexual topics/online sexual activity, or indirect, the adult used grooming strategies such as relationship building), (2) *the maintenance-escalation phase* (e.g., the individual introduces sexual topics, engages the child in sexually explicit chats or online sexual activity, sends explicit material and fantasy enactment, and may arrange an in-person meeting), and (3) *the closure phase* (either results in a meeting or in the victim or adult ceasing any further conversations/interaction). Due to the nature of online sexual grooming, many of the studies to date use relatively small samples/case studies or samples comprised of adults acting as if they are minors (i.e., Perverted Justice), and thus, the validity and generalizability of the models is difficult to establish. Nonetheless, these models of online sexual grooming are promising and continuously developing as more research is conducted, and they will continue to draw research and political attention given the pervasive and global nature of the problem.

2.3.2 *Models of Priest Sexual Grooming*

In the early 2000s following an investigation by the *Boston Globe*, the public became aware of the rampant CSA within the Catholic Church (Rezendes, 2002). Following a large-scale empirical investigation, it was estimated that between 4% and 8% of Catholic clergy in the United States were abusing children (see John Jay College of Criminal Justice, 2004, 2006). While institutional grooming will be further explored in Chap. 8, some researchers have adapted existing models to encompass behaviors unique to certain populations, such as Catholic clergy. Using the John Jay (2004, 2006) data, Tallon and Terry (2008) broadly looked at grooming behaviors used by Catholic priests who were accused of CSA and found that tactics such as threats, enticements, and socializing with family members were used by some of the abusive clergy. Spraitz et al. (2018) proposed a behavioral taxonomy of priest sexual grooming. Using a sample of files describing 16 priests accused of 147 different allegations of CSA obtained from one diocese in Illinois, they identified eight grooming behaviors that were used by the priests. Their frequencies are presented in Table 2.5.

While the first seven behaviors are strategies that have been identified in previous models of child sexual grooming, the eighth behavior is unique to priests. Farrell

Table 2.5 Comparison of frequencies of priest grooming behaviors adapted from Spraitz and Bowen (2019), p. 715

	Spraitz et al. (2018)	**Spratiz and Bowen (2019)**
	n (%)	*n* (%)
Behavioral taxa	***N* = 16**	***N* = 18**
Giving victims, alcohol, cigarettes, and drugs to lower their inhibitions	9 (56.3%)	9 (50%)
Overnight stays and trips	10 (62.5%)	8 (44.4%)
Created a relationship with victims' parents	9 (56.3%)	5 (27.8%)
Used friendship/mentorship to gain trust	8 (50%)	14 (77.8%)
Played favorites	6 (37.5%)	2 (11.1%)
Introduced physical contact to lower inhibitions	5 (31.3%)	8 (44.4%)
Gave victims gifts	4 (25%)	4 (22.2%)
Abuse and misuse of respect by priests to avoid suspicion or detection	6 (37.5%)	15 (83.3%)

and Taylor (2000) first proposed that abusive priests used spiritual manipulation to abuse children through their position *in persona Christi* (in the person of Christ). However, in a replication of their earlier study using the files of 18 monks accused of sexual abuse, Spraitz and Bowen (2019) found that 15 out of the 18 monks (83%) abused the respect and reverence that was innate to their religious role as part of the grooming process. Importantly, the researchers noted that in almost all (94.7%) of the cases in which the misuse of respect and reverence was used as part of the abusive process, it was not used explicitly or purposefully. They only describe one case where a clergyman told two of his victims that reporting his abusive behavior would be a sin. Thus, Spraitz and Bowen (2019) propose that instead of thinking of the priest's position and religious power as a grooming technique, it could instead be conceptualized as religious duress or reverential fear experienced by the victim. However, they highlight that they coded this information from files, and follow-up interviews where abusive clergy members are questioned may help to further elucidate their role in child sexual grooming. Overall, they found that their original (2018) taxonomy held up and that sexual grooming by clergy was very similar to sexual grooming in general, but they noted that more research with larger samples was needed.

More recently, Winters and colleagues (2022) examined SGM behaviors within a large sample (over 10,000) of cases of alleged CSA within the Catholic Church. As further elaborated on in Chap. 8, the findings showed preliminary support for the notion that priests alleged of committing CSA use behaviors throughout the SGM stages of gaining access/isolation, trust development, and desensitization, although further evidence is needed to explore the victim selection and post-abuse maintenance stages.

2.3.3 Model of Adult Sexual Grooming

Almost all research on sexual grooming has examined sexual grooming as it pertains to child or adolescent victims. However, there is growing evidence that sexual grooming may also be used in some cases of sexual abuse against adults (see Chap. 12). Sinnamon (2017) proposed *Sinnamon's seven-stage model of adult sexual grooming*, which is similar to other models of child sexual grooming in that it is stage-based and encompasses many of the same behaviors:

1. *Select*: Selecting the victim. In this stage, individual selects their victim based upon an exploitable vulnerability.
2. *Plan*: Gathering information. In this stage, the individual observes the potential victim and gets to know their needs and vulnerabilities. They then devise a plan on how to satisfy these needs while at the same time enacting the abuse.
3. *Trust*: Gaining personal connection. In this stage individuals use the knowledge they have gained about their target victim to incorporate themselves into their lives and gain their trust. In this stage they may use secrets to develop intimacy, thus blurring the lines between what is and is not appropriate.

4. *Credibility*: Meeting the need and establishing credentials. In this stage, the perpetrator becomes more credible as they fulfill the target victim's needs and establish their credentials as an integral part of the target victim's life.
5. *Prime*: Priming the target. In this stage, the predator uses the credibility they have established to isolate the target victim from family and friends in order to create dependence.
6. *Instigate*: Creating the victim—instigating sexual contact. Here the individual becomes more deliberate with their physical touch in order to habituate the victim to it so that they can begin the abuse.
7. *Maintain*: Controlling the victim. In this seventh and final stage, the individual controls the victim and their environment to continue the abusive relationship, as well as exploits the victim's guilt and shame to prevent detection.

While there is considerable overlap between Sinnamon's (2017) model and the SGM, it is not clear how this model was derived, and to date, there remains a dearth of empirical data on how sexual grooming may manifest itself in adult sexual abuse.

2.4 Conclusion

Knowledge about the sexual grooming process has significantly evolved over the last three decades. One of the limitations in the field has been that researchers have struggled to come to a consensus about what processes and tactics encompass sexual grooming. In reviewing models of CSA generally and then the more specific models of child sexual grooming presented in this chapter, it is clear that there is considerable overlap across models. We believe the SGM is a big step forward as it represents the first model that has been validated by experts in the field, and it addresses some of the omissions and weaknesses identified in previous models. Furthermore, it is straightforward, and observable behaviors and tactics have been generated for each of the five stages. This presents an opportunity for further empirical research using diverse samples to validate the model, but it also presents the opportunity to develop a measure of sexual grooming, which will be discussed in Chap. 13. Having such a measure will lead to additional research with the hope of more accurately identifying grooming behaviors prospectively.

References

Beauregard, E., Leclerc, B., & Lussier, P. (2012). Decision making in the crime commission process: Comparing rapists, child molesters, and victim-crossover sex offenders. *Criminal Justice and Behavior, 39*(10), 1275–1295. https://doi.org/10.1177/0093854812453120

Berliner, L., & Conte, J. R. (1990). The process of victimization: The victims' perspective. *Child Abuse & Neglect, 14*(1), 29–40. https://doi.org/10.1016/0145-2134(90)90078-8

Brackenridge, C. H. (2001). *Spoilsports: Understanding and preventing sexual exploitation in sport*. Routledge.
Budin, L. E., & Johnson, C. F. (1989). Sex abuse prevention programs: Offenders' attitudes about their efficacy. *Child Abuse & Neglect, 13*(1), 77–87. https://doi.org/10.1016/0145-2134(89)90031-8
Canter, D., Hughes, D., & Kirby, S. (1998). Paedophilia: Pathology, criminality, or both? The development of a multivariate model of offence behaviour in child sexual abuse. *Journal of Forensic Psychiatry, 9*(3), 532–555. https://doi.org/10.1080/09585189808405372
Carver, C. S., & Scheier, M. F. (2001). *On the self-regulation of behavior*. Cambridge University Press.
Chinn, P. L., & Kramer, M. K. (2011). *Integrated theory and knowledge development in nursing* (7th ed.). Mosby.
Christiansen, J. R., & Blake, R. H. (1990). The grooming process in father-daughter incest. In A. L. Horton, B. L. Johnson, L. M. Roundy, D. Williams, A. L. Horton, B. L. Johnson, & D. Williams (Eds.), *The incest perpetrator: A family member no one wants to treat* (pp. 88–98). Sage.
Clarke, R. V., & Cornish, D. B. (2001). Rational choice. In R. Paternoster & R. Bahman (Eds.), *Explaining criminals and crime: Essays in contemporary criminological theory* (pp. 23–42). Roxbury Publishing Company.
Conte, J. R., Wolf, S., & Smith, T. (1989). What sexual offenders tell us about prevention strategies. *Child Abuse & Neglect, 13*(2), 293–301. https://doi.org/10.1016/0145-2134(89)90016-1
Cornish, D. B. (1994). The procedural analysis of offender and its relevance for situational prevention. In R. V. Clarke (Ed.), *Crime Prevention Studies* (Vol. 3, pp. 151–196). Criminal Justice Press.
Cornish, D. B. (1998). *Regulating lifestyles: A rational choice perspective*. Paper presented at the 7th international seminar on environmental criminology and crime analysis, Barcelona.
Cornish, D. B., & Clarke, R. V. (1987). Understanding crime displacement: An application of rational choice theory. *Criminology, 25*, 933–947. https://doi.org/10.1111/j.1745-9125.1987.tb00826.x
Craven, S., Brown, S., & Gilchrist, E. (2006). Sexual grooming of children: Review of literature and theoretical considerations. *Journal of Sexual Aggression, 12*(3), 287–299. https://doi.org/10.1080/13552600601069414
Elliott, I. A. (2017). A self-regulation model of sexual grooming. *Trauma, Violence & Abuse, 18*(1), 83–97. https://doi.org/10.1177/1524838015591573
Elliott, M., Browne, K., & Kilcoyne, J. (1995). Child sexual abuse prevention: What offenders tell us. *Child Abuse & Neglect, 19*(5), 579–594. https://doi.org/10.1016/0145-2134(95)00017-3
Farrell, D. P., & Taylor, M. (2000). Silenced by God – An examination of unique characteristics within sexual abuse by clergy. *Counselling Psychology Review, 15*(1), 22–31.
Finkelhor, D. (1984). *Child sexual abuse: New theory and research*. Free Press.
Glanz, K., & Rimer, B. K. (1995). *Theory at a glance: A guide to health promotion practice*. National Cancer Institute.
Gottfredson, M. R., & Hirschi, T. (1990). *A general theory of crime*. Stanford University Press.
Groth, A. N., & Birnbaum, H. J. (1978). Adult sexual orientation and attraction to underage persons. *Archives Of Sexual Behavior, 7*(3), 175–181. https://doi.org/10.1007/BF01542377
Hall, G. N., & Hirschman, R. (1992). Sexual aggression against children: A conceptual perspective of etiology. *Criminal Justice and Behavior, 19*(1), 8–23. https://doi.org/10.1177/0093854892019001003
Hanson, R. K., & Bussiere, M. T. (1998). Predicting relapse: A meta-analysis of sexual offender recidivism studies. *Journal of Consulting and Clinical Psychology, 66*, 348–362. https://doi.org/10.1037/0022-006X.66.2.348
Harms, R., & van Dam, C. (1992). *Child abuse prevention: What the educator needs to know*. Office of the Superintendent of Public Instruction.

Ioannou, M., Synnott, J., Reynolds, A., & Pearson, J. (2018). A comparison of online and offline grooming characteristics: An application of the victim roles model. *Computers in Human Behavior, 85*, 291–297. https://doi.org/10.1016/j.chb.2018.04.011

John Jay College of Criminal Justice. (2004). *The nature and scope of sexual abuse of minors by Catholic priests and deacons in the United States, 1950–2000*. Conference of Catholic Bishops.

John Jay College of Criminal Justice. (2006). *The nature and scope of sexual abuse of minors by Catholic priests and deacons in the United States, Supplementary data analysis*. U.S. Conference of Catholic Bishops.

Kalmar, D. A., & Sternberg, R. J. (1988). Theory knitting: An integrative approach to theory development. *Philosophical Psychology, 1*(2), 153–170. https://doi.org/10.1080/09515088808572934

Kaufman, K. L. (1989). *Modus Operandi Questionnaire*. Children's Hospital.

Klein, V., Schmidt, A. F., Turner, D., & Briken, P. (2015). Are sex drive and hypersexuality associated with pedophilic interest and child sexual abuse in a male community sample? *PLoS One, 10*, e0139533. https://doi.org/10.1371/journal.pone.0129730

Kloess, J. A., Hamilton-Giachritsis, C. E., & Beech, A. R. (2019). Offense processes of online sexual grooming and abuse of children via internet communication platforms. *Sexual Abuse, 31*(1), 73–96. https://doi.org/10.1177/1079063217720927

Lalumiere, M. L., & Quinsey, V. L. (1996). Sexual deviance, antisociality, mating effort, and the use of sexually coercive behaviors. *Personality and Individual Differences, 21*, 33–48. https://doi.org/10.1016/0191-8869(96)00059-1

Lalumiere, M. L., Harris, G. T., Quinsey, V. L., & Rice, M. E. (2005). *The causes of rape: Understanding individual differences in male propensity for sexual aggression*. American Psychological Association.

Lang, R. A., & Frenzel, R. R. (1988). How sex offenders lure children. *Annals of Sex Research, 1*(2), 303–317. https://doi.org/10.1007/BF00852802

Lanning, K. V. (2010). *Child molesters: A behavioral analysis for professionals investigating the sexual exploitation of children*. National Center for Missing & Exploited Children. https://www.ojp.gov/pdffiles1/Digitization/149252NCJRS.pdf

Leclerc, B., Proulx, J., & McKibben, A. (2005). Modus operandi of sexual offenders working or doing voluntary work with children and adolescents. *Journal of Sexual Aggression, 11*(2), 187–195. https://doi.org/10.1080/13552600412331321314

Leclerc, B., Proulx, J., & Beauregard, E. (2009). Examining the modus operandi of sexual offenders against children and its practical implications. *Aggression and Violent Behavior, 14*, 5–12. https://doi.org/10.1016/j.avb.2008.08.001

Leclerc, B., Wortley, R., & Smallbone, S. (2011). Getting into the script of adult child sex offenders and mapping out situational prevention measures. *Journal of Research in Crime and Delinquency, 48*(2), 209–237. https://doi.org/10.1177/0022427810391540

Lynn, M. R. (1986). Determination and quantification of content validity. *Nursing Research, 35*(6), 382–385. https://doi.org/10.1097/00006199-198611000-00017

Marshall, W. L., & Barbaree, H. E. (1990). An integrated theory of the etiology of sexual offending. In *Handbook of sexual assault* (pp. 257–275). Springer.

McAlinden, A. M. (2006). 'Setting 'Em Up': Personal, familial and institutional grooming in the sexual abuse of children. *Social & Legal Studies, 15*(3), 339–362. https://doi.org/10.1177/0964663906066613

Miller, D. C., & Salkind, N. J. (2002). The role of models in research design. In *Handbook of research design & social measurement* (pp. 46–49). Sage. https://doi.org/10.4135/9781412984386

O'Connell, R. (2003). *A typology of child cybersexploitation and online grooming practices*. Cyberspace Research Unit, University of Central Lancashire.

Olson, L. N., Daggs, J. L., Ellevold, B. L., & Rogers, T. K. (2007). Entrapping the innocent: Toward a theory of child sexual predators' luring communication. *Communication Theory, 17*(3), 231–251. https://doi.org/10.1111/j.1468-2885.2007.00294.x

Proulx, J., Ouimet, M., & Lachaine, N. (1995). Criminologie de l'acte et pedophilie. *Revue Internationale de Criminologie et de Police Technique, 48*, 294–310.

Rezendes, M. (2002, January 6). Church allowed abuse by priest for years. *Boston Globe*. https://www.bostonglobe.com/news/special-reports/2002/01/06/church-allowed-abuse-priest-for-years/cSHfGkTIrAT25qKGvBuDNM/story.html

Seto, M. C. (2008). *Pedophilia and sexual offending again children: Theory, assessment, and intervention*. American Psychological Association. https://doi.org/10.1037/11639-000

Seto, M. C. (2013). *Internet sex offenders*. American Psychological Association. https://doi.org/10.1037/14191-000

Seto, M. C. (2019). The motivational-facilitation model of sexual offender. *Sexual Abuse, 31*(1), 3–24. https://doi.org/10.1177/1079063217720919

Seto, M. C., Reeves, L., & Jung, S. (2010). Motives for child pornography offending: The explanations given by the offenders. *Journal of Sexual Aggression, 16*, 169–180. https://doi.org/10.1080/13552600903572396

Sgroi, S. M. (1982). *Handbook of clinical intervention in child sexual abuse*. Lexington Books.

Shoemaker, P. J., Tankard, J., & Lasorsa, D. L. (2004). Theoretical models. In *How to build social science theories* (pp. 107–144). Sage. https://doi.org/10.4135/9781412990110.n7

Sinnamon, G. (2017). The psychology of adult sexual grooming: Sinnamon's seven-stage model of adult sexual grooming. In *The psychology of criminal and antisocial behavior: Victim and offender perspectives* (pp. 459–487). Elsevier/Academic. https://doi.org/10.1016/B978-0-12-809287-3.00016-X

Spraitz, J. D., & Bowen, K. N. (2019). Examination of a nascent taxonomy of priest sexual grooming. *Sexual Abuse, 31*(6), 707–728. https://doi.org/10.1177/1079063218809095

Spraitz, J. D., Bowen, K. N., & Strange, L. (2018). Proposing a behavioral taxonomy of priest sexual grooming. *International Journal for Crime, Justice and Social Democracy, 7*(1), 30–43. https://doi.org/10.5204/ijcjsd.v&i1.387

Tallon, J. A., & Terry, K. J. (2008). Analyzing paraphilic activity, specialization, and generalization in priests who sexually abused minors. *Criminal Justice and Behavior, 35*, 615–628. https://doi.org/10.1177/0093854808314374

van Dam, C. (2001). *Identifying child molesters: Preventing child sexual abuse by recognizing the patterns of the offenders*. Haworth Maltreatment and Trauma Press/The Haworth Press.

Ward, T. (2002). Marshall and Barbaree's integrated theory of child sexual abuse: A critique. *Psychology, Crime & Law, 8*(3), 209–228. https://doi.org/10.1080/10683160208401816

Ward, T., & Beech, A. (2006). An integrated theory of sexual offending. *Aggression and Violent Behavior, 11*(1), 44–63. https://doi.org/10.1016/j.avb.2005.05.002

Ward, T., & Hudson, S. M. (2001). Finkelhor's precondition model of child sexual abuse: A critique. *Psychology, Crime & Law, 7*(4), 291–307. https://doi.org/10.1080/10683160108401799

Ward, T., & Siegert, R. J. (2002). Toward a comprehensive theory on child sexual abuse: A theory of knitting perspective. *Psychology, Crime & Law, 8*(4), 319. https://doi.org/10.1080/10683160208401823

Ward, T., Hudson, S. M., & Keenan, T. (1998). A self-regulation model of the sexual offense process. *Sexual Abuse: A Journal of Research and Treatment, 10*(2), 141–157. https://doi.org/10.1177/107906329801000206

Webster, S., Davidson, J., Bifulco, A., Gottschalk, P., Caretti, V., Pham, T., Grove-Hills, J., Turley, C., Tompkins, C., Ciulla, S., Milazzo, V., Schimmenti, A., & Craparo, G. (2012). *European online grooming project final report*. European Commission Safer Internet Plus Programme, Tech. Rep.

Whittle, H. C., Hamilton-Giachritsis, C. E., & Beech, A. R. (2014). In their own words: Young peoples' vulnerabilities to being groomed and sexually abused online. *Psychology, 5*(10), 1185–1196. https://doi.org/10.4236/psych.2014.510131

Williams, A. (2015). Child sexual victimisation: Ethnographic stories of stranger and acquaintance grooming. *Journal of Sexual Aggression, 21*(1), 28–42. https://doi.org/10.1080/13552600.2014.948085

Windahl, S., & McQuail, D. (1993). *Communication models for the study of mass communications*. Longman.

Winters, G. M., & Jeglic, E. L. (2017). Stages of sexual grooming: Recognizing potentially predatory behaviors of child molesters. *Deviant Behavior, 38*(6), 724–733. https://doi.org/10.1080/01639625.2016.1197656

Winters, G. M., & Jeglic, E. L. (2021). The Sexual Grooming Scale – Victim Version: the development and pilot testing of a measure to assess the nature and extent of child sexual grooming. *Victims & Offenders, 1–22*, 1–22. https://doi.org/10.1080/15564886.2021.1974994

Winters, G. M., Jeglic, E. L., & Kaylor, L. E. (2020). Validation of the sexual grooming model of child sexual abusers. *Journal of Child Sexual Abuse, 29*(7), 855–875. https://doi.org/10.1080/10538712.2020.1801935

Winters, G. M., Jeglic, E. L., & Terry, K. J. (2022). The prevalence of sexual grooming behaviors in a large sample of clergy. *Sexual Abuse : A Journal of Research and Treatment*. https://doi.org/10.1177/10790632211070803

Young, S. (1997). The use of normalization as a strategy in the sexual exploitation of children by adult offenders. *The Canadian Journal of Human Sexuality, 6*(4), 285–295.

Chapter 3
Definitions of Sexual Grooming

Throughout the past several decades, the term sexual grooming has become synonymous with the concept of child sexual abuse (CSA), having been used in popular media and by professionals (e.g., clinicians, criminal justice personnel, researchers). However, despite the common use of this term in the vernacular, there has yet to be a definition of sexual grooming that is widely adopted across fields (e.g., psychology, criminal justice, health care). The term "sexual grooming" has gone by many other names throughout the years, including "entrapment," "engagement," "subjection," "coercive control," or "enticement" (Bennett & O'Donohue, 2014; Conte, 2018; Gallagher, 1998; Howitt, 1995; Kierkegaard, 2008; Salter, 1995). In fact, several experts in the field have argued that the term "seduction" is preferable to grooming, as it closely mirrors the courtship and mating rituals of adults but is misdirected toward children (Dietz, 2018; Lanning, 2018). While the exact wording has varied, the broad conceptualization of the term has remained the same since it was originally coined by the Federal Bureau of Investigation (FBI) in the 1970s. Dietz (2018) reported the word "grooming" became increasingly used in conjunction with CSA following a publication by Conte (1984), who had cited a previous article by Groth and Birnbaum (1979) addressing cases of CSA not committed by a stranger. Groth and Birnbaum pointed out there is "a grooming process in which a combination of kindness, attention, material enticement, special privilege, and coercion are expertly applied" (p. 558). Dietz (2018) described an increase in articles related to the term "grooming" in CSA in the decades that followed these early publications, according to Google Scholar searches. Specifically, Dietz found there were 0–9 yearly publications in the 1980s, 8–63 in the 1990s, 64–277 in the 2000s, and 282–533 in 2010–2016.

Importantly, while the use of the term sexual grooming may have increased throughout the years, it has been well established in the theoretical literature that there is a lack of consensus regarding the true definition of sexual grooming (e.g., Bennett & O'Donohue, 2014; Dietz, 2018; Lanning, 2018; Winters et al., 2021). Lanning (2018) indicated sexual grooming "does not have one official, legal, mental

© The Author(s), under exclusive license to Springer Nature Switzerland AG 2022
G. M. Winters, E. L. Jeglic, *Sexual Grooming*,
https://doi.org/10.1007/978-3-031-07222-2_3

health, or even lay definition" (p. 11). This lack of a definition is problematic, as it can lead to miscommunication across individuals, organizations, and fields in general. As Dietz (2018) aptly pointed out, "we can and should clarify the meaning of the term wherever possible to avoid misuse or misleading of our audiences" (p. 34). Further, in order to study a construct such as sexual grooming, the construct must be defined. It is a necessary task to define sexual grooming in order to clarify the meaning for the range of people who may encounter these behaviors (e.g., caregivers, researchers, clinicians, police officers, court personnel, educators, doctors, and more).

3.1 Difficulty of Defining Sexual Grooming

It is important to acknowledge *why* defining sexual grooming has been difficult. As noted in Chap. 1, sexual grooming may vary depending on the particular circumstances. It has been suggested that the types of sexual grooming behaviors used differ depending on the person seeking to commit the abuse and the intended victim. Factors such as age, sex, and the relationship between the adult and child may impact the grooming behaviors. For example, the behaviors utilized by a 65-year-old male toward a 6-year-old boy may be very different than a 21-year-old male targeting a 16-year-old female. Further, some sexual grooming behaviors may not be applicable for some situations based upon the adult/child relationship, such as a case in which an adult has preexisting access to a potential victim (e.g., a stepfather living with a child they are abusing). In such a case, the adult would not need to engage in victim selection or gaining access behaviors. The context in which the sexual grooming occurs can also impact what the process looks like. For instance, researchers have found that sexual grooming that occurs online may be different in important ways compared to in-person sexual grooming (Davidson & Gottschalk, 2011). Lastly, in-person sexual grooming may occur over a short (days to weeks) or extensive (years) period of time (Craven et al., 2006; McAlinden, 2006), which may in part by due to the "effectiveness" of the tactics used (i.e., if a child is resistant, the individual may have to increase or modify the sexual grooming tactics used). In sum, the fact that sexual grooming varies depending on the particular scenario poses a major obstacle when developing a definition that can broadly encompass all of these scenarios.

A second major obstacle to defining the construct of sexual grooming is that the behaviors can mimic normal interactions between a non-offending adult and child. Indeed, sexual grooming is intended to appear innocuous and innocent, while the underlying goal and intention of these acts is deviant. Research has suggested that people have a difficult time identifying sexual grooming behaviors before the abuse occurs (Winters & Jeglic, 2017), and they tend to overestimate the likelihood they would have recognized these behaviors once they learn the outcome was sexual abuse (Winters & Jeglic, 2016). Thus, when it comes to defining these behaviors, it becomes difficult to establish parameters that differentiate the point at which these seemingly innocent behaviors become deviant.

Third, as noted previously, the definition may vary by field such as mental health, law enforcement, research, and policy. Interestingly, there have been numerous attempts to define sexual grooming in legal terms, the majority of which do not reflect in-person sexual grooming (Bennett & O'Donohue, 2014). In 2017, there were 63 countries that had legislation related to sexual grooming (International Centre for Missing and Exploited Children [ICMEC], 2017), although these laws vastly differed and often focused on online solicitation or sex trafficking, rather than in-person sexual grooming. The varying sexual grooming definitions in the theoretical/empirical literature versus in legislation pose yet another barrier to establishing a universal conceptualization of the term. Legal definitions of sexual grooming will be further explored in Chap. 16.

Despite these notable complexities in developing a definition, it is nonetheless necessary to take on this herculean task given the importance of having a universal definition of this construct.

3.2 Importance of Defining Sexual Grooming

Generally speaking, it is necessary to define a construct in order to better understand it. That is, in order to fully and accurately conceptualize a concept, one must have a concrete and precise definition (Pelz, n.d.). A clear and concise definition of a topic provides information as to what the construct means and what it does not mean. Understandably, this is not easily accomplished for concepts that are abstract, such as sexual grooming, as it becomes difficult to describe this type of nuanced process objectively. The difficulty of this task has been reflected in the literature, legal settings, and clinical settings, as there has yet to be a universally accepted definition for child sexual grooming.

This lack of consensus presents numerous challenges. First, if individuals across different disciplines, and even individuals within the same discipline, are communicating using the same term ("sexual grooming") but with different meanings, there can be misinformation or misunderstanding. For example, if a mental health evaluator utilizes the term sexual grooming in a court-ordered risk assessment, a judge or jury could interpret this concept differently than it was intended, which could lead to an overestimate or underestimate of risk. Alternatively, if a guardian or community member relays concerns regarding potential sexual grooming behaviors to an authority (e.g., child protective services; school official) or law enforcement, these potentially predatory acts may be dismissed, or conversely, innocent behavior may be punished if there is no universal construct for what actually constitutes sexual grooming.

Second, a definition is needed for research purposes. There is already a lack of empirical literature in the field of sexual grooming, and within the studies that have been published, there are varying definitions of what constitutes sexual grooming.

For example, in the two of the early prevalence studies, the researchers conceptualized which offenders were "groomers" differently. Groth and Birnbaum (1978) described sexual grooming as the approaches that utilize "seduction or enticement," including the victims being "bribed, tricked, or pressured into the sexual activity by means of rewards and/or adult authority" (p. 179). Conversely, Canter et al. (1998) identified a group of offenders who sexually groom their victims ("intimate" offenders), who use the following strategies: promise of gifts/treats, reassurance, affection, desensitization, oral sex by offender to victim, and kissing. These two studies clearly operationalized the construct of sexual grooming in very different ways, which will impact the consistency and comparability of findings across studies. In order to further research in this field, a universal definition is needed to promote replicability and accuracy of the empirical data.

Third, a definition is needed to operationalize the construct so that a measure of sexual grooming may be developed and validated. By developing a child sexual grooming measure, researchers can then examine the extent to which grooming may be used during the offense process. However, a measure of assessment cannot be created without a definition. Construct validity refers to the extent to which a measure or test can validly capture the construct it is intended to measure. For example, if one seeks to establish a construct-validated measure of depression, one must first define exactly what depression refers to, which would likely include the symptoms associated with the *Diagnostic and Statistical Manual of Mental Disorders, Fifth Edition* (*DSM-5*; American Psychiatric Association, 2013) and the *International Classification of Diseases 11th Edition* (*ICD-11*; World Health Organization, 2018) diagnostic criteria—as that is how professionals define the construct of depression. In the case of sexual grooming, if there is no clear definition of the term in any field, then construct validity cannot be established as it would be unclear exactly what a measure of sexual grooming should be capturing.

At present, there is no universal definition of child sexual grooming. Most researchers employ variations on a theme when defining sexual grooming, but as noted earlier, there are clear differences across studies and researchers. There have been several calls for an improved definition of sexual grooming (Craven et al., 2006; Dietz, 2018; Lanning, 2018; McAlinden, 2013, Winters et al., 2021) that clearly and precisely identifies the construct. McAlinden (2013) has provided a commentary on the importance of this endeavor but warns that this term cannot be simply a "catch-all" term that overlooks the complex and multifaceted nature of sexual grooming. A proper definition must avoid being too broad so as to label innocent behaviors as deviant (i.e., false positives), but also not too narrow so as to exclude relevant cases (i.e., false negatives; Bennett & O'Donohue, 2014). Bennett and O'Donohue (2014) also argue that a definition should be based on empirical literature and should help inform a valid assessment method for the construct down the line. In sum, there is no question that a definition of sexual grooming is greatly needed, as this has been repeatedly noted over the past several decades as an integral step to move the field forward.

3.3 Prior Definitions of Sexual Grooming

There have been numerous attempts within the literature to provide a definition for sexual grooming. In fact, there are over a dozen previously suggested definitions for this construct. Of note, the present chapter focuses on in-person sexual grooming, whereas Chap. 5 will more explicitly discuss online sexual grooming. In Table 3.1, we provide a list of examples of prior definitions of sexual grooming, which was presented in Winters et al. (2021). These definitions, which span over 20 years, broadly described a pre-offense process of developing a relationship with the victim but vary significantly based on terminology, level of detail provided, and specific aspects involved in the process.

It is important to note that one of the most cited definitions in recent years was provided by Craven and colleagues (2006; see Table 3.1). This definition is based on the authors' conceptualization of sexual grooming involving not only the relationship between the adult and the child but also how the person seeking to commit CSA interacts with the potential victim's family, community, and environment, as well as the cognitive distortions that permit the person to deny or minimize their actions. While this definition has been included in many subsequent publications, it has not become widely accepted across all of the literature, as numerous authors continued to propose new definitions in subsequent years (e.g., Bennett & O'Donohue, 2014, Knoll, 2010; McAlinden, 2012; Sheldon & Howitt, 2007; Winters et al., 2021).

3.4 Recently Proposed Definition of Sexual Grooming

Most recently, we (Winters et al., 2021) sought to contribute a definition that could be widely applicable across disciplines and contexts. This definition was developed based on: (a) a critical analysis of the commonalities and deficits of prior definitions, and (b) the conceptualization of sexual grooming based on the content-validated Sexual Grooming Model (SGM; Winters et al., 2020). This definition was proposed in hopes of serving as a stepping stone toward a more universal understanding of how this construct can be concretely defined.

One strength of the newly proposed definition is that it draws from prior definitions, including both components that seem to be widely included as well as addressing the limitations that are noted in these definitions. Table 3.2 presents a summary of critiques of the prior definitions presented in Winters et al. (2021), with examples.

Ultimately, a critical review of the previous definitions of sexual grooming suggests that a new definition should apply to a broad range of CSA cases, without limiting the definition to only apply to cases:

(a) With a particular type of victim or adult committing the offense
(b) Where the individual was completely conscious of their acts
(c) Where very specific sexual grooming behaviors were present
(d) Involving the relationship-forming aspect of sexual grooming with caretakers and the community

Table 3.1 Definitions of sexual grooming

Source	Definitions of sexual grooming
Salter (1995)	"The establishment (and eventual betrayal) of affection and trust occupies a central role in the child molester's interactions with children" (p. 74)
Howitt (1995)	"Grooming…the steps taken by pedophiles to 'entrap' their victims and is in some way analogous to adult courtship" (p. 176)
Leberg (1997)	"The offender's plan to make the victim less likely to resist, to make others unaware of what he is doing, or even to make them likely to help him, without their knowledge, to molest a child" (p. 25)
Gallagher (1998)	"Entrapment…involves the use of an array of material, illicit and emotional `inducements' to draw children into abusive situations and increases their difficulty in disclosing" (p. 359)
Brackenridge (2001)	"The process by which a perpetrator isolates and prepares an intended victim" (p. 35)
Gillespie (2002)	"The process by which a child is befriended by a would-be abuser in an attempt to gain the child's confidence and trust, enabling them to get the child to acquiesce to abusive activity" (p. 411–412)
Spiegel (2003)	"The process of predisposing a boy to sexual abuse by means of subtle or blatant interactions that lead to boundary diffusion and role confusion" (p. 139)
McAlinden (2006)	"The process by which a would-be abuser skillfully manipulates a child into a situation where he or she can be more readily sexually abused and is simultaneously less likely to disclose" (p. 86)
Craven et al. (2006)	"A process by which a person prepares a child, significant others, and the environment for the abuse of this child. Specific goals include gaining access to the child, gaining the child's compliance, and maintaining the child's secrecy to avoid disclosure. This process serves to strengthen the offender's abusive pattern, as it may be used as a means of justifying or denying their actions" (p. 297)
Sheldon and Howitt (2007)	"The sequence of behaviors employed by the offender in order to make the victim less resistant to the eventual sexual abuse" (p. 58–59)
Knoll (2010)	"Process by which sex offender carefully initiate and maintain sexually abusive relationships with children. Grooming is a conscious, deliberate, and carefully orchestrated approach used by the offender. The goal of grooming is to permit a sexual encounter and keep it a secret" (p. 374)
McAlinden (2012)	"(1) The use of a variety of manipulative and controlling techniques (2) with a vulnerable subject (3) in a range of inter-personal and social settings (4) in order to establish trust or normalise sexually harmful behaviour (5) with the overall aim of facilitating exploitation and/or prohibiting exposure" (p. 11)
Bennett and O'Donohue (2014)	"Antecedent inappropriate behavior that functions to increase the likelihood of future sexual abuse" (p. 969)

Table 3.2 Critique of prior definitions of sexual grooming

Criticism	Justification	Examples
Not specifying sexual grooming is utilized in cases where the ultimate goal is to enact child sexual abuse	Given that sexual grooming is intended to describe cases of child sexual abuse, a definition should explicitly state this in order to avoid any confusion with those who are unfamiliar with the concept.	Brackenridge (2001) and Howitt (1995)—the definitions do not explicitly indicate these behaviors are used with the intention of committing CSA Craven et al. (2006), Gallagher (1998), and Gillespie (2002)—the definitions describe the goal as "abusive" behaviors and do not clearly state the specific type of abuse (sexual)
Stating a specific type of victim or person who commits the sexual offense in the definition	The definition of sexual grooming should be applicable to a wide range of adults and minors, so as not to rule out certain cases that do not meet the overly strict criteria. The terminology should also not include outdated terms, such as "child molester," to describe the person committing the offense.	Howitt (1995)—"steps taken by pedophiles" Salter (1995)—"child molester" Spiegel (2003)—"boy"
Indicating that sexual grooming *must* be a conscious process	While sexual grooming may be conscious in some circumstances, there is a dearth of empirical literature that confidently states that all of the individuals who use these behaviors were cognizant of these acts. Given some offenders have cognitive distortions related to their offending behavior (e.g., minimizing or justifying their acts), it may not be a completely conscious process.	Knoll (2010)—"conscious, deliberate, and carefully orchestrated approach" Leberg (1997)—"The offender's plan" McAlinden (2006)—"skillfully manipulates a child"
Including specific behaviors that may be involved in the broader process of sexual grooming	Sexual grooming may vary depending on the circumstances of the case, and thus, a definition must be general and broad enough to include a range of circumstances. By including very specific behaviors, it may result in a too narrow of a definition.	Gallagher (1998)—"emotional inducements" Gillespie (2002)—"child is befriended" Salter (1995)—"affection"
Suggesting that sexual grooming *must* involve the relationship forming with caretakers or community	A definition of sexual grooming should note that this process may extend beyond the individual child to also manipulate others (e.g., parents, the community). However, these behaviors may not be involved in all cases, so it should not be a requirement in order to meet the definition of sexual grooming.	Craven et al. (2006)—"a person prepares a child, significant others, and the environment" Leberg (1997)—"make others unaware of what he is doing, or even to make them likely to help him"

(continued)

Table 3.2 (continued)

Criticism	Justification	Examples
Not including an acknowledgement that some individuals will continue to sexually groom the child after the abuse	It has been suggested that sexual grooming may continue after the initial sexually abusive incident. Thus, a definition should acknowledge that these strategies may extend to post-abuse maintenance behaviors.	Brackenridge (2001), Knoll (2010), Sheldon and Howitt (2007)—Definitions do not include mention of continued sexual grooming
Use of language that implies the victim consented or complied with the acts	Sexual grooming is process that manipulatively develops a relationship with the victim. As such, a definition should avoid using terminology that could potentially blame the victim or suggest they voluntarily consented or engaged in the behavior.	Craven et al. (2006)—"gaining the victim's compliance"
		Gillespie (2002)—"get the child to acquiesce to abusive activity"
		Howitt (1995)—"adult courtship"
		Knoll (2010)—"permit the sexual encounter"

Additionally, a definition should acknowledge that some individuals who aim to commit sexual abuse will continue to sexually groom the child following the first commission of the abuse. Lastly, the language utilized should be sensitive to the deceptive and manipulative nature of sexual grooming, so as to avoid blaming the victim or implying consent from the minor.

Winters et al. (2021) also acknowledged that many of the definitions provide useful information that could help inform a universal definition of sexual grooming. Table 3.3 presents a summary of commonalities of the prior definitions presented in Winters et al. (2021), with examples.

The analysis of common themes within sexual grooming definitions suggests that it is important to acknowledge that sexual grooming is a deceptive and manipulative process and that it occurs over a period of time rather than as an isolated incident. Additionally, some authors had reported specific stages or steps that should be included in a broad definition, as a means of providing an overarching framework for what the sexual grooming process may look like while not limiting the definition to only apply to *specific* behaviors.

Following the thorough analysis of prior definitions, including both the strengths and weaknesses, Winters et al. (2021) proposed a new definition encompassing these critiques. Importantly, all of the prior definitions were proposed before the content-validated SGM was published. We argued that the SGM has an important role in creating a new definition, as this is the first and only model to have empirical support from experts in the field as to what sexual grooming entails. As such, we

Table 3.3 Commonalities across definitions of sexual grooming

Commonalities	Justification	Examples
Sexual grooming is a process that occurs over time	Sexual grooming is not one singular, isolated act. Rather, these behaviors occur over a period time, and thus, the term "process" accurately captures this notion (i.e., "a systematic series of actions directed to some end," Dictionary.com, n.d.).	Howitt (1995)—"The steps taken"
		Brackenridge (2001); Craven et al. (2006); Gillespie (2002); Knoll (2010); McAlinden (2006); Spiegel (2003)—"The/a process"
		Sheldon and Howitt (2007)—"The sequence"
There are goals of the sexual grooming process	The literature has suggested that sexual grooming has three main goals: (1) facilitate situations in which the abuse can be more readily committed, (2) increase the likelihood the abuse can continue following the initial incident, and (3) decrease the likelihood that the abuse will be disclosed or recognized by others.	Readily commit the abuse
		Knoll (2010) "permit a sexual encounter"
		Leberg (1997)—"make the victim less likely to resist"
		McAlinden (2006)—"he or she can be more readily sexually abused"
		Sheldon and Howitt (2007)–"make the victim less likely to resist"
		Facilitate future abuse
		Bennett and O'Donohue (2014)—"increase the likelihood of future abuse"
		Craven et al. (2006)—"strengthen the abusive pattern"
		Decrease the likelihood of discovery
		Craven et al. (2006)—"avoid disclosure"
		Gallagher (1998)—"increases their difficulty in disclosing"
		Knoll (2010)—"keep it a secret"
		Leberg (1997)—"make others unaware of what he is doing"
		McAlinden (2006)—"less likely to disclose"
		McAlinden (2012)—"prohibiting exposure"

(continued)

Table 3.3 (continued)

Commonalities	Justification	Examples
There are overarching stages involved in the sexual grooming process	As identified in the SGM content validation study, experts in the field agree that there are overarching steps or stages involved in the sexual grooming process. Thus, a definition should include these broader concepts, rather than specific behaviors that may be present. This is consistent with several prior authors who have included broad stages in their definitions.	Victim selection
		McAlinden (2013)—"with a vulnerable subject"
		Gaining access and isolation
		Brackenridge (2001)—"perpetrator isolates…an intended victim"
		Craven et al. (2006)—"gaining access to the child"
		Trust development
		Gillespie (2002)—"gain the child's confidence and trust"
		McAlinden (2012)—"establish trust"
		Salter (1995)—"establishment (and eventual betrayal) of affection and trust"
		Desensitization
		Spiegel (2003)—"subtle or blatant interactions that lead to boundary diffusion"
		McAlinden (2012)—"normalise sexually harmful behaviour"
		Post-abuse maintenance
		Bennett and O'Donohue (2014)—"increase the likelihood of future sexual abuse"
		Craven et al. (2006)—"maintain child's secrecy to avoid disclosure"
		Knoll (2010)—"keep it a secret"
Sexual grooming is a deceptive and manipulative process	It is important to acknowledge that sexual grooming is deceptive in nature and most prior definitions have included language to describe this notion.	Gallagher (1998)—"entrapment"
		McAlinden (2006)—"skillfully manipulates a child"
		McAlinden (2012)—"manipulative and controlling techniques"
		Salter (1995)—"establishment (and eventual betrayal) of affection and trust"

proposed a definition that encompasses both their analysis of prior definitions and the stages of the SGM. The definition reads as follows:

> Sexual grooming is the deceptive process used by sexual abusers to facilitate sexual contact with a minor while simultaneously avoiding detection. Prior to the commission of the sexual abuse, the would-be sexual abuser may select a victim; gain access to and isolate the minor; develop trust with the minor and often their guardians, community, and youth-serving institutions; and desensitize the minor to sexual content and physical contact. Post-abuse, the offender may use maintenance strategies on the victim to facilitate future sexual abuse and/or to prevent disclosure. (p. 7)

3.5 Conclusion

This chapter provided a historical background regarding the term "sexual grooming" and the numerous previously proposed definitions. To date, none of these definitions had been widely adopted across fields. Winters et al. (2021) aimed to provide a new definition of sexual grooming that drew from the decades' worth of definitions that came before it, as well as informed by an empirically supported model of sexual grooming. The next steps will be to establish further empirical evidence for the SGM, as well as the definition based on this model, using real-world cases of CSA (e.g., victim reports, police records, interviews with those who committed CSA). Also, clinical measures of sexual grooming can be developed based on these findings, which can then undergo rigorous evaluation based on the psychometric properties (e.g., inter-rater reliability, test-retest reliability, construct validity). Down the line, it is hoped that a validated definition of sexual grooming will be utilized across relevant stakeholders, such as researchers, clinicians, criminal justice personnel, policy-makers, caregivers, and community members.

References

American Psychiatric Association. (2013). *Diagnostic and statistical manual of mental disorders* (5th ed.). https://doi.org/10.1176/appi.books.9780890425596

Bennett, N., & O'Donohue, W. (2014). The construct of grooming in child sexual abuse: Conceptual and measurement issues. *Journal of Child Sexual Abuse: Research, Treatment, & Program Innovations for Victims, Survivors, & Offenders, 23*(8), 957–976. https://doi.org/10.1080/10538712.2014.960632

Brackenridge, C. H. (2001). *Spoilsports: Understanding and preventing sexual exploitation in sport*. Routledge.

Canter, D., Hughes, D., & Kirby, S. (1998). Paedophilia: Pathology, criminality, or both? The development of a multivariate model of offence behaviour in child sexual abuse. *Journal of Forensic Psychiatry, 9*(3), 532–555. https://doi.org/10.1080/09585189808405372

Conte, J. R. (1984). The justice system and sexual abuse of children. *Social Service Review, 58*, 556–568. https://doi.org/10.1086/644238

Conte, J. R. (2018). Words matter: Introduction to a commentary on grooming. *Journal of Interpersonal Violence, 33*(1), 3–4. https://doi.org/10.1177/0886260517742039

Craven, S., Brown, S., & Gilchrist, E. (2006). Sexual grooming of children: Review of literature and theoretical considerations. *Journal of Sexual Aggression, 12*(3), 287–299. https://doi.org/10.1080/13552600601069414

Davidson, J., & Gottschalk, P. (2011). Characteristics of the Internet for criminal child sexual abuse by online groomers. *Criminal Justice Studies: A Critical Journal of Crime, Law & Society, 24*(1), 23–36. https://doi.org/10.1080/1478601X.2011.544188

Dictionary.com. (n.d.). *The definition of process*. Retrieved November 7, 2020, from http://www.dictionary.com/browse/process

Dietz, P. (2018). Grooming and seduction. *Journal of Interpersonal Violence, 33*(1), 28–36. https://doi.org/10.1177/0886260517742060

Gallagher, B. (1998). *Grappling with smoke: Investigating and managing organised abuse – A good practice guide*. NSPCC.

Gillespie, A. A. (2002). Child protection on the internet: Challenges for criminal law. *Child & Family Law Quarterly, 14*(4), 411–425.

Groth, A. N., & Birnbaum, H. J. (1978). Adult sexual orientation and attraction to underage persons. *Archives of Sexual Behavior, 7*(3), 175–181. https://doi.org/10.1007/BF01542377

Groth, A. N., & Birnbaum, H. J. (1979). *Men who rape: The psychology of the offender*. Plenum Press.

Howitt, D. (1995). *Paedophiles and sexual offences against children*. Wiley.

International Centre for Missing & Exploited Children [ICMEC]. (2017). *Online grooming of children for sexual purposes: Model legislation & global review*. https://www.icmec.org/wp-content/uploads/2017/09/Online-Grooming-of-Children_FINAL_9-18-17.pdf

Kierkegaard, S. (2008). Cybering, online grooming and ageplay. *Computer Law & Security Review, 24*(1), 41–55. https://doi.org/10.1016/j.clsr.2007.11.004

Knoll, J. (2010). Teacher sexual misconduct: Grooming patterns and female offenders. *Journal of Child Sexual Abuse: Research, Treatment, & Program Innovations for Victims, Survivors, & Offenders, 19*(4), 371–386. https://doi.org/10.1080/10538712.2010.495047

Lanning, K. (2018). The evolution of grooming: Concept and term. *Journal of Interpersonal Violence, 33*(1), 5–16. https://doi.org/10.1177/0886260517742046

Leberg, E. (1997). *Understanding child molesters: Taking charge*. Sage.

McAlinden, A. M. (2006). Setting 'em up': Personal, familial and institutional grooming in the sexual abuse of children. *Social & Legal Studies, 15*(3), 339–362. https://doi.org/10.1177/0964663906066613

McAlinden, A. M. (2012). *'Grooming' and the sexual abuse of children: Institutional, internet and familial dimensions* (Clarendon Series in Criminology). Oxford University Press.

McAlinden, A. M. (2013, January 10). *'Grooming' and the sexual abuse of children*. http://blog.oup.com/2013/01/grooming-child-abuse/

Pelz, P. B. (n.d.). *Research methods for the social sciences*. https://courses.lumenlearning.com/suny-hccc-research-methods/chapter/chapter-6-measurement-of-constructs/

Salter, A. C. (1995). *Transforming trauma: A guide to understanding and treating adult survivors of child sexual abuse*. Sage.

Sheldon, K., & Howitt, D. (2007). *Sex offenders and the Internet*. Wiley.

Spiegel, J. (2003). *Sexual abuse of males: The SAM model of theory and practice*. Brunner-Routledge.

Winters, G. M., & Jeglic, E. L. (2016). I knew it all along: The sexual grooming behaviors of child molesters and the hindsight bias. *Journal Of Child Sexual Abuse: Research, Treatment, & Program Innovations For Victims, Survivors, & Offenders, 25*(1), 20–36. https://doi.org/10.1080/10538712.2015.1108945

Winters, G. M., & Jeglic, E. L. (2017). Stages of sexual grooming: Recognizing potentially predatory behaviors of child molesters. *Deviant Behavior, 38*(6), 724–733. https://doi.org/10.1080/01639625.2016.1197656

Winters, G. M., Jeglic, E. L., & Kaylor, L. E. (2020). Validation of the sexual grooming model of child sexual abusers. *Journal of Child Sexual Abuse: Research, Treatment, & Program Innovations for Victims, Survivors, & Offenders*. https://doi.org/10.1080/10538712.2020.1801935
Winters, G. M., Kaylor, L. E., & Jeglic, E. L. (2021). Toward a universal definition of child sexual grooming. *Deviant Behavior*, 1–13. https://doi.org/10.1080/01639625.2021.1941427
World Health Organization. (2018). *International classification of diseases for mortality and morbidity statistics (11th revision)*. https://icd.who.int/browse11/l-m/en

Chapter 4
Consequences of Sexual Grooming

Child sexual abuse (CSA) is an adverse childhood experience that has significant long-term impact on those who experience it (Centers for Disease Control [CDC], 2019). Not only are there psychological consequences, but longitudinal research has found that CSA also results in negative health, psychosocial and socioeconomic outcomes for victims. While we know that a large portion of CSA involves sexual grooming (Canter et al., 1998; Winters & Jeglic, 2021), there is no research to our knowledge that examines whether those who experience sexual grooming-based CSA have different long-term consequences as opposed to those who do not experience these behaviors. Thus, this chapter will provide an overview of the long-term consequences of CSA generally, and then we will present some preliminary findings and hypotheses on how sexual grooming specifically may impact individuals, families, communities, and institutions.

4.1 Consequences of Child Sexual Abuse

4.1.1 *Psychological*

There is a wealth of research examining the long-term psychological impact of CSA. A recent umbrella review of 19 meta-analyses, including data from over four million participants, examined the long-term outcomes of CSA (Hailes et al., 2019) Using odds ratios[1] (see Table 4.1), results showed the psychological disorders with the strongest associations to CSA were conversion disorder, borderline personality

[1] Odds ratios mathematically quantify the relationship between the exposure to an event (in this case CSA) and the subsequent disease or disorder. It compares those who were exposed to CSA and those who were not (controls) and shows how much higher the odds of developing a disorder are for someone who experienced CSA as compared to someone who did not.

© The Author(s), under exclusive license to Springer Nature Switzerland AG 2022

G. M. Winters, E. L. Jeglic, *Sexual Grooming*,
https://doi.org/10.1007/978-3-031-07222-2_4

Table 4.1 Psychological outcomes of CSA

Disorder	Odds ratio
Conversion disorder	3.3
Borderline personality disorder	2.9
Anxiety	2.7
Depression	2.7
Post-traumatic stress disorder	2.3
Eating disorders	2.2
Somatoform disorders	1.9
Schizophrenia	1.4
Suicide attempt	2.43–2.65

disorder (BPD), anxiety, depression, post-traumatic stress disorder (PTSD), and eating disorders. Associations between psychiatric disorders and CSA were also found for somatoform disorders and schizophrenia (Hailes et al., 2019).

Some studies have examined the relationship between suicide and CSA. One meta-analysis of seven longitudinal studies and two twin studies found that CSA increased the odds of making a suicide attempt between 2.43 and 2.65 times (Devries et al., 2014). Similarly, in a retrospective study of over 17,000 Health Maintenance Organization (HMO) members in San Diego, California, both men and women who reported a history of CSA were more than twice as likely as those without a history of CSA to have reported making a suicide attempt (Dube et al., 2005). Overall, findings suggest that CSA should be considered a general nonspecific risk factor for suicide and that the type, duration, or severity of the CSA was not related to increased suicide risk.

It should be noted that many of the sequelae of CSA may not emerge immediately. For example, one study found that the average time of onset between the CSA and the major depressive episode was 11.5 years and 8.0 years for PTSD (Teicher et al., 2009). It is postulated that child abuse prior to the onset of puberty results in decreased hippocampal volume and synaptic density post-puberty, thus accounting for delayed onset of depressive symptoms (Teicher, 2009).

More recently there have been several studies examining the impact of CSA on personality disorders, such as BPD and antisocial personality disorder. Using archival data from a sample of 865 federally incarcerated inmates (86% male), a history of CSA significantly increased the risk of an antisocial personality disorder diagnosis and was significantly related to a history of conduct disorder and earlier age of arrest (DeLisi et al., 2019). A systematic review of 40 studies examining the association between CSA, adult sexual assault, and BPD concluded that CSA was an important risk factor for BPD and individuals with BPD who had experienced sexual abuse either in childhood or adulthood had a more severe presentation (increased suicidal and self-harm behavior) and poorer prognosis compared to those without a history of sexual abuse (de Aquino Ferreira et al., 2018). CSA was also found to be robustly associated with substance abuse for both males and females even after controlling for mental health status. Specifically, CSA was associated with both heavy and hazard drinking, marijuana use, and use of other illicit and off-label prescription drugs in adulthood (Tonmyr & Shields, 2017).

4.1.2 Physical

The long-term effects of CSA on physical health have also been well documented. In a meta-analysis of 31 studies comparing the health outcomes of those with and without histories of CSA, Irish and colleagues (2010) found that adults who experienced CSA were 1.35–2.12 times more likely to report health problems across multiple domains (including, but not limited to, general overall health, pain, gastrointestinal symptoms, gynecological symptoms, cardiopulmonary symptoms, and obesity) than adults who did not experience CSA. Another umbrella review of 28 meta-analyses found that adults who experience CSA were more likely to be obese, have human immunodeficiency virus (HIV), experience pain, and have a diagnosis of fibromyalgia (Hailes et al., 2019). Consequently, adults with a history of CSA use health care more frequently than those without a history of CSA, spending on average 16% more per year on healthcare which equates to about $472 in 2015 dollars (Kamiya et al., 2016; Letourneau et al., 2018). Notably, however, a history of CSA is also associated with lower odds of having health insurance and receiving a general checkup (preventative care) in past year (Alcalá et al., 2018).

4.1.3 Psychosocial

Research has demonstrated that the sequelae of CSA have numerous psychosocial impacts. In a longitudinal study of maltreated children and matched controls, Colman and Widom (2004) found that individuals who experienced CSA were more likely to experience relationship disruption in adulthood (e.g., walking out, divorce), and women who experienced CSA were also more likely to report dissatisfaction with their relationships, sexual unfaithfulness, and infidelity. Another review of the sexual health literature found that women who experienced CSA experienced a lack of positive emotions related to sexuality which was often related to increased sexual dysfunction (Pulverman et al., 2018).

One study examined breastfeeding among women with CSA histories and compared them to matched aged mothers without a CSA history, and they found that while rates of breastfeeding were comparable between the two groups, women with a CSA history reported more complications, such as mastitis and pain. One-fifth of women with CSA histories also said that breastfeeding served as a trigger for their abuse (Elfgen et al., 2017).

Sadly, there is considerable evidence to suggest that those who have experienced CSA are also likely to be revictimized. A recent meta-analysis of 80 studies involving 12,252 survivors of CSA found that 47.5% were sexually victimized again later in life (Walker et al., 2019). Similarly, a review of 108 qualitative studies of mothering practices of women who experienced CSA found that in 45% of the studies, the children of these mothers also experienced sexual abuse themselves (Lange et al., 2020), suggesting that the cycle of abuse may continue into the next generation.

4.1.4 Socioeconomic

From an economic perspective, Fang et al. (2012) estimated the average lifetime cost of nonfatal child maltreatment (including CSA) per victim in 2010 US dollars is $210,012. Then, in 2018, using updated quality-adjusted life years methodology, Peterson and colleagues suggested that the cost of childhood maltreatment (including CSA) was in fact $830,928 in 2015 US dollars. The breakdown for lifetime costs is shown in Table 4.2.

Further, male victims of CSA are almost three times more likely to be out of the labor force due to sickness and disability, have significantly lower incomes, and live alone compared to men who did not experience CSA (Barrett et al., 2014). In a longitudinal study of individuals with documented histories of maltreatment in childhood and matched controls, Currie and Widom (2010) found that those with a history of CSA had lower educational attainment and intelligence testing scores, were less likely to have a skilled job, and were 14% less likely to be employed at middle age compared to non-abused adults. Those who experienced CSA in childhood earned on average $8000 per year less than non-abused controls and were also less likely to have a bank account or own stock, a vehicle, or home compared to non-abused adults (Currie & Widom, 2010).

Table 4.2 Lifetime cost of childhood maltreatment per victim

Item	Cost in 2010 US dollars (Fang et al., 2012)	Cost in 2015 US dollars (Peterson et al., 2018)
Childhood health care	$32,648	$35,162
Adult medical	$10,530	$11,341
Productivity	$144,360	$8399
Child welfare	$7728	$8399
Criminal justice	$6747	$7333
Special education	$7999	$8696
Quality-adjusted life years	n/a	$760,000
Total	$210,012	$830,928

4.2 Consequences of Sexual Grooming

While the long-term consequences of sexual abuse in general have been extensively studied, there is almost no research specifically examining whether individuals who have experienced sexual grooming-based CSA may have differential outcomes as compared to those who experience CSA without sexual grooming. Based upon the CDC socio-ecological model of violence prevention (CDC, 2021), we will discuss how sexual grooming may impact the child, family, institutions, and society (see Fig. 4.1).

4.2.1 Consequences to the Child

There are several reasons to postulate that there may be differences in outcomes between those who experience CSA with grooming and those who experience CSA without grooming. Because of the manipulation and deception involved in the sexual grooming process, children may be less likely to disclose or formally report the CSA, or there may be a significant delay between the time of the abuse and the time of the disclosure (Bennett & O'Donohue, 2016). While the data on the relationship between disclosure, time to disclosure, and mental health outcomes is not entirely consistent across studies, the majority of research has found that among nonclinical samples of both men and women, early disclosure (i.e., within one year of the CSA) and in-depth discussion of the abuse is protective against negative psychological outcomes in adulthood (Easton, 2014, 2019; O'Leary et al., 2010; Ullman, 2007; Ullman & Filipas, 2005). The few studies that found no relationship or a negative

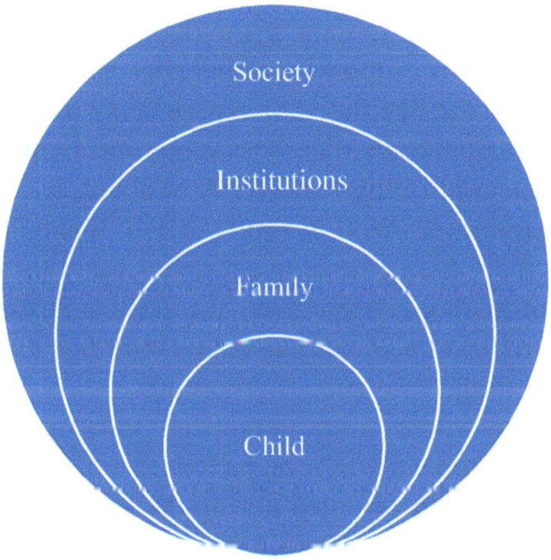

Fig. 4.1 The impact of sexual grooming

relationship between disclosure and mental health outcomes had some methodological limitations. For example, Ullman and Filipas (2005) found that in their sample of undergraduate students, women who disclosed CSA had fewer symptoms of PTSD; however, no relationship was found among males who disclosed and PTSD symptoms. This could be because their sample was predominantly female (71%) and that comparably fewer males reported a CSA history (13%); thus, they may not have had a large enough sample of males who did or did not disclose to properly analyze the question. In another study, O'Leary et al. (2010) found that disclosure within a year was related to increased mental health problems, but an in-depth discussion of the abuse with a family member, friend, counselor, or other health profession in the year following the CSA was related to better mental health functioning. While it was not assessed in the study, the authors speculate that those who disclosed and did not have in-depth discussion about the abuse received an inadequate response to their disclosure, meaning that they were either not believed or nothing was done. Similarly, Swingle et al. (2016) found that in a clinical sample of survivors of CSA, those who disclosed but had the abuse continue experienced the most severe psychiatric symptoms compared to those who did not disclose or those who disclosed and for whom the abuse stopped. As will be discussed in Chap. 7 when familial grooming is reviewed, along with grooming the minor, the perpetrator may also groom significant adults in the child's life in order to prevent detection. It is possible that because of familial grooming, adults are less likely to suspect or believe the minor when the abuse is reported, thus leading to more negative outcomes. While this has yet to be studied empirically, it is a plausible hypothesis.

Wolf and Pruitt (2019) have conducted the only known quantitative analysis of the relationship between sexual grooming tactics and adult trauma symptoms. Using a sample of 277 adult survivors of CSA (86% female), the authors administered the verbal coercion, drug/alcohol grooming, and threatening/violent grooming subscales of the *Computer Assisted Maltreatment Inventory* (*CAMI*; DiLillo et al., 2010). Overall, they found that CSA involving these select sexual grooming behaviors increased the severity of trauma symptoms among adult CSA survivors. Moreover, while each type of grooming (verbal coercion, drug/alcohol, and threatening/violence) increased the likelihood of experiencing trauma symptoms in adulthood, it was only the threatening/violent grooming that significantly contributed to trauma symptoms when controlling for severity of abuse, age of onset of the abuse, and relationship to perpetrator (Wolf & Pruitt, 2019). It should be noted that while many of the items in the *CAMI* grooming subscales were also among those identified by recent literature (e.g., Winters et al., 2020's Sexual Grooming Model [SGM]), this conceptualization is not exhaustive and not theoretically derived or validated as belonging to the construct of grooming.

Two other qualitative studies were conducted assessing the impact of sexual grooming on victims. Plummer (2018) conducted interviews with 11 male survivors of CSA. Common themes that emerged during the sexual grooming process were confusion, self-blame, feeling responsible for the abuse, shame, and fear, which made them feel that they could not leave the abusive situation or disclose. Survivors also described how the manipulation and emotional coercion used in the sexual grooming process resulted in enduring feelings of self-blame, guilt, and responsibility. Whittle et al. (2013) conducted interviews with eight adolescents (aged 13–18; two males and six females) who had experienced online sexual grooming. They concluded that there was no difference in the negative consequences to those who experienced online grooming followed by offline CSA compared to those who experienced only online CSA (i.e., sexual chats, sending of sexual pictures and/or videos). Similar to other studies on the impact of CSA in general, the adolescents who experienced online sexual grooming followed by CSA in the Whittle et al. (2013) study reported psychological difficulties, shame, embarrassment, and aggression.

Taken together, these preliminary studies suggest that individuals who experience sexual grooming-based CSA may be at risk for experiencing more severe long-term consequences than those who do not experience sexual grooming in their CSA. It appears that as a consequence of the psychological manipulation and coercion that are innate to the sexual grooming process, the victim may experience more confusion, guilt, and shame, which have been related to increased PTSD and suicidal behavior among trauma survivors (Cunningham, 2020). These feelings of guilt, shame, and culpability can also lead to decreased levels of disclosure, which has also been linked to more negative outcomes. Finally, if the individual has also sexually groomed the minor's parents and/or guardians and the minor does disclose the CSA, they may not be believed, or the abuse may be minimized or ignored. Ultimately, an inadequate or inappropriate response to CSA disclosure can lead to more severe trauma symptoms stemming from the CSA (Swingle et al., 2016).

4.2.2 Consequences to the Family

As part of the grooming process, perpetrators may groom not only the minor but also significant others in the child's life, such as parents or caregivers to gain their trust. This enables the perpetrator to access and abuse the minor without suspicion (Craven et al., 2006; Winters et al., 2020). As described in the SGM, perpetrators also select potential victims based upon vulnerabilities, such as a lack of parental supervision or that the minor lives in a single-parent home and may need a father-like figure (Winters et al., 2020). Van Dam (2001) proposed that when a parent has brought the perpetrator into the minor's life because they believe them to be warm, likeable, and trustworthy, they may experience cognitive dissonance if the perpetrator's behaviors become suspicious, and consequently, they may disregard or explain away their concerns. When the perpetrator is a member of the family, they may work to isolate the minor from the non-abusing parent and other siblings. Strategies may include encouraging the mother to have a life outside of the home so that they can be alone with the child, isolating the non-abusing parent so that they do not have anyone to share their concerns with, encouraging the mother to develop a substance abuse problem, or question the mother's parenting in front of others so that any disclosures may lack credibility (Craven et al., 2006; Leberg, 1997). Consequently, when the abuse is discovered, it is not only the child who is impacted but also their parents and family as well.

While there has not been any research specifically assessing the impact of sexual grooming on families, multiple studies have looked at how disclosure of CSA impacts parents and the family system. Most of the research on parental response to CSA has found that parents experience a multitude of reactions and emotions once the abuse of their child has been revealed. The research that focused on parents of CSA victims found that parents experienced guilt regarding their failure as parents, emotional distress, PTSD, marital distress, loss of trust in adults, and anger at the perpetrator (Davies, 1995; Manion et al., 1996; Regehr, 1990; Tsang et al., 2020).

One long-term study of parents of young children abused by a daycare worker in Amsterdam, the Netherlands (the Amsterdam Sexual Abuse Case), found that while feelings of sadness, fear, and anger over the CSA decreased across time, PTSD symptoms continued to fluctuate over the eight-year follow-up period (Tsang et al., 2020). Tsang and colleagues postulated that it was possible that this was a result of ongoing involvement with the legal system, which could have been retraumatizing. Further, they found that behavioral problems (both internalizing and externalizing) persisted for the children who had experienced the abuse across time, which may also cause additional stress for parents. However, another longitudinal study that assessed 124 parents (92 mothers) of children who experienced CSA at 12- and 18-months post-disclosure found that physical and psychological trauma, including PTSD symptoms, peaked at one-year post-disclosure, but that only PTSD symptoms had significantly decreased by 18 months post-disclosure (Cyr et al., 2018). It is possible that as noted by Tsang et al. (2020), symptoms of PTSD may wax and wane over time and that longer-term follow-up may reveal a different clinical presentation.

The majority of participants in the collateral CSA impact research were mothers, and many studies only examined mothers' reactions. One study examining mothers of CSA victims who themselves had experienced CSA found that once the abuse of their own child was revealed, this negatively impacted the mothers' own psychological well-being (Daignault et al., 2018). Specifically, mothers who were exposed to interparental violence in childhood were more likely to experience dissociation and PTSD, while having a history of CSA was directly related to dissociation-only post-disclosure. Recent exposure to intimate partner violence in the mother's current relationship was also related to more trauma among mothers of CSA victims (Daignault et al., 2018). A qualitative study of 20 mothers of CSA victims found strain in the parent-child relationship both leading up to and following the disclosure of CSA (Plummer & Eastin, 2007). The mothers reported feeling insecure prior to the disclosure of CSA as they knew something was not right, but they were not sure what. Following disclosure, mothers reported strain resulting from child behavioral problems stemming from the abuse; feelings of guilt, shame, and self-blame for not protecting their child; and overall feelings of physical and emotional exhaustion (Plummer & Eastin, 2007). Across the board, when compared to fathers of children who disclosed CSA, mothers of children who disclose CSA report more symptoms of trauma, distress, PTSD, and general negative impact (e.g., Cyr et al., 2018; Manion et al., 1996).

A further complicating factor in many revelations of abuse is that the perpetrator is a family member and potentially a parent (usually the father). This has serious impact on family relationships, the structure of the family, and the family financial situation, as the offending family member may be incarcerated and thus no longer able to help financially. Further, there is the guilt, shame, and stigma that is associated with intrafamilial abuse and incest (e.g., Wallis & Woodworth, 2021). One study of 100 CSA victims (63 intrafamilial, 37 extrafamilial) found that it was not the type of abuse (i.e., intrafamiliar or extrafamilial) that predicted negative psychological outcomes, but rather the degree of family cohesion prior to the abuse (Bal et al., 2004).

Finally, while much of the research on the family impact of CSA focuses on the disclosure itself, there are also other stressors such as police, court, and the involvement of child protective services that may also contribute to outcomes. Another study that examined parental responses to alleged incidents of CSA at a daycare center found that the sequalae of CSA disclosure, such as testifying in court, hearing the verdict, and the media coverage of a high-profile event, cause parents significant stress (Dyb et al., 2003). This is consistent with Tsang et al.'s (2020) postulation that the fluctuations they noted in the PTSD symptoms of the parents in the study could be related to ongoing legal system involvement and the high-profile media coverage of the abuse.

4.2.3 Consequences to Institutions and Community

Over the past 20 years, child abuse within many institutions such as the Catholic Church, Boy Scouts of America, and major sporting organizations in the United States (US; i.e., USA Gymnastics) has been revealed (see Chap. 8). The scope of the abuse within these organizations was widespread. For example, it was estimated that between 1950 and 2002, 4% (or 4392) of all active priests within the US Catholic church had allegations of sexual abuse (Terry, 2008). By the 2020 filing deadline, nearly 95,000 claims of sexual abuse were filed against the Boy Scouts of America in civil court (Baker, 2020). It was believed that institutional sexual abuse involved sexual grooming (McAlinden, 2006)—an assertion later supported by a wealth of empirical data (e.g., Spraitz & Bowen, 2019; Spraitz et al., 2018; Winters et al., 2022).

To date, the US Catholic Church has paid out 3.2 billion dollars in settlements (Coffman, 2020), and it is estimated that that figure will increase with additional claims. The Boy Scouts of America have declared bankruptcy because of the lawsuits filed against them (Wamsley & Goodwyn, 2020). However, these institutional costs are infinitesimal when compared to the societal costs of sexual abuse, including child and adult healthcare costs, lost productivity, child welfare, and criminal justice costs, to name a few. It is estimated that lifetime costs incurred annually from confirmed cases of child maltreatment were $428 billion and up to two trillion dollars using the incidence of investigated cases (Peterson et al., 2018).

The fallout to institutions from abuse revelations has been immense, not only in terms of financial liability but also in terms of public trust and confidence in these organizations and their leadership. For example, Rossetti (1995) surveyed Catholics in the US and Canada and found that those who were victimized by clergy had significantly more negative opinions of the Catholic church, "highlighting the spiritual damage caused by child sexual abuse" (p. 1469). Another study examining Catholic school enrollment following abuse revelations showed substantial decline (Dills & Hernández-Julián, 2012). The authors speculated this could have been due to parents' negative perceptions of church attendance or the decreased number of placements following significant financial ramifications. Institutional trust was further eroded when it became clear that institutions were aware of the abuse and covered it up, thus endangering more minors (O'Brien, 2020). Similarly, in the "Penn State Scandal" with Jerry Sandusky, when it became known that multiple people had previously reported Sandusky's behavior to coach Paterno and others at the University, there was a serious erosion of trust in the institution and its leadership, and the University continues to work to rebuild public support (O'Brien, 2012).

If there was some good that came out of these high-profile cases of institutional abuse, it was the recognition that some perpetrators use their positions within youth-serving organizations to gain access to children for abuse using sexual grooming strategies. Consequently, almost all youth-serving organizations have now implemented policies and procedures to minimize opportunities for perpetration. These include but are not limited to universal background checks for all employees and volunteers; staff training on boundaries, reporting, and red flags for abuse; not allowing one adult alone with minors (two person rule); keeping doors open whenever an adult is in a room with a child; windows in all doors so there is always a clear line of sight; and policies and procedures about out of program contact and program excursions (see Saul & Audage, 2007). However, increased research on grooming tactics within youth-serving organizations is needed to ensure proper safeguards are in place.

4.3 Conclusion

The effects of CSA are serious and long lasting. CSA negatively impacts not only the victim, but their families, communities, institutions, and society at large. While the long-term psychological, physical, psychosocial, and socioeconomic impact of CSA is well documented, we know little about how the sexual grooming process may differentially impact outcomes. Based upon the little that is known, it is likely that individuals who experience sexual grooming-based CSA have experienced more psychological manipulation, thus leading to more feelings of confusion, culpability for the abuse, guilt, and shame. It is also likely that because of the sexual grooming, CSA victims who experience grooming tactics will be less likely to disclose—or disclose after a long period of time—thus preventing intervention and exacerbating distress. Once disclosed, parents of victims experience significant distress which is also apt to be magnified if they themselves were groomed and thus did not suspect abuse. On a community and institutional level, grooming that has not been adequately prevented or disclosed breeds public distrust and anger. What remains clear is that more research on the impact of child sexual grooming, especially from a socioecological perspective, is needed to better understand the needs of victims, families, and communities in the healing process.

References

Alcalá, H. E., Valdez-Dadia, A., & von Ehrenstein, O. S. (2018). Adverse childhood experiences and access and utilization of health care. *Journal of Public Health, 40*(4), 684–692. https://doi.org/10.1093/pubmed/fdx155

Baker, M. (2020, November 15). Sex-abuse claims against Boy Scouts now surpass 82,000. *The New York Times.* https://www.nytimes.com/2020/11/15/us/boy-scouts-abuse-claims-bankruptcy.html

Bal, S., De Bourdeaudhuij, I., Crombez, G., & Van Oost, P. (2004). Differences in trauma symptoms and family functioning in intra-and extrafamilial sexually abused adolescents. *Journal of Interpersonal Violence, 19*(1), 108–123. https://doi.org/10.1177/0886260503259053

Barrett, A., Kamiya, Y., & O'Sullivan, V. (2014). Childhood sexual abuse and later-life economic consequences. *Journal of Behavioral and Experimental Economics, 53*, 10–16. https://doi.org/10.1016/j.socec.2014.07.001

Bennett, N., & O'Donohue, W. T. (2016). Child abuser's threats and grooming techniques. In W. T. O'Donohue & M. Fanetti (Eds.), *Forensic interviews regarding child sexual abuse: A guide to evidence-based practice* (pp. 307–316). Springer.

Canter, D., Hughes, D., & Kirby, S. (1998). Paedophilia: Pathology, criminality, or both? The development of a multivariate model of offence behaviour in child sexual abuse. *Journal of Forensic Psychiatry, 9*(3), 532–555. https://doi.org/10.1080/09585189808405372

Centers for Disease Control and Prevention [CDC]. (2019). *Preventing adverse childhood experiences: Leveraging the best available evidence.* https://www.cdc.gov/violenceprevention/pdf/preventingACES.pdf

CDC. (2021). *The social-ecological model: A framework for prevention.* https://www.cdc.gov/violenceprevention/about/social-ecologicalmodel.html

Coffman, K. (2020, December 1). Catholic Church pays $7 million to victims in Colorado of sexual abuse by priests. *Reuters.* https://www.reuters.com/article/us-colorado-priests-sexabuse/catholic-church-pays-7-million-to-victims-in-colorado-of-sexual-abuse-by-priests-idUSKBN28C01C

Colman, R. A., & Widom, C. S. (2004). Childhood abuse and neglect and adult intimate relationships: A prospective study. *Child Abuse & Neglect, 28*(11), 1133–1151. https://doi.org/10.1016/j.chiabu.2004.02.005

Craven, S., Brown, S., & Gilchrist, E. (2006). Sexual grooming of children: Review of literature and theoretical considerations. *Journal of Sexual Aggression, 12*(3), 287–299. https://doi.org/10.1080/13552600601069414

Cunningham, K. C. (2020). Shame and guilt in PTSD. In *Emotion in posttraumatic stress disorder* (pp. 145–171). Academic. https://doi.org/10.1016/B978-0-12-816022-0.00006-5

Currie, J., & Widom, C. S. (2010). Long-term consequences of child abuse and neglect on adult economic well-being. *Child Maltreatment, 15*(2), 111–120. https://doi.org/10.1177/1077559509355316

Cyr, M., Frappier, J. Y., Hébert, M., Tourigny, M., McDuff, P., & Turcotte, M. E. (2018). Impact of child sexual abuse disclosure on the health of nonoffending parents: A longitudinal perspective. *Journal of Child Custody, 15*(2), 147–167. https://doi.org/10.1080/15379418.2018.1460649

Daignault, I. V., Hébert, M., Cyr, M., Pelletier, M., & McDuff, P. (2018). Correlates and predictors of mothers' adaptation and trauma symptoms following the unveiling of the sexual abuse of their child. *Journal of Interpersonal Violence*. https://doi.org/10.1177/0886260518808849

Davies, M. G. (1995). Parental distress and ability to cope following disclosure of extra-familial sexual abuse. *Child Abuse & Neglect, 19*(4), 399–408. https://doi.org/10.1016/0145-2134(95)00010-6

de Aquino Ferreira, L. F., Pereira, F. H. Q., Benevides, A. M. L. N., & Melo, M. C. A. (2018). Borderline personality disorder and sexual abuse: A systematic review. *Psychiatry Research, 262*, 70–77. https://doi.org/10.1016/j.psychres.2018.01.043

DeLisi, M., Drury, A. J., & Elbert, M. J. (2019). The etiology of antisocial personality disorder: The differential roles of adverse childhood experiences and childhood psychopathology. *Comprehensive Psychiatry, 92*, 1–6. https://doi.org/10.1016/j.comppsych.2019.04.001

Devries, K. M., Mak, J. Y., Child, J. C., Falder, G., Bacchus, L. J., Astbury, J., & Watts, C. H. (2014). Childhood sexual abuse and suicidal behavior: A meta-analysis. *Pediatrics, 133*(5), e1331–e1344. https://doi.org/10.1542/peds.2013-2166

DiLillo, D., Hayes-Skelton, S. A., Fortier, M. A., Perry, A. R., Evans, S. E., Moore, T. L. M., Walsh, K., Nash, C., & Fauchier, A. (2010). Development and initial psychometric properties of the Computer Assisted Maltreatment Inventory (CAMI): A comprehensive self-report measure of child maltreatment history. *Child Abuse & Neglect, 34*(5), 305–317. https://doi.org/10.1016/j.chiabu.2009.09.015

Dills, A. K., & Hernández-Julián, R. (2012). Negative publicity and Catholic schools. *Economic Inquiry, 50*(1), 143–152. https://doi.org/10.1111/j.1465-7295.2010.00342.x

Dube, S. R., Anda, R. F., Whitfield, C. L., Brown, D. W., Felitti, V. J., Dong, M., & Giles, W. H. (2005). Long-term consequences of childhood sexual abuse by gender of victim. *American Journal of Preventive Medicine, 28*(5), 430–438. https://doi.org/10.1016/j.amepre.2005.01.015

Dyb, G., Holen, A., Steinberg, A. M., Rodriguez, N., & Pynoos, R. S. (2003). Alleged sexual abuse at a day care center: Impact on parents. *Child Abuse & Neglect, 27*(8), 939–950. https://doi.org/10.1016/s0145-2134(03)00141-8

Easton, S. D. (2014). Masculine norms, disclosure, and childhood adversities predict long-term mental distress among men with histories of child sexual abuse. *Child Abuse & Neglect, 38*(2), 243–251. https://doi.org/10.1016/j.chiabu.2013.08.020

Easton, S. D. (2019). Childhood disclosure of sexual abuse and mental health outcomes in adulthood: Assessing merits of early disclosure and discussion. *Child Abuse & Neglect, 93*, 208–214. https://doi.org/10.1016/j.chiabu.2019.04.005

Elfgen, C., Hagenbuch, N., Goerres, G., Block, E., & Leeners, B. (2017). Breastfeeding in women having experienced childhood sexual abuse. *Journal of Human Lactation, 33*(1), 119–127. https://doi.org/10.1177/0890334416680789

Fang, X., Brown, D. S., Florence, C. S., & Mercy, J. A. (2012). The economic burden of child maltreatment in the United States and implications for prevention. *Child Abuse & Neglect, 36*(2), 156–165. https://doi.org/10.1016/j.chiabu.2011.10.006

Finkelhor, D. (1984). *Child sexual abuse: New theory and research*. Free Press.

Hailes, H. P., Yu, R., Danese, A., & Fazel, S. (2019). Long-term outcomes of childhood sexual abuse: An umbrella review. *The Lancet Psychiatry, 6*(10), 830–839. https://doi.org/10.1016/S2215-0366(19)30286-X

Hall, G. N., & Hirschman, R. (1992). Sexual aggression against children: A conceptual perspective of etiology. *Criminal Justice and Behavior, 19*(1), 8–23. https://doi.org/10.1177/0093854892019001003

Irish, L., Kobayashi, I., & Delahanty, D. L. (2010). Long-term physical health consequences of childhood sexual abuse: A meta-analytic review. *Journal of Pediatric Psychology, 35*(5), 450–461. https://doi.org/10.1093/jpepsy/jsp118

Kamiya, Y., Timonen, V., & Kenny, R. A. (2016). The impact of childhood sexual abuse on the mental and physical health, and healthcare utilization of older adults. *International Psychogeriatrics, 28*(3), 415–422. https://doi.org/10.1017/S1041610215001672

Lange, B. C., Condon, E. M., & Gardner, F. (2020). Parenting among mothers who experienced child sexual abuse: A qualitative systematic review. *Qualitative Health Research, 30*(1), 146–161. https://doi.org/10.1177/1049732319882914

Leberg, E. (1997). *Understanding child molesters: Taking charge*. Sage.

Letourneau, E. J., Brown, D. S., Fang, X., Hassan, A., & Mercy, J. A. (2018). The economic burden of child sexual abuse in the United States. *Child Abuse & Neglect, 79*, 413–422. https://doi.org/10.1016/j.chiabu.2018.02.020

Manion, I. G., McIntyre, J., Firestone, P., Ligezinska, M., Ensom, R., & Wells, G. (1996). Secondary traumatization in parents following the disclosure of extrafamilial child sexual abuse: Initial effects. *Child Abuse & Neglect, 20*(11), 1095–1109. https://doi.org/10.1016/0145-2134(96)00098-1

McAlinden, A. (2006). "Setting 'em up": Personal, familial and institutional grooming in the sexual abuse of children. *Social & Legal Studies, 15*(3), 339–362. https://doi.org/10.1177/0964663906066613

O'Brien, G. (2012, January 23). After Paterno, Penn State's struggle to rebuild trust. *Business Ethics*. https://business-ethics.com/2012/01/23/8828-after-paterno-penn-states-struggle-to-rebuild-trust/

O'Brien, P. M. (2020). Transparency as a means to rebuild trust within the Church: A case study in how Catholic dioceses and eparchies in the United States have responded to the clergy sex abuse crisis. *Church, Communication and Culture, 5*(3), 456–483. https://doi.org/10.1080/23753234.2020.1827962

O'Leary, P., Coohey, C., & Easton, S. D. (2010). The effect of severe child sexual abuse and disclosure on mental health during adulthood. *Journal of Child Sexual Abuse, 19*(3), 275–289. https://doi.org/10.1080/10538711003781251

Peterson, C., Florence, C., & Klevens, J. (2018). The economic burden of child maltreatment in the United States, 2015. *Child Abuse & Neglect, 86*, 178–183. https://doi.org/10.1016/j.chiabu.2018.09.018

Plummer, M. (2018). Lived experiences of grooming among Australian male survivors of child sexual abuse. *Journal of Interpersonal Violence, 33*(1), 37–63. https://doi.org/10.1177/0886260517732539

Plummer, C. A., & Eastin, J. (2007). The effect of child sexual abuse allegations/investigations on the mother/child relationship. *Violence Against Women, 13*(10), 1053–1071. https://doi.org/10.1177/1077801207305931

Pulverman, C. S., Kilimnik, C. D., & Meston, C. M. (2018). The impact of childhood sexual abuse on women's sexual health: A comprehensive review. *Sexual Medicine Reviews*, 1–13. https://doi.org/10.1016/j.sxmr.2017.12.002

Regehr, C. (1990). Parental responses to extrafamilial child sexual assault. *Child Abuse & Neglect, 14*(1), 113–120. https://doi.org/10.1016/0145-2134(90)90086-9

Rossetti, S. J. (1995). The impact of child sexual abuse on attitudes toward God and the Catholic Church. *Child Abuse & Neglect, 19*(12), 1469–1481. https://doi.org/10.1016/0145-2134(95)00100-1

Saul, J., & Audage, N. C. (2007). *Preventing child sexual abuse within youth-serving organizations: Getting started on policies and procedures*. Atlanta, GA: Centers for Disease Control and Prevention; National Center for Injury Prevention and Control.

Spraitz, J. D., & Bowen, K. N. (2019). Examination of a nascent taxonomy of priest sexual grooming. *Sexual Abuse, 31*(6), 707–728. https://doi.org/10.1177/1079063218809095

Spraitz, J. D., Bowen, K. N., & Strange, L. (2018). Proposing a behavioral taxonomy of priest sexual grooming. *International Journal for Crime, Justice and Social Democracy, 7*(1), 30–43. https://doi.org/10.5204/ijcjsd.v7i1.387

Swingle, J. M., Tursich, M., Cleveland, J. M., Gold, S. N., Tolliver, S. F., Michaels, L., Kupperman-Caron, L. N., Garcia-Larrieu, M., & Sciarrino, N. A. (2016). Childhood disclosure of sexual abuse: Necessary but not necessarily sufficient. *Child Abuse & Neglect, 62*, 10–18. https://doi.org/10.1016/j.chiabu.2016.10.009

Teicher, M. H., Samson, J. A., Polcari, A., & Andersen, S. L. (2009). Length of time between onset of childhood sexual abuse and emergence of depression in a young adult sample: A retrospective clinical report. *The Journal of Clinical Psychiatry, 70*(5), 684–691. https://doi.org/10.4088/jcp.08m04235

Terry, K. J. (2008). Stained glass: The nature and scope of child sexual abuse in the Catholic Church. *Criminal Justice and Behavior, 35*(5), 549–569. https://doi.org/10.1177/0093854808314339

Tonmyr, L., & Shields, M. (2017). Childhood sexual abuse and substance abuse: A gender paradox? *Child Abuse & Neglect, 63*, 284–294. https://doi.org/10.1016/j.chiabu.2016.11.004

Tsang, V. M., Verlinden, E., van Duin, E. M., Twisk, J. W., Brilleslijper-Kater, S. N., Gigengack, M. R., Verhoeff, A. P., & Lindauer, R. J. (2020). The Amsterdam sexual abuse case: What scars did it leave? Long-term course of psychological problems for children who have been sexually abused at a very young age, and their parents. *Child Psychiatry & Human Development*, 1–12. https://doi.org/10.1007/s10578-020-01067-5

Ullman, S. E. (2007). Relationship to perpetrator, disclosure, social reactions, and PTSD symptoms in child sexual abuse survivors. *Journal of Child Sexual Abuse, 16*(1), 19–36. https://doi.org/10.1300/J070v16n01_02

Ullman, S. E., & Filipas, H. H. (2005). Gender differences in social reactions to abuse disclosures, post-abuse coping, and PTSD of child sexual abuse survivors. *Child Abuse & Neglect, 29*(7), 767–782. https://doi.org/10.1016/j.chiabu.2005.01.005

van Dam, C. (2001). *Identifying child molesters: Preventing child sexual abuse by recognizing the patterns of the offenders*. Haworth Maltreatment and Trauma Press/The Haworth Press.

Walker, H. E., Freud, J. S., Ellis, R. A., Fraine, S. M., & Wilson, L. C. (2019). The prevalence of sexual revictimization: A meta-analytic review. *Trauma, Violence, & Abuse, 20*(1), 67–80. https://doi.org/10.1177/1524838017692364

Wallis, C. R., & Woodworth, M. (2021). Non-offending caregiver support in cases of child sexual abuse: An examination of the impact of support on formal disclosures. *Child Abuse & Neglect, 113*, 104929. https://doi.org/10.1016/j.chiabu.2021.104929

Wamsley, L., & Goodwyn, W. (2020, February 18). Boy Scouts of America files for bankruptcy as it faces hundreds of sex-abuse claims. *NPR*. https://www.npr.org/2020/02/18/806721827/boy-scouts-of-america-files-for-bankruptcy-as-it-faces-hundreds-of-sex-abuse-cla#:~:text=The%20Boy%20Scouts%20of%20America%20has%20filed%20for%20bankruptcy%2C%20a,to%20provide%20compensation%20to%20victims

Ward, T., & Siegert, R. J. (2002). Toward a comprehensive theory on child sexual abuse: A theory of knitting perspective. *Psychology, Crime & Law, 8*(4), 319–351. https://doi.org/10.1080/10683160208401823

Whittle, H. C., Hamilton-Giachritsis, C., & Beech, A. R. (2013). Victims' voices: The impact of online grooming and sexual abuse. *Universal Journal of Psychology, 1*(2), 59–71. https://doi.org/10.13189/ujp.2013.010206

Williams, A. (2015). Child sexual victimisation: Ethnographic stories of stranger and acquaintance grooming. *Journal of Sexual Aggression, 21*(1), 28–42. https://doi.org/10.1080/13552600.2014.948085

Winters, G. M., Jeglic, E. L., & Kaylor, L. E. (2020). Validation of the sexual grooming model of child sexual abusers. *Journal of Child Sexual Abuse, 29*(7), 855–875. https://doi.org/10.1080/10538712.2020.1801935

Winters, G. M., Jeglic, E. L., & Terry, K. J. (2022). The prevalence of sexual grooming behaviors in a large sample of clergy. *Sexual Abuse: A Journal of Research and Treatment*. https://doi.org/10.1177/10790632211070803

Wolf, M. R., & Pruitt, D. K. (2019). Grooming hurts too: The effects of types of perpetrator grooming on trauma symptoms in adult survivors of child sexual abuse. *Journal of Child Sexual Abuse, 28*(3), 345–359. https://doi.org/10.1080/10538712.2019.1579292

Chapter 5
Online Sexual Grooming

The use of the Internet by youth has been increasing with easy access to devices (e.g., computers and laptops, smart phones, gaming systems) at home, school, and many other locations. In 2019, 95% of children aged 3–18 had Internet access at home (National Center for Education Statistics, 2021). While there are many benefits to the Internet, such as for socialization and educational purposes, this increase has also produced a heightened risk for sexual solicitation from adults. The *Triple A–Engine* theory suggests that the easy accessibility, affordability, and anonymity of the Internet promotes a setting in which adults can more readily commit online sexual offenses against children (Cooper, 1998). These deviant sexual behaviors can include sending or receiving child sexual exploitation material (CSEM), communicating with other adults about sexual interests in children, or communicating with minors in a sexual manner (Durkin, 1997). In the United States (US), the National Center for Missing and Exploited Children (NCMEC, 2021) reviewed 21.7 million reports of online child sexual exploitation in 2020. These reports included over 21 million reports of CSEM, as well as nearly 38,000 cases of online sexual solicitation. Given the wide reach of the Internet, the online sexual abuse of children is a global problem, making these crimes especially difficult to identify and prosecute as they span across different jurisdictions (e.g., challenges associated with prosecuting an adult who sexually solicits a child from a different country; UNICEF, 2011).

As noted above, there are various types of online sexual abuse of children. Of relevance to the present book, adults have used the Internet to locate and communicate with minors for the purposes of engaging in online or offline sexual abuse. This is generally referred to as the *online sexual solicitation* of youth, which involves the use of the Internet to interact with children or adolescents for sexual purposes (Schulz et al., 2015; Seto et al., 2012), including various cybersexual activities (i.e., sexualized conversations or activities for the purpose of sexual gratification, such as sending or receiving sexual images or videos; Doring, 2000). Sexual solicitation of minors may occur soon after the initial contact with a minor online (Dehart et al., 2017; Winters et al., 2017); however, some individuals may engage in a lengthier

© The Author(s), under exclusive license to Springer Nature Switzerland AG 2022

G. M. Winters, E. L. Jeglic, *Sexual Grooming*,
https://doi.org/10.1007/978-3-031-07222-2_5

online sexual grooming process in order to form a relationship before proceeding to the sexual content or acts (Broome et al., 2018). Greene-Colozzi et al. (2020) describe the difference between these two terms (which are often incorrectly used interchangeably in the literature), indicating that "online sexual grooming differs from online sexual solicitation in that solicitation is a behavior, which may occur only once, whereas grooming is a process, the outcome of which is an intimate relationship" (p. 838). Thus, the present chapter aims to provide an overview of online solicitation and sexual grooming of minors via the Internet, including information on the victims and individuals who commit these offenses, as well as the proposed models and behaviors involved in the process. Finally, the chapter will conclude with a brief description of areas of prevention and intervention.

5.1 Online Sexual Solicitation

The online sexual solicitation of youth has increased over the past two decades (Mitchell et al., 2014). Overall, meta-analytic evidence suggests 20% of youth have experienced unwanted sexual contact online, with 11% endorsing having been sexually solicited via the Internet (Madigan et al., 2018). In one large-scale study, Mitchell et al. (2014) investigated the rates of online sexual solicitation, as defined by "requests to engage in sexual activities or sexual talk, or give personal sexual information that were unwanted or, whether wanted or not, made by an adult" (p. 1). Through telephone interviews with youth, they found that 1 in 11 (9%) minors who used the Internet had experienced online sexual solicitation in the past year. Moreover, 3% of youth reported "aggressive" sexual solicitation (i.e., attempted or actual offline contact via mail, telephone, or in-person). Other studies have shown that between 17% and 32% of minors who use the Internet have been sexually solicited online (e.g., Finkelhor et al., 2000; Greene-Colozzi et al., 2020; Shannon, 2008; Ybarra et al., 2004).

It has been suggested that these rates are underestimating the extent of the problem (Staksrud, 2013). Due to young age and vulnerabilities of the victim, there may be feelings of embarrassment or shame about their experience or a lack of understanding that they have been victimized (Martellozzo, 2019). Additionally, the Internet provides access to multiple victims at a single given time, permitting an adult to cast a wide net for possible victims in this setting. Many of these studies are several years old and thus may not account for the increased use of the Internet by youth and the developments in Internet-related activities for youth (e.g., online gaming, social media; Bowles & Keller, 2019; Interpol, 2020; Silva, 2019; Stiggers, 2020). Ultimately, there are likely higher rates of online sexual solicitation than are being reported. Also of note, the instances of online sexual abuse of children have been reportedly increasing following the onset of the global coronavirus pandemic in 2020. The Federal Bureau of Investigation (FBI) and the United Nations International Children's Emergency Fund (UNICEF) issued warnings that the instances of online sexual offenses may be multiplying (Jeglic, 2020). Indeed,

NCMEC reported a significant rise in cybertips for online child sexual abuse (CSA) during that time. For example, NCMEC received 1 million reports on its CyberTipline in April 2019 versus 4.1 million in April 2020 (Alfonso, 2020). There was a 97.5% increase from 2019 to 2020 in the number of reports of online sexual solicitation of minors (19,174 cases in 2019 vs 37,8772 cases in 2020; O'Donnell, 2021), which highlights that this is a pervasive and growing problem.

5.2 Online Sexual Grooming

Similar to the in-person sexual grooming literature, there is no universal definition of online sexual grooming. Generally speaking, literature on online sexual grooming relies upon the same definitions as those proposed in the in-person sexual grooming literature (Kloess et al., 2014), in that they emphasize the importance of the emotional connection developed with the potential victim in the online setting in preparation for the sexual abuse (Broomie et al., 2018). While some adults may seek contact with minors online to progress to in-person sexual contact, there are many offenders who seek to solely engage in online activities (e.g., sexual chats, sending or receiving CSEM). While there are similarities between online and in-person sexual grooming (e.g., Marcum, 2007; Wolak et al., 2010), there are unique aspects of the online setting that warrant an in-depth investigation. As Martellozzo (2015) notes, "the Internet does not create new stages of the cycle of abuse, but allows the cycle of abuse to be quickened" (p. 66).

5.3 Individuals Who Sexually Solicit and Groom Minors Online

In order to garner an understanding of online sexual grooming, it is important to explore the types of individuals who commit these types of offenses. Researchers have identified characteristics of those who commit sexual solicitation and/or sexual grooming in online settings, as well as offense typologies specific to this group.

5.3.1 General Characteristics

In general, when comparing individuals who commit online versus in-person sexual offenses, evidence has shown those with online offenses tend to be younger, White, unemployed males with fewer offense supportive attitudes/beliefs and less emotional identification with minors, as well as have higher levels of victim empathy and sexually deviant interests (Babchishin et al., 2011;

Mitchell et al., 2014; Wolak et al., 2008). In regard to online sexual solicitation, evidence has shown that two-thirds of self-reported incidents by youth were committed by a stranger the minor met online (Mitchell et al., 2014). While many cases of online solicitation are committed by adults, as many as half of the cases (42%) may be committed by other youth aged 18 or younger. There may be some instances of adults posing as children to sexually solicit the minor, but contrary to popular belief, most of the adults accurately portray their age and identity (Wolak et al., 2008). For example, Wolak et al. (2004) found that only 5% of offenders posed as minors, and Winters et al. (2017) found that while one-third lied about their age to some degree (97% presenting as younger than their actual age), none presented as minors.

5.3.2 Typologies

There have been many proposed typologies of the individuals who commit sexual solicitation and/or sexual grooming of minors online. In Table 5.1, we present a summary of the most commonly cited typologies of online solicitation offenders.

In a general conceptualization of individuals who commit online offenses, McLaughlin (1998) suggested there are *travelers* who use the Internet to locate victims for in-person sexual encounters and *chatters* who use the guise of mentorship to engage the minor in sexualized conversations or cybersexual activity and do not typically seek to commit an in-person offense. McLaughlin also included two other categories who utilize or distribute (*collectors/traders*) or produce (*manufacturers*) CSEM content online. In a sample of 200 law enforcement cases of online offending, 24% were travelers, and only one case was classified as a chatter; the remaining cases fell under the categories related to CSEM (McLaughlin, 1998).

More recently, Briggs et al. (2011) expanded upon McLaughlin's (1998) online offending typologies. In their study of 51 individuals convicted of an online sexual offense, they found distinct subgroups of individuals based on their ultimate goal of the inappropriate online contact. *Contact-driven offenders* ($n = 30$; 59%) aimed to converse with minors online with the ultimate goal of moving to an offline setting to engage in sexual behaviors. On the other hand, *fantasy-driven offenders* ($n = 21$; 41%) sought to solely engage in cybersexual activities and did not have the intention of moving the sexual contact offline. Briggs et al. (2011) found that contact-driven offenders were younger, had less formal education, and were more likely to be employed, and fewer were married compared to fantasy-driven offenders. Regarding the sexualized behaviors, the contact-driven offenders engaged in fewer online sexual behaviors (e.g., sending nude photographs, engaging the victim in cybersex), although the groups did not differ in terms of their use of online grooming. Notably, in a later systematic review of 22 studies of contact-driven versus fantasy-driven internet offenders (Broome et al., 2018), there were no clear patterns

Table 5.1 Typologies of individuals who commit online sexual solicitation

Authors	Typology	Description
McLaughlin (1998)	*Travelers*	Use the Internet to meet victims for in-person sexual contact
	Chatters	Communicate with minors online for sexual discussions or acts, but typically do not move to in-person contact
	Collectors/ traders	Use or distribute CSEM online
	Manufacturers	Produce online child pornography
Briggs et al. (2011)	*Contact-driven*	Use the Internet to meet minors with the ultimate goal of moving to in-person sexual contact
	Fantasy-driven	Use the Internet to meet minors to engage in cybersexual activities only
European Online Grooming Project (2012)	*Intimacy-seeking*	Spend a significant amount of time talking to the minor before introducing sexual behaviors or an in-person meeting
	Adaptable style	Adapt their identity and sexual grooming style based on the minor's presentation and reaction
	Hyper-sexualized	Highly sexualized in the communication and escalate to sexual content quickly
Martellozzo (2015)	*Hyperconfident*	Openly shared sexual interests/intent
	Hypercautious	Cautiously engages in online sexual behavior by establishing closeness with the minor over time
DeHart et al. (2017)	*Cybersex only*	Engaged in or encouraged masturbation and did not attempt to schedule an offline meeting
	Cybersex/ schedulers	Engaged in or encouraged masturbation and attempted to schedule an offline meeting
	Schedulers	Attempted to schedule an offline meeting and did not engage in offline masturbation
	Buyers	Engaged in a third-party chats for the purposes of child sexual trafficking

of behavior that differentiated the two groups in terms of the use of relationship building strategies, deceptive identities, assessment of risk, sexualized content, or threatening behaviors.

The European Online Grooming Project (EOGP; Webster et al., 2012) was a research consortium of European experts who used a range of methods (e.g., review of police files, interviews with key stakeholders, interviews with perpetrators) to develop a typology of those who sexually groom online. They suggested there are three types of online groomers: *intimacy-seeking*, *adaptable style*, and *hyper-sexualized*. These were based on eight behavioral characteristics: (1) prior sexual offense convictions, (2) deceptive identity, (3) nature and extent of explicit image use, (4) contact with other offenders online, (5) offense-supportive attitudes, (6) length of contact with the minor, (7) how contact was initiated and maintained, and (8) outcome of the offense. The intimacy-seeking group view their offense as a "consenting" relationship and thus spent significant amounts of time talking with the minor before engaging in sexual behaviors or meeting in-person. They tend to present as themselves online, and they did not have criminal histories, possess CSEM, or contact other offenders. The adaptable style mold their identity and sexual grooming strategies to the presentation and reaction of the minor. They tended to have prior sexual convictions, held offense-supportive attitudes, and possessed some indecent images of children. Lastly, the hyper-sexualized group were highly sexual and moved quickly in their interactions with minors. They tended to misrepresent their identity, had large amounts of CSEM, and contacted other people engaged in inapropriate online sexual activity. The EOGP report does not provide empirical, quantitative data associated with these typologies.

One typology specific to online sexual grooming was proposed by Martellozzo (2015). Using 160 transcripts from undercover policing operations in the United Kingdom, she proposed a spectrum of "groomers" based on level of openness, ranging from *hyperconfident* to *hypercautious*. Those who are hyperconfident openly share their sexual interests and explicit material (e.g., nude photographs of themselves), while those who are hypercautious spend time establishing relationships with whom they interact and do not readily share sexual content. Martellozzo (2015) suggests the hypercautious group is more dangerous, in that they are not easily identifiable and maintain a passive role until they are confident that they will remain undetected.

Testing Briggs et al. (2011) distinction between contact- and fantasy-driven typologies, DeHart et al. (2017) examined chatroom logs, social media content, and emails of 179 individuals who committed online offenses. The results supported the distinction between the Briggs et al. (2011) categories, but the authors suggested a more nuanced typology containing four subgroups based on: (1) whether they engaged in or encouraged masturbation online in real time, (2) whether they attempted to schedule an offline meeting (e.g., specific times and places), and (3) whether they involved a third-party (e.g., pimp, family member) for sex trafficking purposes. These groups were labeled as: *cybersex only*, *cybersex/schedulers*, *schedulers*, and *buyers*. Qualitative analyses of the typologies showed the cybersex only group (n = 48; 27%) tended to chat with the minor for long periods of time (e.g., months), during which they often asked about the physical appearance of the child, coached the child on masturbation, and vaguely mentioned a future meeting without scheduling one. The cybersex/schedulers (n = 64; 36%) also chatted for months and focused on the physical sex features of the minor but then scheduled an in-person meeting. The schedulers (n = 44; 25%) attempted to schedule meetings within a comparatively shorter period of time (i.e., 1 week). The buyers (n = 23; 13%) focused on scheduling a meeting and negotiating terms (e.g., cost, type of sexual activity) with the third party, such as a pimp or family member; these cases often began with a classified advertisement, and the minor was asked to confirm their identity through photographs.

5.4 Minors Who Experience Sexual Solicitation Online

Research has shown girls were more frequently impacted by online solicitation than boys, with 75% of girls compared to 25% of boys reporting unwanted sexual solicitation (Mitchell et al., 2014). A self-report study of youth showed victims of online sexual solicitation are often ages 16 or 17 (54% of cases), although victimization has been reported as young as 8 years old (Marcum, 2007; Shannon, 2008). When looking at sexual grooming more specifically, the average age of minors having lengthy conversations with adult strangers was 16 years according to one self-report victimization study (Greene-Colozzi et al., 2020).

The EOGP (Webster et al., 2012) categorized victims in to two groups: *vulnerable victims* and *risk-taking victims* (see Fig. 5.1). They further identified an interaction between the type of offender (see EOGP "Typologies" section above) and the preferred victim type. Specifically, they indicated the intimacy-seeking typology will seek out vulnerable victims, the adaptable group can meet the needs of either victim group, and the hypersexual group will prefer interactions with the risk-taking victims.

Similar to the above conceptualization of youth vulnerability and risk-taking, through a thematic analysis of interviews with eight victims of online sexual grooming, Whittle et al. (2014) proposed there are situations that place minors at risk. These three scenarios that result in vulnerability for a child include: (1) multiple long-term risk factors (e.g., difficult family situations), (2) trigger events (e.g., loss of friendships, difficulty in school), and (3) online behavioral risks (e.g., talking to strangers). They found various risk factors for online sexual grooming as it relates to the child (e.g., low self-esteem, loneliness), as well as the family (e.g., separated parents, fights at home), friends (e.g., bullying), school (e.g., no Internet safety education, disliking school), living area (e.g., boredom), and Internet use (e.g., talking to strangers, Internet used in bedroom). The above findings have been supported by empirical data from victim reports of online sexual grooming. Indeed,

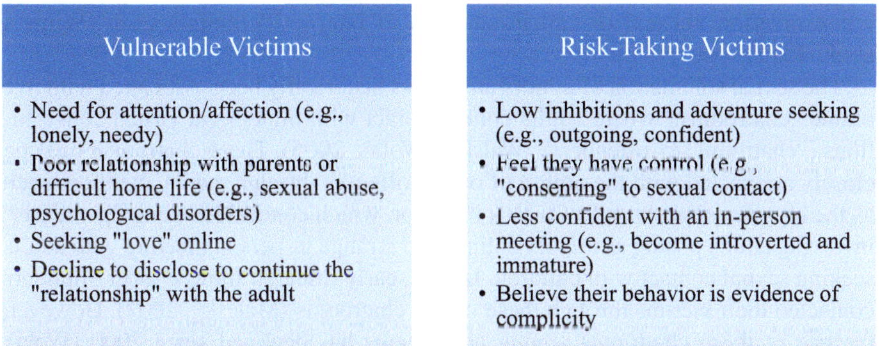

Fig. 5.1 EOGP victim typology

Greene-Colozzi et al. (2020) found that minors chat with adult strangers due to feeling bored, lonely, or curious.

Youth who are sexually solicited online may experience negative emotions as a result of the solicitation, such as feelings of being afraid or upset (Mitchell et al., 2014). Victims are more likely to have current and lifetime post-traumatic stress disorder diagnoses, as well as other mental health issues (e.g., depression, anxiety, phobias, suicidal ideation, or attempts; Wells & Mitchell, 2007). It should also be noted, however, that some victims may not perceive their experience to be abusive. In a survey of 489 adolescents, Villacampa and Gomez (2017) found of the 10% of youth who endorsed having been sexually groomed online, only between 42% and 52% of these youth described being offended or upset from the experience. Similarly, Greene-Colozzi et al. (2020) found only a small portion of participants who were sexually groomed as a minor endorsed feeling unsafe (11%) or found the adult to be aggressive (8%), angry (8%), or threatening (5%). The authors suggest this is likely a result of the sexual grooming strategies used to increase compliance and develop a seemingly consensual relationship.

5.5 Vulnerable Platforms

The Internet has become widely available across electronic devices that most children have ready access to, such as smartphones, tablets, laptops, desktop computers, and gaming consoles. Thus, when considering vulnerable platforms, it is important to note that these Internet services can be accessed through a range of means. As one example, 95% of teenagers aged 13–17 in the US either have a smartphone or have access to one (Anderson & Jiang, 2018). Given these connections to the Internet, the children may be contacted by adults either known to them or strangers for the purposes of sexual grooming. Moreover, after contact is established online, there may be instances of texting or telephone conversations afterward. In fact, one study found that 83% of adults who solicited minors online had a conversation via text or call in addition to Internet communication (Winters et al., 2017).

The sexual solicitation of minors online has historically been associated with live online "chatrooms," where adults could interact with minors via virtual conversations ("chatroom sex offenders"; Walsh & Wolak, 2005). These chatrooms became closely associated with the notion of online offenses through media attention, such as the hit television show To Catch a Predator, which conducted "sting operations" involving adults posing as minors online who arrange in-person meeting with adults seeking sexual contact with children. Indeed, early research showed most offenders contacted their victims through these online chatrooms (Malesky, 2007). However, the use of these chatrooms among adolescents has declined since 2000 (Wolak et al., 2006), and there have been a new wave of Internet platforms that facilitate easy and accessible contact with minors online.

5.5.1 *Social Media*

A survey of adolescents (ages 13–17) in the US revealed high percentages of youth using social media platforms, including Instagram (72%), Snapchat (69%), Facebook (51%), and Twitter (32%; Anderson & Jiang, 2018). These types of social media platforms, among others (e.g., TikTok, Kik, LiveMe, MeetMe, WhatsApp), are now being used for the sexual solicitation of minors (Silva, 2019; Stiggers, 2020). In the United Kingdom, over a period of 6 months, there were 1,317 cases of online sexual solicitation reported by police, including cases on Instagram (32%), Facebook (23%), and Snapchat (14%; British Broadcasting Corporation [BBC], 2019). These social media websites allow for the user to post images or messages and have "followers" or "friends" respond to these either publicly or privately. Therefore, an adult seeking to sexually groom a minor online may have easy access to information about the child and an ability to initiate and maintain communication with them.

5.5.2 *Gaming*

In the US, 84% of teenagers aged 13–17 have access to a video game console at home, with 83% of girls and 97% of boys endorsing playing video games (either by computer, game console, or smartphone; Anderson & Jiang, 2018). There have been more recent reports of online sexual solicitation of minors through multiplayer video games (Bowles & Keller, 2019; Interpol, 2020), in which individuals can communicate with one another via the Internet during game play. For example, online games such as Fortnite permit individuals to form a team to compete, which promotes forming relationships and communication in order to win. These gaming platforms (e.g., Minecraft, Roblox) include built-in functions that allow for text or voice chats, thus normalizing conversing with strangers (Bowles & Keller, 2019). Equally concerning is the ability to "gift" across these platforms, such as sending money or game rewards/credit, which can be a tactic used by adults in the online sexual grooming process. There have also been chatrooms developed for gaming, the most popular being Discord, where players can video or text chat about games—which provides a setting in which adults can contact children and discuss shared interests such as gaming (Defend Young Minds, 2021).

5.6 Models of Online Sexual Grooming

Similar to the in-person sexual grooming literature, there have been numerous proposed models of the processes involved in online sexual grooming. In Table 5.2, we present the most commonly referenced models within the literature.

Table 5.2 Models of online sexual grooming

Authors	Stages/phases	Description
O'Connell (2003)	*Friendship-forming stage*	Getting to know the minor
	Relationship-forming stage	Developing a closer relationship through personal conversations
	Risk assessment stage	Assessing the level of risk of being detected by others
	Exclusivity stage	Developing a strong sense of mutual respect and trust
	Sexual stage	Gradually increasing sexualized conversations and content
Webster et al. (2012)	*Vulnerability*	Relationships and situations
	Scanning	Mapping and appraisal
	Identity	Own and extent changed
	Contact	Model, extent, style, timing
	Intensity	Images, language, incentives
	Outcome	Online contact, physical meetings
Staksrud (2013)	*Introduction phase*	(a) Observing (b) Identify potential target (c) Engage targeted minor in conversation (d) Establish a personal and private conversation with the minor
	Grooming phase	Create a personal, trusting relationship with the minor through strategic communication
Williams et al. (2013)	*Rapport building*	Creating a friendship/relationship with the minor through: (a) Coordination (b) Mutuality (c) Positivity
	Sexual content	Engage the child in sexualized conversations: (a) Introduction (b) Maintenance
	Assessment	Assessing risk of detection: (a) Of child (b) Of environment
Lorenzo-Dus et al. (2016)	*Access*	Making initial online contact with victims
	Entrapment phase	Series of overlapping processes: (a) Deceptive trust development (b) Isolation (c) Sexual gratification (d) Compliance testing
	Approach	Use of verbal "lead-ins" to request to meet the child in-person for sexual contact

(continued)

Table 5.2 (continued)

Authors	Stages/phases	Description
Kloess et al. (2019)	*Approach*	Two types of approaches: (a) Indirect—engage in sexual grooming to develop a relationship with the victim (b) Direct—explicitly, immediately, and directly introduces sexual content
	Maintenance-escalation	Introduction and escalation of sexualized content and behaviors
	Closure	The outcome and closure of the encounter. This may include terminations of the interaction, or an attempted or actual in-person meeting.

As described in Chap. 2, one of the most widely cited models of online sexual grooming is one proposed by O'Connell (2003), which provides a nuanced description of strategies involved. First, the *friendship-forming stage* involves the adult getting to know the minor, often including exchanging nonsexual photographs. Second, the *relationship-forming stage* involves developing increased closeness with the child through conversations about the child, such as their life at school or home. Third, the *risk assessment stage* is used to establish the level of risk involved based on the child's environment, such as who else has access to the computer, parental supervision, etc. Fourth, in the *exclusivity stage*, the adult aims to establish a trusting and intimate relationship with the minor, through the guise of empathy and understanding for the child's circumstance. The fifth and final stage, *sexual stage*, the adult may introduce sexual content into conversations, which escalates to more sexualized discussions and behaviors (e.g., sending or receiving nude images, arranging a meeting for in-person sexual contact). O'Connell (2003) further described the methods used to terminate a sexual encounter, including damage limitation (e.g., encouragement, praise, and affection toward the minor to prevent disclosure) and the "hit-and-run" tactic (i.e., immediately removing themselves from the interaction). Black et al. (2015) empirically examined O'Connell's (2003) model using content analysis of transcripts from 44 cases of online sexual solicitation. Overall, the authors concluded the strategies employed were consistent with the stages of O'Connell's model, but the progression and order may not be as linear as previously proposed. They found a number of key sexual grooming tactics, such as the assessment of risk and introduction of sexual content, were often used early in conversations.

Nearly one decade later, Staksrud (2013) proposed a two-phase model of online sexual grooming. During the *introduction phase*, the individual will observe online activities of potential victims (e.g., view chatrooms without interacting) in order to identify a potential target, and then they seek to engage the targeted minor and proceed to a more personal, private conversation. Next, during the *grooming phase*, the core sexual grooming strategies (e.g., sharing personal information, learning about the child's life) are employed to develop an emotional connection with the child. This model has not been empirically examined in a qualitative or quantitative manner.

A more comprehensive model was introduced the same year by Williams et al. (2013). The authors developed a three-stage model by analyzing eight transcripts from a publicly available database of online chatroom communications of offenders communicating with decoy victims. In the first stage, *rapport building*, the offender develops a close relationship with the child through three tactics: coordination (i.e., aligning their language and behaviors with the child's), mutuality (i.e., identifying similar interests, attitudes, and circumstances), and positivity (i.e., portraying themselves in a positive light, such as being trustworthy and nice). The second stage, *sexual content*, involves the introduction of sexualized content in conversations (i.e., sexual content as a game, providing sex advice, engaging in "mutual fantasy," or by force), which is then later maintained afterward (i.e., repetition over time or by force). Third, in the *assessment* stage, the adult aims to evaluate the dangers of detection by assessing the child (i.e., assessing their level of trust, vulnerability, and receptiveness) and the environment (i.e., assessing obstacles, opportunity, and avoiding disclosing identifiable information). Given the authors based the model on qualitative analyses, they stressed the model requires further validation using quantitative data.

The EOGP (Webster et al., 2012) proposed there were six features to the online grooming process: *vulnerability*, *scanning*, *identity*, *contact*, *intensity*, and *outcome*. Vulnerability refers to circumstances that triggered the adult to engage in the online contact with the minor, such as problems in relationships (e.g., end of a romantic relationship) or situational factors (e.g., loss of a job). The individual may then engage in scanning, in which they observe the online environment and appraise the characteristics of the minor involved (e.g., virtual-sexual content in the profile, looking for idealistic/romantic traits, identifying desired physical traits). Next, identity is the process whereby the individual creates their online identity, which may include minor (e.g., name, marital status) or major (e.g., pretending to by a minor) changes. In the contact stage, they aim to communicate with the minor, including the mode (e.g., chatrooms, phones, gaming platforms, web camera), extent (i.e., the amount of time spent talking with the minor), style (e.g., compliments, mentorship, sharing similar interests), and timing (i.e., the length of time spent talking with the minor) of conversations. Subsequently, intensity refers to the increasing use of images (e.g., sending or receiving explicit photographs), incentives (e.g., providing gifts, threatening the child), and sexualized language (e.g., sexual conversations, requesting suggestive images, describing sex as fun). Lastly, the ultimate outcome will depend on the individual's goals, whether it be an in-person physical meeting or solely online contact.

Lorenzo-Dus et al. (2016) identified a three-phased model based on Computer-Mediated Discourse Analyses of 24 transcripts of online sexual grooming. First, the *access* phase involves the adult initiating contact with the minor in an online setting. Second, during the *entrapment* phase, the bulk of the sexual grooming process occurs through four interconnected strategies: deceptive trust development (i.e., exchanging personal information, engagement in activities, praise/compliments, sociability and small talk), sexual gratification (i.e., explicit [commands] and implicit [suggestions/requests] desensitization; reframing to emphasize the benefits of sexual content), isolation (i.e., both mental and physical), and compliance testing (i.e., strategic withdrawal by giving the minor control of the relationship, role reversal by adopting attitudes of a child, reverse psychology by challenging the child's decisions about sexual behavior). Lastly, in the *approach* phase, the adult seeks to initiate an in-person meeting for sexual contact through online conversations.

Most recently, Kloess et al. (2019) proposed an offense process model of online sexual grooming to reflect the potentially dynamic nature of movement between the stages. They conducted a qualitative thematic analysis of five cases (involving 29 transcripts) of online sexual grooming. According to the diagram proposed by the authors, the offense process occurs across three broad categories: (1) *approach*, (2) *maintenance-escalation*, and (3) *closure*. The approach phase includes both indirect (e.g., using sexual grooming strategies to develop a relationship) and direct (e.g., quickly introducing sexual topics/activity) approaches. The maintenance-escalation phase involves the commencement and maintenance of sexual activity, which may occur after relationship building tactics (grooming) in some cases. The sexual activities may escalate over time and include various behaviors (e.g., discussing sexual topics, fantasy enactment, online sexual activities). Lastly, the closure phase can include the termination of online conversations (by the adult, victim, or both) or an attempted or actual in-person meeting.

5.7 Online Sexual Grooming Tactics

While the Sexual Grooming Model (SGM; Winters et al., 2020) has not been validated for the online grooming setting, the progression of stages largely mirrors those of the aforementioned models. In Table 5.3, we identify how the previously proposed stages/phases of online sexual grooming models fit in to the overarching framework of the SGM.

As there has yet to be a universal or validated model of online sexual grooming, the SGM may be helpful in elucidating the specific behavioral tactics that may be observed in the online setting. We suggest that viewing online grooming through the lens of the SGM may be helpful in integrating numerous prior conceptualizations in to a single, more parsimonious model. In the section below, we provide examples of types of strategies that may be used throughout the online grooming process using the SGM stages (see Table 5.4).

5.8 Prevention and Intervention

While general sexual grooming prevention strategies will be discussed more in-depth in Chap. 14, there are some online specific prevention and intervention efforts that will be addressed below pertaining to child education, parental education and supervision, law enforcement, policy efforts, and treatment.

Table 5.3 The online sexual grooming model stages that correspond to the Sexual Grooming Model

SGM stage	Corresponding model stages
Victim selection	Webster et al.'s (2012) scanning stage Staksrud's (2013) introduction phase (observing and identifying a target) O'Connell's (2003) risk assessment stage Williams et al.'s (2013) assessment stage Lorenzo-Dus et al.'s (2016) access phase
Gaining access and isolation	Staksrud's (2013) introduction phase (engaging the targeted minor in conversation and establishing a private conversation) Lorenzo-Dus et al.'s (2016) entrapment phase (isolation)
Trust development	Webster et al.'s (2012) contact stage Staksrud's (2013) grooming phase O'Connell's (2003) friendship forming, relationship forming, and exclusivity stages Williams et al.'s (2013) rapport building stage Lorenzo-Dus et al.'s (2016) entrapment phase (deceptive trust development, compliance testing) Kloess et al.'s (2019) indirect approach
Desensitization to sexual content and physical contact	Webster et al.'s (2012) intensity stage O'Connell's (2003) sexual stage Williams et al.'s (2013) sexual content stage Lorenzo-Dus et al.'s (2016) entrapment phase (sexual gratification) Kloess et al.'s (2019) maintenance-escalation phase
Post-abuse maintenance	Webster et al.'s (2012) outcome stage O'Connell's (2003) damage limitation and "hit-and-run" tactic Lorenzo-Dus et al.'s (2016) approach stage Kloess et al.'s (2019) closure phase

5.8.1 Child Education

In an effort to prevent the online sexual solicitation and grooming of minors, it is imperative to educate youth about the risks online. They should be advised about the dangers of sharing personal information and photographs/videos with strangers and what content is appropriate to post or share with known individuals (Jeglic, 2020). For example, children would benefit from a greater understanding of how intimate, personal details (e.g., age, interests, hobbies, photographs) can be used by strangers or persons known to them, as these details can be used to develop a deceptively trusting relationship with a minor. Moreover, minors should be informed of how these risks can span multiple online platforms, including chatrooms, gaming platforms, and social media. Children should understand that it is never appropriate to send photographs to or speak with an adult stranger online, and under no circumstances should they agree to an in-person meeting. While caregivers and other adults in the child's life should openly discuss these concepts with the child, it may be helpful to incorporate online educational resources on Internet safety (e.g., Commonsense.org, Oh, 2020; missingkids.org/education, NCMEC, 2020;

Table 5.4 The online sexual grooming model behaviors or characteristics

SGM stage	Behaviors or characteristics
Victim selection	Observes chatroom and assesses ongoing conversation (O'Connell, 2003; Staksrud, 2013) Observes profile content (e.g., age, sex location, hobbies; Greene-Colozzi et al., 2020; Marcum, 2007; Malesky, 2007) and screen names (e.g., younger or sexually suggestive names; Marcum, 2007) Using "vetting" questions to determine a target (O'Connell, 2003) Difficult family circumstances, such parental neglect or conflict (Malesky, 2007) Lacks supervision on the Internet (Malesky, 2007) Target multiple victims at one time to select the most vulnerable target (Marcum, 2007)
Gaining access and isolation	Establishes a private conversation with the minor (Black et al., 2015; Staksrud, 2013) Offender may ask about the victim's parents' schedule or other contextual risk factors (e.g., whether the victim is alone) to ensure they are alone (Black et al., 2015) Encouraging the victim to hide the relationship from family and friends (Greene-Colozzi et al., 2020)
Trust development	Victim's shared personal information with the adult, including name, age, interests, hobbies, and location (Greene-Colozzi et al., 2020) Develop a friendship or flirty/dating relationship with the victim, or in some situations a romantic/loving or sexually driven relationship (Greene-Colozzi et al., 2020; Malesky, 2007) Compliment the victim on their personality, intelligence, and maturity (Lorenzo-Dus & Izura, 2017; Greene-Colozzi et al., 2020) Personal conversations about life, school, and relationships (Greene-Colozzi et al., 2020) Discuss similarities with the victim, such as their likes, dislikes, and interests (Williams et al., 2013; Greene-Colozzi et al., 2020) Promises of love and companionship (Marcum, 2007) Some discussed marriage, having children, and running away together with the victims (Greene-Colozzi et al., 2020) Claims to want to meet the victim's friends and family (Greene-Colozzi et al., 2020) Giving money or gifts (tickets, day trips, cell phone, games; CEOP, 2008)
Desensitization to sexual content and physical contact	Introducing sexual content in conversation, often very quickly (e.g., within the first day of conversation; Malesky, 2007; Winters et al., 2017) Normalize sexual behaviors between an adult and child, through sending adult pornography or nude photographs of themselves (Malesky, 2007) Broach the topic on an in-person meeting soon in conversation (e.g., within 3 days of conversation; Winters et al., 2017)
Post-abuse maintenance	Maintaining trust to prevent disclosure (Martellozzo, 2015) Threats or blackmail (Greene-Colozzi et al., 2020)

thinkuknow.co.uk, National Crime Agency, 2021). Knowledge of these educational messages have been shown to decrease over time, and thus ongoing and repeated education for children is recommended (Davidson et al., 2009).

5.8.2 Parental Education and Supervision

Research has shown that many youth (40%) do not have supervision over their online activities (Greene-Colozzi et al., 2020), which can increase their risk since an adult may purposely select these children (Malesky, 2007). First and foremost, there should be established household rules as to when and where online devices can be used and for what purposes. For example, a parent could place limits on how long their child can spend on these devices and that they should only be used in common areas of the house. Even then, parents should regularly monitor all devices that children use with Internet access, including computers, laptops, tablets, smart phones, and gaming systems, and be aware of who the child is communicating with and what type of information they are sharing. Caregivers can create user agreements with their children for Internet-related devices, which includes these aforementioned rules and provides the caregiver with all usernames and passwords for these devices. Of note, the majority of apps and games (e.g., Roblox) offer optional privacy settings and parental controls that can limit the user's ability to chat with strangers, as well as block offensive and sexual content. These should be appropriately utilized to ensure online safety based on the age and maturity of the child. There are also omnibus protection services (e.g., Bark, FamiSafe, Qustodio) that can be installed on Internet devices to permit monitoring of content on online platforms (Staples, 2020). Lastly, and perhaps most importantly, there should be ongoing and open communication about Internet use between parents and children. It may be beneficial to set aside family meeting times to discuss these topics and relay to children that they should feel open and comfortable discussing any inappropriate online behavior. Furthermore, the child should know they are not to blame. If a child is to disclose an event to parents, they should be careful to validate the child's feelings and avoid punishing the behavior (e.g., restricting video game or social media use).

5.8.3 Law Enforcement

Proactive investigations are used by law enforcement to attempt to locate and arrest adults who are seeking inappropriate sexual contact with minors by posing as youth online. One study found as many as one-quarter of arrests for online sexual offenses of minors was a result of proactive investigations (Mitchell et al., 2005). Krone (2005) interviewed law enforcement officers who conducted these types of investigations, which found that they generally resulted in the arrest of an individual and often lasted more than 1 year (14 months on average). It has been suggested that proactive investigations are beneficial for several reasons, including that many of those arrested also had in-person victims (13%) and possessed CSEM (41%), and a large portion sought to meet the "child" for in-person contact (43%; Mitchell et al., 2005). Overall, proactive investigations are commonly used in an effort to prevent online and offline sexual abuse, deter those who may consider engaging in inappropriate online behaviors, and provide a method for law enforcement to gather substantial, concrete evidence. Indeed, there are high rates of guilty pleas, and few dropped cases that are involved in proactive investigations.

5.8.4 *Policy*

As will be described further in Chap. 16, there has been a range of legislation targeting online sexual grooming in an effort to charge and convict adults seeking to contact children for sexual purposes even in the absence of physical sexual contact. One study by the ICMEC (2017) investigated the global legislation on online sexual grooming and provided recommendations for developing a comprehensive law. Out of 196 countries in the study, 63 had legislation related to online sexual grooming, with 24 countries having legislation that was deemed thorough and complete. Notably, there were only 34 countries that criminalized the pre-offense online sexual behaviors in the absence of an attempt to meet the child in-person for sexual contact. As described above, there are some adults who contact minors for sexual contact that remains solely online; thus, legislation should include the criminalization of these behaviors, as the unwanted sexual conversations or content may be harmful to victims even in the absence of sexual contact in-person. Of concern, there were 133 countries with no online sexual grooming legislation, suggesting there needs to be movement toward including these laws in all jurisdictions, given the ability for strangers to contact children online anywhere in the world. Given the lack of laws across many countries, combined with the incomplete laws in other jurisdictions, the authors propose a model for creating legislation, involving: (1) definitions, (2) offenses, and (3) sanctions/sentencing. First, they recommend including clear definitions for "child," as well as "grooming" or "online grooming." Second, the type of offenses that should be criminalized include the process of online sexual grooming, with or without the intent to meet the child in-person. Third, the authors recommend the types of sanctions and sentencing be clearly outlined, including minimum penalties or increased sentencing with the presence of aggravating factors while also considering including treatment or services for victims. Overall, it is evident there is a greater need for clear and accurate definitions within online sexual grooming legislation and that these types of laws need to be widely adopted across jurisdictions.

5.8.5 *Treatment*

There is a lack of research on the treatment strategies that are most effective for victims of Internet-facilitated sexual offenses. It has been suggested that for children who do not view their experience as abuse, the typical trauma-focused cognitive-behavioral interventions may not be appropriate (Wolak et al., 2008). Rather, a treatment provider must therefore assess the child's specific needs and develop strategies accordingly, including strong rapport building. Family interventions may be helpful in some cases, especially in situations involving a lack of parental supervision or the presence of family conflict or strain.

For offenders, those who commit online solicitation or sexual grooming offenses may benefit from the standard treatment modalities for those who committed sexual offenses, including cognitive-behavioral therapy and relapse prevention (Wolak et al., 2008). These are designed to help online offenders identify maladaptive cognitions and other factors that lead to their offending behaviors, as well as strategies to prevent this pattern from occurring again. Also of note, there have been services online for individuals who have sexual thoughts (or acts) involving children. For example, Johns Hopkins Bloomberg School of Public Health (2020) created a website including options for anonymous counseling, confidential helplines, online self-help courses, referrals, and consultations. Similarly, an institute in Sweden offers the program "Prevent It," which has online cognitive-behavioral services that can be offered anonymously to those who utilized CSEM materials (Parks et al., 2020).

5.9 Conclusion

While there is a vast amount of information on online offending, this chapter sought to identify some key characteristics of these types of offenses in the context of online sexual solicitation and sexual grooming of youth. As was discussed throughout the chapter, there are unique characteristics of these online sexual grooming offenses, but there are many similarities to in-person sexual grooming. It appears that sexual grooming in the online setting may utilize similar processes as in-person cases, involving selecting a vulnerable victim, gaining access and isolating the child online, using a variety of trust development techniques, gradually introducing sexual content and images, and potentially using some ongoing maintenance behaviors following online or offline sexual contact. However, the process may be quickened in the online setting due to anonymity and the vast number of potential victims. There are many areas that are ripe for prevention in the online sexual grooming realm, including education for children and parents, law enforcement investigations, implementation of legislation, and treatment. Future research can help shed light on differences between sexual grooming in the online and offline setting, as well as how we can implement the most effective prevention strategies.

References

Alfonso, F. (2020, May 25). *The pandemic is causing an exponential rise in the online exploitation of children, experts say.* CNN. https://www.cnn.com/2020/05/25/us/child-abuse-online-coronavirus-pandemic-parents-investigations-trnd/index.html\

Anderson, M., & Jiang, J. (2018). *Teens, social media and technology 2018.* The Pew Research Center. https://www.pewresearch.org/internet/2018/05/31/teens-social-media-technology-2018/

Babchishin, K. M., Hanson, R. K., & Hermann, C. A. (2011). The characteristics of online sex offenders: A meta-analysis. *Sexual Abuse: Journal of Research and Treatment, 23*, 92–123. https://doi.org/10.1177/1079063210370708

Black, P. J., Wollis, M., Woodworth, M., & Hancock, J. T. (2015). A linguistic analysis of grooming strategies of online child sex offenders: Implications for our understanding of predatory sexual behavior in an increasingly computer-mediated world. *Child Abuse & Neglect, 44*, 140–149. https://doi.org/10.1016/j.chiabu.2014.12.004

Bowles, N., & Keller, M. H. (2019). Video games and online chats are 'hunting grounds' for sexual predators. *The New York Times.* https://www.nytimes.com/interactive/2019/12/07/us/video-games-child-sex-abuse.html

Briggs, P., Simon, W. T., & Simonsen, S. (2011). An exploratory study of internet-initiated sexual offenses and the chat room sex offender: Has the internet enabled a new typology of sex offender? *Sexual Abuse: Journal of Research and Treatment, 23*(1), 72–91. https://doi.org/10.1177/1079063210384275

British Broadcasting Corporation [BBC]. (2019, March 01). *Instagram biggest for child grooming online—NSPCC finds.* https://www.bbc.com/news/uk-47410520

Broome, L. J., Izura, C., & Lorenzo-Dus, N. (2018). A systematic review of fantasy driven vs. contact driven internet-initiated sexual offences: Discrete or overlapping typologies? *Child Abuse & Neglect, 79*, 434–434. https://doi.org/10.1016/j.chiabu.2018.02.021

Child Exploitation and Online Protection Centre [CEOPC]. (2008). *Strategic overview 2007–2008.* http://ceop.police.uk/Publications/

Cooper, A. (1998). Sexuality and the Internet: Surfing into the new millennium. *Cyber Psychology & Behavior, 1*(2), 187–193. https://doi.org/10.1089/cpb.1998.1.187

Davidson, J., Martellozzo, E., & Lorenz, M. (2009). *Evaluation of CEOP ThinkUKnow internet safety programme and exploration of young people's internet safety knowledge*. WorldCat.org.

Defend Young Minds. (2021). *Dangers of Discord: 6 steps for safeguarding teens on the popular chat app.* https://www.defendyoungminds.com/post/dangers-of-discord-6-steps-safeguarding-teens-on-popular-chat-app

DeHart, D., Dwyer, G., Seto, M. C., Moran, R., Letourneau, E., & Schwarz-Watts, D. (2017). Internet sexual solicitation of children: A proposed typology of offenders based on their chats, e-mails, and social network posts. *Journal of Sexual Aggression, 23*(1), 77–89. https://doi.org/10.1080/13552600.2016.1241309

Doring, N. (2000). Feminist views of cybersex: Victimization, liberation, and empowerment. *CyberPsychology and Behavior, 3*, 863–884. https://doi.org/10.1089/10949310050191845

Durkin, K. F. (1997). Misuse of the Internet by pedophiles: Implications for law enforcement and probation practice. *Federal Probation, 61*(3), 14–18.

Finkelhor, D., Mitchell, K. J., & Wolak, J. (2000). *Online victimization: A report on the nation's youth (No. 6-00-020).* National Center for Missing & Exploited Children.

Greene-Colozzi, E. A., Winters, G. M., Blasko, B., & Jeglic, E. L. (2020). Experiences and perceptions of online sexual solicitation and grooming of minors: A retrospective report. *Journal of Child Sexual Abuse, 29*(7), 836–854. https://doi.org/10.1080/10538712.2020.1801938

International Centre for Missing & Exploited Children [ICMEC]. (2017). *Online grooming of children for sexual purposes: Model legislation & global review.* https://www.icmec.org/wp-content/uploads/2017/09/Online-Grooming-of-Children_FINAL_9-18-17.pdf

Interpol. (2020). *Threats and trends of child sexual exploitation and abuse*. Retrieved 18 Sept 2020 from https://www.interpol.int/content/download/15611/file/COVID19%20-%20Child%20Sexual%20Exploitation%20and%20Abuse%20threats%20and%20trends.pdf?inLanguage=eng-GB

Jeglic, E. L. (2020, April 09). Keeping your child safe online during the pandemic. *Psychology Today.* https://www.psychologytoday.com/us/blog/protecting-children-sexual-abuse/202004/keeping-your-child-safe-online-during-the-pandemic

John Hopkins Bloomberg School of Public Health. (2020, June 10). *COVID-19 CSA prevention.* https://www.jhsph.edu/research/centers-and-institutes/moore-center-for-the-prevention-of-child-sexual-abuse/resources/covid-19-csa-prevention/index.html

Kloess, J. A., Beech, A. R., & Harkins, L. (2014). Online child sexual exploitation: Prevalence, process, and offender characteristics. *Trauma, Violence & Abuse, 15*(2), 126–139. https://doi.org/10.1177/1524838013511543

Kloess, J. A., Hamilton-Giachritsis, C. E., & Beech, A. R. (2019). Offense processes of online sexual grooming and abuse of children via internet communication platforms. *Sexual Abuse, 31*(1), 73–96. https://doi.org/10.1177/1079063217720927

Krone, T. (2005). Queensland police stings in online chat rooms. *Trends and Issues in Crime and Criminal Justice, 301*, 1–6. https://www.ojp.gov/ncjrs/virtual-library/abstracts/queensland-police-stings-online-chat-rooms

Lorenzo-Dus, N., & Izura, C. (2017). "Cause ur special": Understanding trust and complimenting behaviour in online grooming discourse. *Journal of Pragmatics, 112*, 68–82. https://doi.org/10.1016/j.pragma.2017.01.0040378-2166

Lorenzo-Dus, N., Izura, C., & Pérez-Tattam, R. (2016). Understanding grooming discourse in computer-mediated environments. *Discourse, Context and Media, 12*, 40–50. https://doi.org/10.1016/j.dcm.2016.02.004

Madigan, S., Villani, V., Azzopardi, C., Laut, D., Smith, T., Temple, J. R., Browne, D., & Dimitropoulos, G. (2018). The prevalence of unwanted online sexual exposure and solicitation among youth: A meta-analysis. *Journal of Adolescent Health, 63*(2), 133–141. https://doi.org/10.1016/j.jadohealth.2018.03.012

Malesky, L. A. (2007). Predatory online behavior: Modus operandi of convicted sex offenders in identifying potential victims and contacting minors over the internet. *Journal of Child Sexual Abuse, 16*, 23–32. https://doi.org/10.1300/J070v16n02_02

Marcum, C. D. (2007). Interpreting the intentions of internet predators: An examination of online predatory behaviour. *Journal of Child Sexual Abuse, 16*(4), 99–114. https://doi.org/10.1300/J070v16n04_06

Martellozzo, E. (2015). Policing online child sexual abuse—The British experience. *European Journal of Policing Studies, 3*(1), 32–52.

McLaughlin, J. (1998). Technophilia: A modern day paraphilia. *Knight Stick, 51*(Spring/Summer 98), 47–51. https://www.iletsbeiforumjournal.com/images/Issues/FreeIssues/ILEEF%202002-2.3.pdf

Mitchell, K., Wolak, J., & Finkelhor, D. (2005). Police posing as juveniles online to catch sex offenders: Is it working? *Sexual Abuse: A Journal of Research and Treatment, 17*(3), 241–267. https://doi.org/10.1007/s11194-005-5055-2

Mitchell, K., Jones, L., Finkelhor, D., & Wolak, J. (2014). *Trends in unwanted sexual solicitations: Findings from the youth internet safety studies*. Crimes Against Children Research Center.

National Center for Education Statistics. (2021). *Children's Internet access at home.* https://nces.ed.gov/programs/coe/pdf/2021/cch_508c.pdf

National Center for Missing and Exploited Children [NCMEC]. (2021). *CyberTipline.* https://www.missingkids.org/gethelpnow/cybertipline#bythenumbers

National Crime Agency. (2021). *Thinkuknow*. www.thinkuknow.co.uk/

O'Connell, R. (2003). *A typology of child cybersexploitation and online grooming practices*. Cyberspace Research Unit, University of Central Lancashire.

O'Donnell, B. (2021). *Rise in online enticement and other trends: NCMEC releases 2020 exploitationstats.* https://www.missingkids.org/blog/2021/rise-in-online-enticement-and-other-trends%2D%2Dncmec-releases-2020-
Oh, E. W. (2020, February 07). *Help kids practice smart internet habits and stay safe online.* Commonsense. https://www.commonsense.org/education/articles/23-great-lesson-plans-for-internet-safety
Parks, A., Sparre, C., Söderquist, E., Arver, S., Andersson, G., Kaldo, V., Gorts-Oberg, K., & Rahm, C. (2020). Illegal online sexual behavior during the COVID-19 pandemic: A call for action based on experiences from the ongoing Prevent It research study. *Archives of Sexual Behavior, 49*(5), 1433–1435. https://doi.org/10.1007/s10508-020-01750-7
Schulz, A., Bergen, E., Schuhmann, P., Hoyer, J., & Santtila, P. (2015). Online sexual solicitation of minors: How often and between whom does it occur? *Journal of Research in Crime and Delinquency, 53*(2), 165–188. https://doi.org/10.1177/0022427815599426
Seto, M. C., Wood, J. M., Babchishin, K. M., & Flynn, S. (2012). Online solicitation offenders are different from child pornography offenders and low risk contact sexual offenders. *Law and Human Behaviour, 36*(4), 230–320. https://doi.org/10.1037/h0093925
Shannon, D. (2008). Online sexual grooming in Sweden—Online and offline sex offenses against children as described in Swedish police data. *Journal of Scandinavian Studies in Criminology and Crime Prevention, 9*, 160–180. https://doi.org/10.1080/14043850802450120
Silva, M. (2019, April 05). Video app TikTok fails to remove online predators. *BBC News.*
Staksrud, E. (2013). Online grooming legislation: Knee-jerk regulation? *European Journal of Communication, 28*(2), 152–167. https://doi.org/10.1177/0267323112471304
Staples, M. (2020). *Online child predators are using these social media apps to contact kids.* https://thevoiceofblackcincinnati.com/fight-online-child-predators/
Stiggers, L. (2020, March 18). *Mobile apps that may be unsafe for your child.* The Voice of Black Cincinnati. https://thevoiceofblackcincinnati.com/fight-online-child-predators/
UNICEF. (2011). *Child safety: Online global challenges and strategies.* https://www.unicef-irc.org/publications/pdf/ict_eng.pdf
Villacampa, C., & Gomez, M. J. (2017). Online child sexual grooming: Empirical findings on victimisation and perspectives on legal requirements. *International Review of Victimology, 23*(2), 105–121. https://doi.org/10.1177/0269758016682585
Walsh, W. A., & Wolak, J. (2005). Nonforcible internet-related sex crimes with adolescent victims: Prosecution issues and outcomes. *Child Maltreatment, 10*(3), 260–271. https://doi.org/10.1177/1077559505276505
Webster, S., Davidson, J., Bifulco, A., Gottschalk, P., Caretti, V., Pham, T., Grove-Hills, J., Turley, C., Tompkins, C., Ciulla, S., Milazzo, V., Schimmenti, A., & Craparo, G. (2012). *European online grooming project final report.* European Commission Safer Internet Plus Programme, Tech. Rep.
Wells, M., & Mitchell, K. J. (2007). Youth sexual exploitation on the Internet: *DSM-IV* diagnoses and gender differences in co-occurring mental health issues. *Child and Adolescent Social Work Journal, 24*, 235–260. https://doi.org/10.1007/s10560-007-0083-z
Whittle, H. C. (2014). *An exploration of young people's vulnerabilities to online grooming and sexual abuse* (Doctoral dissertation, University of Birmingham).
Williams, R., Elliott, I. A., & Beech, A. R. (2013). Identifying sexual grooming themes used by internet sex offenders. *Deviant Behavior, 34*(2), 135–152. https://doi.org/10.1080/01639625.2012.707550
Winters, G. M., Kaylor, L. E., & Jeglic, E. L. (2017). Sexual offenders contacting children online: An examination of transcripts of sexual grooming. *Journal of Sexual Aggression, 23*(1), 62–76. https://doi.org/10.1080/13552600.2016.1271146
Winters, G. M., Jeglic, E. L., & Kaylor, L. E. (2020). Validation of the sexual grooming model of child sexual abusers. *Journal of Child Sexual Abuse: Research, Treatment, & Program Innovations for Victims, Survivors, & Offenders.* https://doi.org/10.1080/10538712.2020.1801935

Wolak, J., Finkelhor, D., & Mitchell, K. J. (2004). Internet-initiated sex crimes against minors: Implications for prevention based on findings from a national study. *Journal of Adolescent Health, 35*, 424.e11–424.e20. https://doi.org/10.1016/j.jadohealth.2004.05.006

Wolak, J., Mitchell, K. J., & Finkelhor, D. (2006). *Online victimization of youth: Five years later*. National Center for Missing and Exploited Children. http://unh.edu/ccrc/pdf/CV138.pdf

Wolak, J., Finkelhor, D., Mitchell, K. J., & Ybarra, M. L. (2008). Online "predators" and their victims: Myths, realities, and implications for prevention and treatment. *American Psychologist, 63*(2), 111–128. https://doi.org/10.1037/0003-066X.63.2.111

Wolak, J., Finkelhor, D., Mitchell, K. J., & Ybarra, M. L. (2010). Online "predators" and their victims: Myths, realities, and implications for prevention and treatment. *Psychology of Violence, 1*(S), 13–35. https://doi.org/10.1037/2152-0828.1.S.13

Ybarra, M. L., Leaf, P., & Diener-West, M. (2004). Sex differences in youth-reported depressive symptomatology and unwanted internet sexual solicitation. *Journal of Medical Internet Research, 6*, e5. https://doi.org/10.2196/jmir.6.1.e5

Chapter 6
Self-Grooming

It has been broadly established that to gain access to a minor and prevent detection of the abuse, perpetrators may engage in the sexual grooming of the child, their family, the community, and/or institutions. Craven et al. (2006) further theorized that individuals who sexually abuse children may also engage in what they termed *self-grooming*. They explained that "self-grooming is likely to play a part in the move from being motivated to sexually abuse a child to the subsequent targeting of a child, through the justification or denial of the steps child sexual offenders take towards abusing a child" (Craven et al., 2006, p. 292). They developed the term self-grooming based upon van Dam's (2001) observation that during treatment, individuals who committed a sexual offense discussed how they would "groom themselves," which aligns with already established literature exploring cognitive constructs related to sexual offending. Craven et al. (2006) suggested that self-grooming may not be the best term to describe the process of self-justification and denial in offending, yet the term appears to have persisted, and it is now often included as part of the sexual grooming literature. This chapter will explore what is known about self-grooming and how it fits into the child sexual grooming process, as well as how it may overlap with existing research on neutralization techniques, cognitive distortions, implicit theories of sexual offending, and overcoming internal barriers to offending. The chapter will conclude with a discussion of the importance of understanding self-grooming for the prevention of child sexual abuse (CSA) and the treatment of individuals who commit these offenses.

6.1 Self-Grooming and Related Terms

Self-grooming has been described as part of the sexual grooming process, along with grooming the child, significant others, and the environment (Craven et al., 2006). While the sexual grooming literature in general lacks empirical studies, the

© The Author(s), under exclusive license to Springer Nature Switzerland AG 2022

G. M. Winters, E. L. Jeglic, *Sexual Grooming*,
https://doi.org/10.1007/978-3-031-07222-2_6

concept of self-grooming in particular has been almost completely neglected both theoretically and empirically. Although Craven and colleagues first coined the term self-grooming in 2006, there has been little to no development of the construct in subsequent literature. One possible reason for this could be the apparent overlap between self-grooming and the existing research on other cognitive constructs related to sexual offending, including: (1) neutralization techniques, (2) cognitive distortions, (3) implicit theories of sexual offending, and (4) overcoming internal barriers to offending. As will be described in the sections below, these areas of research speak to the justifications, minimizations, and distortions that individuals make in order to engage in CSA, which is broadly how Craven et al. (2006) defined the construct of self-grooming.

6.1.1 Neutralization Techniques

Self-grooming has also been described as a *neutralization technique* which prevents the individual committing the abuse from feeling bad about themselves before, during, and after CSA (Craven et al., 2006; McAlinden, 2013). According to Maruna and Copes (2005), neutralizations are the reasons or excuses individuals use to justify deviant behavior. The concept of neutralizations (also referred to interchangeably as rationalizations) originated in the criminological literature in the 1950s as a way to explain how people justified their criminal behavior (Kaptein & van Helvoort, 2019). One of the first models of neutralization techniques was developed by Sykes and Matza (1957) to explain juvenile offending. They described five techniques (later known as the "famous five") to explain the rationalization of crime:

1. Denial of responsibility
2. Denial of injury
3. Denial of the victim
4. Condemnation of the condemners
5. Appeal to higher loyalties

While there was criticism that neutralization theory was not theoretical sound or empirically validated (Maruna & Copes, 2005), it became one of the most universally used theories to explain how those who commit crime justify their behavior. There have been other additions to neutralization theory (see Kaptein and Van Helvoort (2019) for one of the more recent models of neutralizations); however, despite modifications, the theory has continued to be criticized for not offering a parsimonious explanation as to how and when the five neutralization techniques are utilized (Maruna & Copes, 2005).

While neutralizations have been applied to crime in general, there have been a few studies applying the neutralization theory specifically to those who sexually offend and how, if it all, it relates to sexual grooming. In her book, van Dam (2001) discussed how those who sexually offend against children overcome their inhibitions to offend in the sexual grooming process using such neutralization techniques (although she does not label it as self-grooming). Based upon the work of De Young (1988), van Dam (2001) listed four steps that perpetrators use in the grooming process to "redefine reality" so that they can overcome cognitive barriers and engage in sexual abuse (van Dam, 2001, p. 92; see Fig. 6.1).

As noted, there has been little empirical support for neutralization theory in general (Maruna & Copes, 2005), and De Young's version was largely grounded in writings from the North American Man/Boy Love Association (NAMBLA), whose perspectives are not representative of CSA in general. However, there appears to be some overlap between the concept of "denial of victimization" and the child sexual grooming process. As is outlined in the third stage of the Sexual Grooming Model (SGM; Winters et al., 2020; see Chap. 2)—developing trust with the minor—the perpetrator works to gain the trust of the often vulnerable and neglected minor by developing a caring relationship with them. It is this relationship that is thought to be at the core of the sexual grooming process, since the fear of losing the relationship may prevent the child from disclosing the abuse (Winters et al., 2020). Since the minor is often seeking emotional closeness, the fact that they are spending time with the perpetrator may lead the individual to believe that the minor may want a sexual relationship, especially if they tolerate the desensitization that is initiated in the fourth stage of the SGM. Similarly, it may be the fact that the child does not report the abuse and continues the relationship that convinces the individual engaging in sexual grooming that the child is a "willing participant," thus minimizing their guilt about the abuse—and potentially serving the function of self-grooming. As noted by Craven et al. (2006), it may be the "success" of the child and/or family

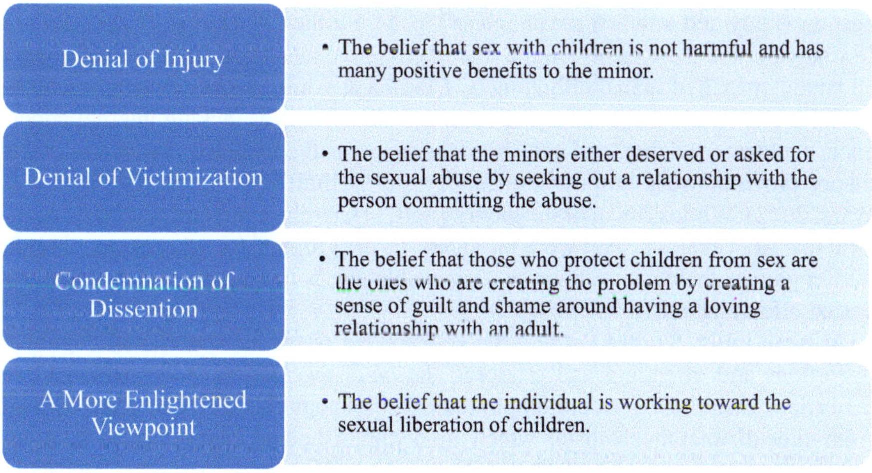

Fig. 6.1 Four steps individuals use to redefine reality in the grooming process. (Van Dam, 2001)

sexual grooming process that then further establishes and reinforces the person's abusive motivations and behaviors.

6.1.2 Cognitive Distortions

The term *cognitive distortion* was first used by Beck in 1963 to describe thoughts and beliefs that may distort reality for individuals with depression and anxiety. Subsequently, Abel et al. (1989) applied the term to individuals who commit child sexual offenses, suggesting that targeting distorted thoughts and beliefs about sexual offending formed the basis of cognitive behavior therapy for individuals who have committed a sexual offense (see Moster et al., 2008 for review). Historically, when the term cognitive distortions was first applied to sexual offending, it was defined as the incorrect attitudes and beliefs that support offending behavior (Marshall et al., 1999) and covered three main types of distortions:

1. Attitudes and beliefs that minimize and justify offending behavior (Abel et al., 1989; Blumenthal et al., 1999).
2. Misperception of cues (Beckett et al., 1994).
3. Denial and minimization of sexual offenses themselves (Schneider & Wright, 2004).

However, there has been significant critique of the research on cognitive distortions as it has been applied to those who offend sexually. While there is considerable evidence that those who sexually abuse children have thoughts and beliefs that enable them to abuse children, Ó Ciardha and Ward (2013) argue that the term cognitive distortions as it pertains to sex offenders "is vague and so broad that it is at best unwieldy and at worst meaningless" (p. 5). Further, Abel et al. (1989) did not formally outline their theory on the role of cognitive distortions in the development and maintenance of sexual offending (Ó Ciardha & Ward, 2013). As such, researchers have criticized Abel's theory of cognitive distortions as lacking internal coherence, explanatory depth, and external consistency and concluded that overall, their theory provides weak empirical adequacy and is limited in scope (Ó Ciardha & Ward, 2013). While critical of the theory itself, Ó Ciardha and Ward (2013) do highlight that Abel et al.'s (1989) work provided "fertile ground" for subsequent research into cognitive factors that may be responsible for both causing and maintaining sexual offending behavior.

Most recently, Szumski et al. (2018) expanded on earlier theories of cognitive distortions and offending and proposed the *multi-mechanism theory of cognitive distortions* (MMT-CD). According to their theory, cognitive distortions are derived from three distinct mechanisms which are distinguished by their temporal relationship to the offense (see Fig. 6.2). While the role of distorted cognitions appears to be well accepted among those who study sexual offending behavior, the exact mechanisms in which they contribute to and maintain sexual offending behavior remain debated.

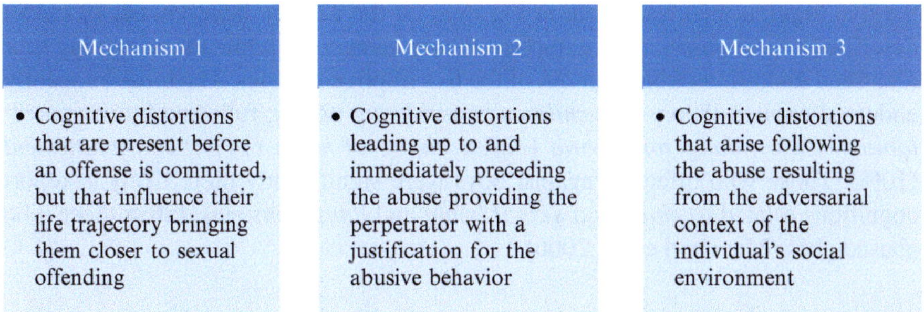

Fig. 6.2 The multi-mechanism theory of cognitive distortions (MMT-CD; Szumski et al., 2018)

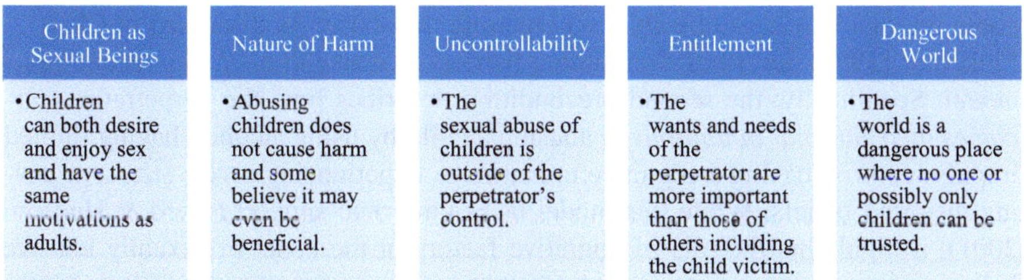

Fig. 6.3 Common implicit theories among those who offend against children

6.1.3 Implicit Theories of Sexual Offending

Ward and his colleagues (1999, 2000) examined the role of cognitive factors in the onset and maintenance of offending. They postulated that those who offend against children had a set of beliefs they termed *implicit theories of sexual offending* that allowed perpetrators to "explain, predict and interpret interpersonal phenomena" (Ward, 2000, p. 494). Ward (2000) likened these beliefs to cognitive schema, which are a core set of beliefs that are used by individuals to understand and interpret both their own behaviors and responses as well as those of others across various contexts (see Dozois & Beck, 2008). Ward and Keenan (1999) proposed five of these implicit theories that were most common among those who offended against children (see Fig. 6.3).

Ward (2000) highlights the implicit nature of these beliefs, underscoring that those who commit sexual offenses may not be consciously aware of these beliefs. Consequently, they may not be cognizant of the bias present in the way that they process information, particularly as it pertains to sexual offending. Marziano et al. (2006) interviewed 22 adult males convicted of sex crimes against children about their offense process and their life circumstances before the offending, the day of the offense, and the days and weeks following the offense. From the interviews, researchers identifying 2660 cognitive distortions that were then categorized into the five implicit theories shown in Fig. 6.3. Of the 22 men interviewed, 18 (82%) described cognitions in all five implicit theory categories, while the remaining four identified distortions from four out of the five implicit theories. The most frequently endorsed explicit theory was *child as sexual being* (28%), followed by *uncontrollability* (26%), *dangerous world* (22%), *nature of harm* (14%), and *entitlement* (10%). Those who offended against boys were significantly more likely to report cognitions related to *child as a sexual being* and *dangerous world* than those who abused girls (Marziano et al., 2006).

6.1.4 Overcoming Internal Barriers to Offending

There has also been some research examining how those who abuse children overcome internal barriers to be able to perpetrate the abuse. As discussed in Chap. 2, Finkelhor (1984) describes overcoming barriers to abuse in his *four preconditions model*. Specifically, the second precondition describes how the perpetrator *overcomes their internal inhibitions* to abusing a child by using alcohol, having limited impulse control, having a cognitive impairment, experiencing severe stress, or having distorted beliefs. While this model lacks empirical support (Ward & Hudson, 2001), it highlights the role of cognitive factors in the onset of sexually abusive behaviors.

Petruccelli et al. (2017a, b) and D'Urso and colleagues (2018, 2019) examined the role of *moral disengagement* in order to "break free from the ethical codes imposed by society" (D'Urso et al., 2019, p. 415). For example, the ethical, moral, and legal codes of society prohibit adults from engaging in sexual relationships with children. Should an adult want to engage in sexual contact with a child, this desired behavior would then cause cognitive dissonance between their beliefs and their behavior. In an effort to dissipate the dissonance, one strategy could be moral disengagement. According to Bandura (1986), moral disengagement involved restructuring or reframing cognitive schema so that the behavior (in this case child abuse) is now morally acceptable, and thus they can engage in the behavior without guilt. Mechanisms of moral disengagement as described by Bandura (1999) include the following:

1. Reconstruing the behavior so that it is no longer perceived to be immoral.
2. Dehumanizing or devaluing the victim so that they can be blamed for what is being done to them.
3. Disregarding or misrepresenting the harmful consequences that may result from the actions.
4. Displacement of responsibility such that the perpetrator can minimize their role in causing harm.

Petruccelli, Simonelli, and colleagues (2017b) found those who perpetrate sex crimes use more moral disengagement strategies than non-offenders. In another study of those who committed sexual crimes again children, they found a relationship between moral disengagement and cognitive distortions about children as sexual objects which they postulated helped overcome the moral barriers to abuse (D'Urso et al., 2019).

6.2 Self-Grooming in the Context of Sexual Grooming

As has been shown in this chapter, the construct of self-grooming has not been well developed, and conceptually, it has significant overlap with neutralizations, cognitive distortions, implicit theories, and the research on overcoming barriers to abuse. It is in fact debatable whether these constructs are indeed different at all. This is an empirical question that needs to be examined as the research on sexual grooming becomes more empirically developed. As depicted in Fig. 6.4, regardless of what it is called, it appears that self-grooming does have its own place within the sexual grooming process. In the *preparation* phase, perpetrators must take some actions on a cognitive level to overcome social, moral, ethical, and legal barriers to be able to engage in the grooming process, and then once the grooming has begun, the second phase involves the *justification* to themselves of their actions, so that they minimize and discount to themselves the impact and potential nefarious nature of their behaviors. In the final phase, *maintenance,* the abuse has already occurred, and the individual then rationalizes the abuse to themselves to reduce any feelings of guilt, shame, or culpability so that the abusive process can continue without detection.

Interestingly, some definitions of sexual grooming describe it as a planned and purposeful process (see Winters et al., 2021 and Chap. 3 for a review). For example, McAlinden (2007) describes how a perpetrator "skillfully manipulates the child" in the grooming process. Leberg (1997) states that in grooming the child, perpetrators are enacting a "plan", and Knoll (2010) defines sexual grooming to be a "conscious, deliberate, and carefully orchestrated approach." Based upon these definitions it would seem that some believe that sexual grooming is a conscious process. This is

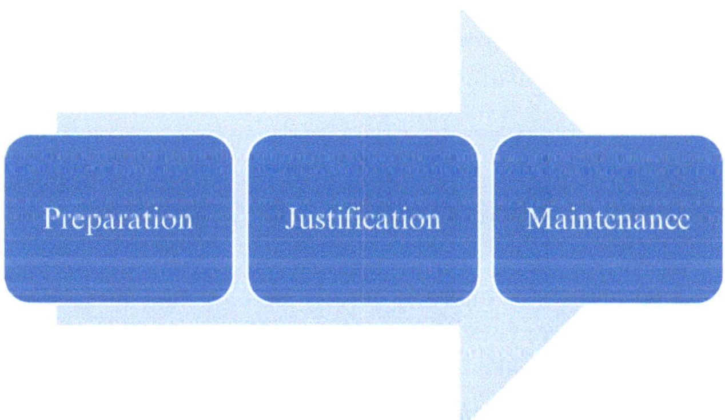

Fig. 6.4 Proposed model of self-grooming in child sexual abuse

somewhat supported by the work of Elliott et al. (1995) who interviewed 91 men convicted of sexual offenses against children about the methods they used to during the offense process. The men were asked to describe the characteristics of the children they targeted and recruited as victims, as well as the strategies they used to gain the trust of the victims, desensitize them to sexual content and touch, and what they did or told the children after the abuse so that they would avoid detection. While this study was conducted before much of the research on sexual grooming was developed, it is clear that much of what is described involves the stages of sexual grooming as described in the SGM (Winters et al., 2020). The findings showed the men appear to have considerable insight into their abuse strategy, as 84% reported that once they developed strategies that were effective in perpetrating sexual abuse, they approached future victims in the same way, suggesting that sexual grooming was indeed planful. The researchers also asked how the perpetrators chose the strategies they did to abuse the children and avoid detection. Most reported they had no idea, 30% said they had success in the past which then reinforced those strategies, and 14% said they were influenced by pornography, television, movies, or other media sources (Elliott et al., 1995).

In contrast, Ward (2000) and Smallbone (n.d.) have suggested that the abuse may not be an entirely conscious process and the sexual motivations may not become evident to the perpetrator until right before the abuse occurs. For example, in Szumski and colleagues' MMT-CD (2018), *Mechanism 1* describes cognitive distortions that are formed earlier in life but that influence an individual's life course, goals, and decision-making, thus putting them on a path toward offending. While the MMT-CD does not explicitly state whether *Mechanism 1* is a conscious process, it can be surmised that these types of distortions may not be evident to the individual prior to the perpetration of the abuse. In reviewing the extant literature, it is likely that those who engage in sexual grooming have developed conscious strategies that they use to perpetrate the abuse—and for many repeat offenders these strategies can become like an abuse playbook. However, drawing from the research on cognitive distortions, implicit theories, and schemas, there are also likely cognitive processes that are less conscious or planful, such as minimization, justification, and denial that enable the individual to begin the abusive process and then to continue it, therein minimizing their cognitive dissonance regarding the abuse and its impact on the child and diminishing their distress.

6.3 Importance of Understanding Self-Grooming

At present, self-grooming is relatively poorly defined and understood. However, based upon this review there is evidence to suggest that those who engage in sexual grooming of minors may partake in a process that is both conscious and unconscious in order to abuse the child. This underscores the importance of better understanding what constitutes self-grooming from a prevention and treatment perspective. For example, it appears that the initial barrier to abuse is high and that those who engage in CSA may have to undergo a process of moral disengagement or cognitive restructuring in order to overcome established moral, ethical, and legal prohibitions to sexual contact with a minor. This is a potential target for prevention and falls in line with the work that is currently being done to support minor attracted persons (MAPs)—those with identified pedophilic sexual interests but who chose not to act on them. Organizations such as the Global Prevention Project provide resources and access to anonymous online supports groups for these MAPs such as Virped and B4U-ACT. Stop-It-Now is a confidential helpline for those who want help in coping with their minor attraction and in Germany Project Dunkelfeld (see Beier et al., 2015 for a description and summary of findings) provides an anonymous and confidential cognitive behavioral treatment program for MAPs. Given the stigma in society surrounding sexual attraction to minors, many individuals who have sexual attraction to prepubescent and pubescent children do not seek support or treatment due to a legitimate fear of rejection and potential legal involvement. Thus, from a public health perspective, identifying those at increased risk for perpetration and providing services to help them cope with the dissonance that arises between societal and legal perspectives on CSA and their sexual urges and desires prior to any offending (i.e., to change the beliefs before the behavior occurs) may prove tremendously beneficial.

A better understanding of the role of self-grooming in the grooming process may also be important for treatment. For example, according to the *risk, needs, responsivity model* of offender rehabilitation (see Chap. 13), treatment programs for incarcerated individuals should be based upon a cognitive behavioral framework (Andrews et al., 1990). As such, addressing distorted thinking and schema related to sexual offending are integral to this process (see Moster et al., 2008; Schaffer et al., 2010). Further, understanding the grooming process, how that relates to distorted thinking and abuse perpetration may prove to be integral to treatment. In addition, identifying where in the offense chain self-grooming may occur and how it is manifested may be invaluable to self-management and relapse prevention strategies. For example, the service provider can work with the individual to identify cognitions or schema that permit them to abuse children and develop effective restructuring strategies (Moster et al., 2008).

6.4 Conclusion

Self-grooming is not a well-defined, developed, or researched construct, and it remains unclear if it even exists as a separate construct from neutralization, cognitive distortions, implicit theories, and surmounting internal barriers to abuse. Researchers have studied the cognitive processes of those who sexually offend and have identified thought processes and cognitions that are shared by many who abuse children to justify their behavior and minimize and deny the harm they cause. It is likely that this is what some researchers have described as self-grooming. While there is evidence that there may be conscious planful aspects to the abusive behaviors used in sexual grooming, the ability to overcome social, moral, and legal barriers may require less conscious control. Thus, it is proposed that individuals who engage in sexual grooming also employ self-grooming strategies that encompass preparation, justification, and maintenance that permit them to surmount these barriers and perpetrate the abuse. However, more research is needed to determine how the self-grooming of those who engage in sexual grooming may differ (or not) from those perpetrators who do not use grooming tactics and how such knowledge can inform prevention and intervention.

References

Abel, G. G., Gore, D. K., Holland, C. L., Camps, N., Becker, J. V., & Rathner, J. (1989). The measurement of the cognitive distortions of child molesters. *Annals of Sex Research, 2*(2), 135–152. https://doi.org/10.1007/BF00851319

Andrews, D. A., Bonta, J., & Hoge, R. D. (1990). Classification for effective rehabilitation: Rediscovering psychology. *Crim Justice Behav, 17*(1), 19–52. https://doi.org/10.1177/0093854890017001004

Bandura, A. (1986). The explanatory and predictive scope of self-efficacy theory. *J Soc Clin Psychol, 4*(3), 359–373. https://doi.org/10.1521/jscp.1986.4.3.359

Bandura, A. (1999). Moral disengagement in the perpetration of inhumanities. *Personal Soc Psychol Rev, 3*, 193–209. https://doi.org/10.1207/s15327957pspr0303_3

Beckett, R., Beech, A., Fisher, D., & Fordham, A. S. (1994). *Community-based treatment for sex offenders: An evaluation of seven treatment programmes*. Home Office Publications Unit.

Beier, K. M., Grundmann, D., Kuhle, L. F., Scherner, G., Konrad, A., & Amelung, T. (2015). The German Dunkelfeld project: A pilot study to prevent child sexual abuse and the use of child abusive images. *J Sex Med, 12*(2), 529–542. https://doi.org/10.1111/jsm.12785

Blumenthal, S., Gudjonsson, G., & Burns, J. (1999). Cognitive distortions and blame attribution in sex offenders against adults and children. *Child Abuse & Neglect, 23*(2), 129–143. https://doi.org/10.1016/S0145-2134(98)00117-3

Craven, S., Brown, S., & Gilchrist, E. (2006). Sexual grooming of children: Review of literature and theoretical considerations. *J Sex Aggress, 12*(3), 287–299. https://doi.org/10.1080/13552600601069414

D'Urso, G., Petruccelli, I., & Pace, U. (2018). Drug use as a risk factor of moral disengagement: A study on drug traffickers and offenders against other persons. *Psychiatry Psychol Law, 25*(3), 417–424. https://doi.org/10.1080/13218719.2018.1437092

D'Urso, G., Petruccelli, I., Costantino, V., Zappulla, C., & Pace, U. (2019). The role of moral disengagement and cognitive distortions toward children among sex offenders. *Psychiatry Psychol Law, 26*(3), 414–422. https://doi.org/10.1080/13218719.2018.1506718

De Young, M. (1988). The indignant page: Techniques of neutralization in the publications of pedophile organizations. *Child Abuse Negl, 12*(4), 583–591. https://doi.org/10.1016/0145-2134(88)90076-2

Dozois, D. J., & Beck, A. T. (2008). Cognitive schemas, beliefs and assumptions. *Risk Factors in Depression, 119–143*. https://doi.org/10.1016/B978-0-08-045078-0.00006-X

Elliott, M., Browne, K., & Kilcoyne, J. (1995). Child sexual abuse prevention: What offenders tell us. *Child Abuse Negl, 19*(5), 579–594. https://doi.org/10.1016/0145-2134(95)00017-3

Finkelhor, D. (1984). *Child sexual abuse: New theory and research*. Free Press.

Hudson, S. M., Ward, T., & McCormack, J. C. (1999). Offense pathways in sexual offenders. *Journal of Interpersonal Violence, 14*(8), 779–798. https://doi.org/10.1177/088626099014008001

Kaptein, M., & Van Helvoort, M. (2019). A model of neutralization techniques. *Deviant Behav, 40*(10), 1260–1285. https://doi.org/10.1080/01639625.2018.1491696

Knoll, J. (2010). Teacher sexual misconduct: Grooming patterns and female offenders. *Journal of Child Sexual Abuse, 19*(4), 371–386. https://doi.org/10.1080/10538712.2010.495047

Leberg, E. (1997). *Understanding child molesters: Taking charge*. Sage.

Maruna, S., & Copes, H. (2005). What have we learned from five decades of neutralization research? *Crime Justice, 32*, 221–320. https://doi.org/10.1086/655355

Marziano, V., Ward, T., Beech, A. R., & Pattison, P. (2006). Identification of five fundamental implicit theories underlying cognitive distortions in child abusers: A preliminary study. *Psychol Crime Law, 12*(1), 97–105. https://doi.org/10.1080/10683160500056887

McAlinden, A. M. (2007). *The shaming of sexual offenders: Risk, retribution and reintegration*. Hart Publishing.

McAlinden, A. M. (2013). 'Grooming' and the sexual abuse of children: Implications for sex offender assessment, treatment and management. *Sexual Offender Treatment, 8*(1). http://www.sexual-offender-treatment.org/118.html

Moster, A., Wnuk, D. W., & Jeglic, E. L. (2008). Cognitive behavioral therapy interventions with sex offenders. *Journal of Correctional Health Care, 14*(2), 109–121. https://doi.org/10.1177/1078345807313874

Ó Ciardha, C., & Ward, T. (2013). Theories of cognitive distortions in sexual offending: What the current research tells us. *Trauma Violence Abuse, 14*(1), 5–21. https://doi.org/10.1177/1524838012467856

Petruccelli, I., Barbaranelli, C., Costantino, V., Gherardini, A., Grilli, S., Craparo, G., & D'Urso, G. (2017a). Moral disengagement and psychopathy: A study on offenders in Italian jails. *Psychiatry Psychol Law, 24*(5), 670–681. https://doi.org/10.1080/13218719.2017.1291291

Petruccelli, I., Simonelli, C., Barbaranelli, C., Grilli, S., Tripodi, M. F., & D'Urso, G. (2017b). Moral disengagement strategies in sex offenders. *Psychiatry Psychol Law, 24*(3), 470–480. https://doi.org/10.1080/13218719.2016.1252291

Schaffer, M., Jeglic, E. L., Moster, A., & Wnuk, D. (2010). Cognitive behavioral therapy in the treatment and management of sex offenders. *J Cogn Psychother, 24*(2), 92–103. https://doi.org/10.1891/0889-8391.24.2.92

Schneider, S. L., & Wright, R. C. (2004). Understanding denial in sexual offenders: A review of cognitive and motivational processes to avoid responsibility. *Trauma Violence Abuse, 5*(1), 3–20. https://doi.org/10.1177/1524838003259320

Smallbone, S. (n.d.). *Sexual abuse in schools: Analysis (3 of 5)*. http://www.ucl.ac.uk/jdibrief/documents/sexual-abuse-in-schools/SEXUAL_ABUSE_IN_SCHOOLS__3-Analysis_pdf

Sykes, G., & Matza, D. (1957). Techniques of neutralization: A theory of delinquency. *Am Sociol Rev, 22*(6), 664–670. https://doi.org/10.2307/2089195

Szumski, F., Bartels, R. M., Beech, A. R., & Fisher, D. (2018). Distorted cognition related to male sexual offending: The multi-mechanism theory of cognitive distortions (MMT-CD). *Aggress Violent Behav, 39*, 139–151. https://doi.org/10.1016/j.avb.2018.02.001

van Dam, C. (2001). *Identifying child abusers: Preventing child sexual abuse by recognizing the patterns of offenders*. The Haworth Press.

Ward, T. (2000). Sexual offenders' cognitive distortions as implicit theories. *Aggression and Violent Behavior, 5*(5), 491–507. https://doi.org/10.1016/S1359-1789(98)00036-6

Ward, T., & Hudson, S. M. (2001). Finkelhor's precondition model of child sexual abuse: A critique. *Psychol Crime Law, 7*(4), 291–307. https://doi.org/10.1080/10683160108401799

Ward, T., & Keenan, T. (1999). Child molesters' implicit theories. *Journal of Interpersonal Violence, 14*(8), 821–838. https://doi.org/10.1177/088626099014008003

Winters, G. M., & Jeglic, E. L. (2017). Stages of sexual grooming: Recognizing potentially predatory behaviors of child molesters. *Deviant Behav, 38*(6), 724–733. https://doi.org/10.1080/01639625.2016.1197656

Winters, G. M., Jeglic, E. L., & Kaylor, L. E. (2020). Validation of the sexual grooming model of child sexual abusers. *Journal of Child Sexual Abuse: Research, Treatment, & Program Innovations for Victims, Survivors, & Offenders*. https://doi.org/10.1080/10538712.2020.1801935

Winters, G. M., Kaylor, L. E., & Jeglic, E. L. (2021). Toward a universal definition of child sexual grooming. *Deviant Behav, 1–13*. https://doi.org/10.1080/01639625.2021.1941427

Chapter 7
Families and Communities and Sexual Grooming

Sexual grooming typically refers to the process by which an adult develops a relationship with their potential child victim before enacting the sexual abuse. Notably, it has been suggested the adult may also seek to spend time and effort grooming the family (*familial grooming*) and community (*community grooming*). As part of this process, the adult will use strategies to become close with the child's family and establish themselves as a respected, trusted member of the community. These tactics are used in order to find and gain access to potential victims, while simultaneously eluding detection or discovery of their deviant behaviors. In this chapter, we will first provide the theoretical framework for understanding family/community in the context of child sexual abuse (CSA) and review the role of the family and community as both risk and protective factors for CSA. Then, we provide an overview of what is known about familial and community grooming and how it fits within the stages of the Sexual Grooming Model (SGM; Winters et al., 2020), followed by recommendations for prevention.

7.1 Family and Community as Risk and Protective Factors in Child Sexual Abuse

7.1.1 Theoretical Framework

The importance of the family system and community in criminal behavior has long been theorized in the literature. From an environmental criminology perspective, the *routine activities theory* (Cohen & Felson, 1979) purports that a crime, such as CSA, is facilitated by the presence of three elements: (1) an individual motivated to commit an offense, (2) a suitable victim target, and (3) the absence of a capable

© The Author(s), under exclusive license to Springer Nature Switzerland AG 2022
G. M. Winters, E. L. Jeglic, *Sexual Grooming*,
https://doi.org/10.1007/978-3-031-07222-2_7

guardian. The term a "capable guardian" was proposed as a broad construct (e.g., police officers, neighbors, video surveillance), which can encompass both the supervision from caregivers as well as vigilance from the community at large. This theory suggests that the presence of capable guardians can reduce the likelihood of CSA by minimizing access to vulnerable children.

Moreover, Belsky's (1980) *theory of child maltreatment*, which is based on Bronfenbrenner's (1979) ecological perspective, suggests that CSA victimization is impacted by risk or protective factors that may occur at different levels of proximity to the child (Belsky, 1980). Specifically, the four interacting levels as shown in Fig. 7.1 include (1) ontogenic development (the individual), (2) microsystem (the family), (3) exosystem (the community), and (4) macrosystem (culture).

This theory encompasses the importance of the child's family at the ontogenic and microsystem levels. Ontogenic development includes the aspects of a caregiver's upbringing that may impact their parenting practices and the family system, while the microsystem addresses how dysfunctional patterns of family interactions can lead to child maltreatment. At the community level, Belsky addresses the impact employment and neighborhood relations has on child maltreatment; that is, fewer job opportunities within the community and poor social supports can increase a child's risk for victimization. As outlined in these theories, a child's family and community cannot be overlooked as both risk and protective factors for CSA.

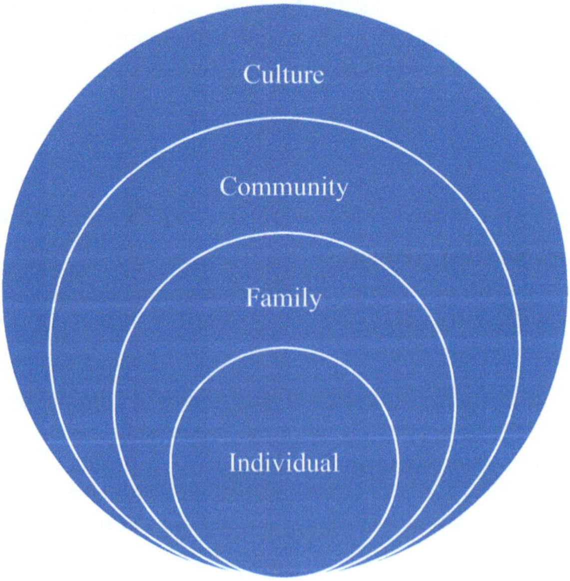

Fig. 7.1 Belsky's (1980) theory of child maltreatment

7.1.2 Family Factors

In addition to the proposed theoretical framework regarding the impact of families on CSA, the empirical research has long supported the notion that a child's family situation impacts the likelihood of a child experiencing CSA. For example, children are at lower risk for CSA if they reside with both biological parents (Sedlak et al., 2010). Conversely, children who live in foster care or live with a single parent are 10 and 20 times, respectively, more likely to experience sexual abuse compared to children living with both biological parents. More specifically, children who resided with two married parents were abused at a rate of 0.5 per 1000, with higher rates found for children living with a single parent with a partner (9.9 per 1000), single parent without a partner (2.4 per 1000), and neither parent (5.3 per 1000). Assink et al. (2019) conducted a meta-analysis of 72 studies that examined risk factors for CSA across 35 different domains. Of those risk domains, there were 23 variables that had a significant mean effect on rates of CSA—16 of which were related to the parental or family risk factors. See Table 7.1 for a summary of the results from

Table 7.1 Summary of findings from Assink et al. (2019)

	Risk domain	**Effect size**[a]
Parental-related risk factors ($n = 9$)		*r value*
	Parental history of child abuse victimization	.272
	Parental overprotection	.215
	Intimate partner violence between a child's caretakers	.190
	Parental relationship problems (excluding intimate partner violence)	.177
	Parental substance (ab)use	.173
	Parental mental/psychiatric or physical problems	.171
	Low level of parental education	.152
	Low parental care/affection (excluding forms of child neglect)	.150
	Low (sense of) parenting competences	.137
Family-related risk factors ($n = 7$)		
	Prior sexual abuse victimization of child or sibling	.377
	Prior or concurrent forms of (nonsexual) child abuse in the home environment	.291
	Problems in the family system functioning	.197
	Child grew up in a nonnuclear family structure (excluding having a stepfather)	.193
	Sibling(s) experienced child abuse (other than sexual abuse)	.166
	Child has a stepfather	.119
	Low family socioeconomic status	.101

[a]Effect sizes interpreted as small (.1), medium (.3), and large (.5)

Assink et al. (2019). Overall, the findings suggest that a range of both parental- and family-related variables can serve as risk factors for a child experiencing CSA.

While parents and family systems may pose risks for children, these variables may also serve as protective factors; that is, when certain factors are present, they may help reduce the risks of victimization. According to the Child Welfare Information Gateway (2004), these protective factors include:

1. Secure attachment, positive and warm parent-child relationship
2. Supportive family environment
3. Household rules/structure, parental monitoring of child
4. Extended family support and involvement, including caregiving help
5. Stable relationship with parents
6. Parents have a model of competence and good coping skills
7. Family expectations of pro-social behavior
8. High parental education

7.1.3 Community Factors

In addition to the family, there are community-based risk and protective factors for CSA. When looking at child abuse or neglect more broadly, the Centers for Disease Control and Prevention (CDC, 2021) identified the following community risk factors:

1. High rates of violence and crime
2. High rates of poverty
3. Fewer educational and economic opportunities
4. High unemployment rates
5. Easy access to drugs and alcohol
6. Low community involvement
7. Few community-based activities for youth
8. Unstable housing
9. Food insecurity

Black et al. (2001) conducted a review of risk factors for CSA specifically, finding that children residing in impoverished neighborhoods are at higher risk. Other studies have shown children may be at increased risk for CSA if they lack a community, such as being socially isolated from those around them or they have problems in or dissatisfaction with school (Olson et al., 2007; Whittle et al., 2013). Conversely, the CDC (2021) reported the following protective community factors: safe and stable housing, high-quality preschool education, safe and nurturing childcare, afterschool programs and activities, access to mental health and medical services, economic assistance, and employment with family-friendly policies.

7.2 Familial Grooming

Given the significant role that parents and families play as a risk or protective factor for CSA, some adults seeking to commit sexual offenses against children may engage in what has been termed *familial grooming* as part of the offense process. As examples, Leberg (1997), Salter (2003), Craven et al. (2006), McAlinden (2006), and Bennett and O'Donohue (2014) have identified one subtype of sexual grooming that involves the grooming of the victim's family or significant others. While there is no universal definition of the construct, familial grooming generally refers to the process by which an adult develops a trusting, close relationship with a potential victim's family. By doing so, the adults in the child's life are "primed and controlled for victimization in similar ways to children" (McAlinden, 2006; p. 348). Salter (2003) describes this as a skillful and premeditated process, by which the adult uses social skills and deception techniques to avoid suspicion from the family. The goals of familial grooming are twofold (McAlinden, 2006; Salter, 2003):

1. Facilitate easy and frequent access to the child
2. Minimize the likelihood of disclosure or discovery from others

The extent of familial grooming may differ depending on the age of the child. That is, adolescents have more autonomy and independence outside of their family; thus, familial grooming may not be necessary to have contact with older victims (Sanderson, 2004).

Broadly, the process of familial grooming can be conceptualized through the stages of *victim selection* and *gaining access and isolation* in the SGM (Winters et al., 2020); see Fig. 7.2.

First, the adult may seek to select a victim based on family vulnerabilities (Conte et al., 1989; Elliott et al., 1995). As outlined in the SGM, experts indicated that children may be targeted if they are not close to their parents, they come from a

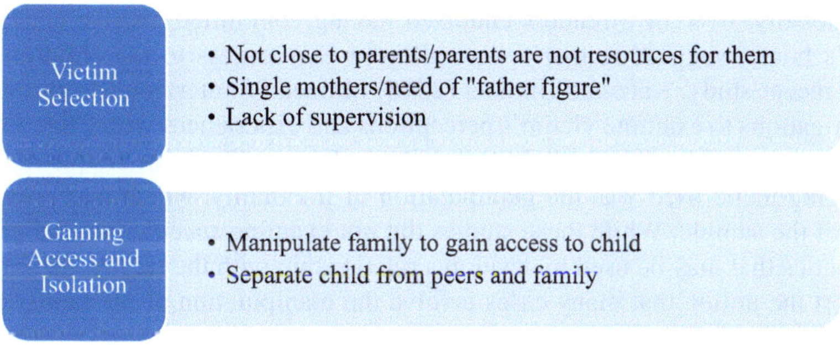

Fig. 7.2 SGM items relevant to familial grooming

single mother household or lack a father figure, or they lack supervision. Family vulnerabilities may include the presence of marital problems between parents (Finkehor, 1984; Gruber & Jones, 1983), a parent with a medical illness (Herman & Hirschman, 1981; Finkelhor, 1984), or poor interpersonal relationships within family (Berliner & Conte, 1990). Additionally, a child who has experienced neglect or abuse within the home may be more likely to be targeted (Bagley & Ramsey, 1986; Craven et al., 2006).

Once a victim is selected, the adult may seek to gain access to the child by developing a trusting relationship with the family, such as forming a friendship or romantic relationship with the caregiver(s). Indeed, experts on sexual grooming reported that an individual may attempt to manipulate the family to gain access to the child (Winters et al., 2020). Once the relationship has formed, the adult may use that familial trust to have access to the minor so that they can then emotionally and physically isolate the child from the family. By using these tactics, the adult is able to create situations in which they can be alone with the child, such as taking them on overnight stays or outings without the suspicion of the parents and in many instances with parental consent. The successful use of family to select and gain access to a victim can in turn facilitate subsequent steps in the sexual grooming process, such as developing trust with the child and those around them.

7.2.1 *Prevalence*

While no studies have explicitly studied familial grooming, research on tactics used by perpetrators of CSA suggest that in about two thirds of the cases, perpetrators develop or exploit relationships with the family in order to get access to the minors. For example, Elliott et al. (1995) conducted interviews with 91 adults who committed a child sexual offense. Most of the offenders (66%) knew the victims through family, friends, or a caretaking role (e.g., babysitting). For extrafamilial offenders, results showed that 33% worked toward being welcome in the victim's home, and 20% reported they obtained the trust of the entire family. Additionally, 61% of offenders endorsed having committed abusive acts in the child's home, suggesting many were allowed easy access to the children. In a more recent study, Katz and Barnetz (2016) utilized 95 interviews from forensic investigations to examine victim's perceptions and experiences with CSA. Results from a thematic analysis of the interviews showed the most frequent sexual grooming tactic used was the manipulation of the family, which was present in 68% of the sample. While these studies did not examine *specific* familial grooming tactics that may be used to develop a relationship with the family, the findings support the notion that many cases involve the manipulation of the family in the sexual grooming process.

7.3 Familial Grooming by Offender Type

Individuals who commit sexual offenses against children are commonly categorized as either an *intrafamilial offender* or *extrafamilial offender*. Intrafamilial offenders are those who are related to the victim and often (but not always) reside in the same home. This may include parents, stepparents, siblings, or other blood relatives. Extrafamilial offenders are those who are outside of the child's family, such as family friends, babysitters, teachers, strangers, or others unrelated to the victim. Overall, prior literature demonstrated that intrafamilial and extrafamilial offenders may differ (see for example Fischer & McDonald, 1998; Seto et al., 2015), which may be particularly necessary to explore in the instance of familial grooming as these groups have differential access to the family system of potential victims.

7.3.1 Extrafamilial Offending

The use of familial grooming may be especially important for cases of extrafamilial offending. These individuals may choose potential victims based on vulnerabilities of the child's family, such as those outlined in Fig. 7.2. In order to gain access to a victim, it may be necessary to present as "nice men who simply like children" (p. 119; McAlinden, 2012). Familial grooming can be used to create a trusting friendship with a child's parents, so they can establish legitimate access to the child once the caregiver feels comfortable with the adult being around their child. They may offer to provide childcare for the parents (e.g., babysitting) or teach the children games or coach sports, and then escalate to more isolated activities such as overnight stays (McAlinden, 2012). Once access is gained, they can more readily develop a close relationship with the potential victim and distance the child from caregivers or other significant people.

7.3.2 Intrafamilial Offending

The familial grooming process is unique in cases involving intrafamilial offending. That is, these adults already have a position of trust and power in the family, as well as the ability to readily access victims and create situations in which they are alone with the child (Craven et al., 2006). In a study of over 500 cases of CSA, Sas and Cunningham (1995) found that sexual grooming was most common in cases of intrafamilial abuse, especially when the offender was serving in a caretaking role (two-thirds of the intrafamilial cases).

In terms of the selecting a victim, McAlinden (2006) indicated, "one of the easiest ways to make contact with a child is to live with one" (p. 349). Single-parent households (typically a single mother) have been notable targets according to prior literature (McAlinden, 2006), especially if there are comorbid emotional, economic, or substance use problems (Bagley & Ramsey, 1986; Herman & Hirschman, 1981; Salter, 1995). In these households, the mother and child may be seeking out a "father figure" for the family, and thus, the mother may form a romantic relationship in hopes of marriage and cohabitation (NCIS, 2003). In the most extreme cases, an adult interested in committing CSA may seek out a romantic partner with the long-term plan to have children with the person who can then be victimized (Salter, 2003).

The intrafamilial offenders have gained access to, and are able to isolate, the victim and significant others by being or becoming a part of the family. Especially in the case of single parent households, the adult has the ability to create situations alone with the child without raising concern. The intrafamilial offender may seek to emotionally and physically isolate the child from the non-abusive parents, siblings, or friends (Craven et al., 2006). This creates a more exclusive, tight-knit relationship with the child. The adult may manipulatively encourage the non-abusing parent to have hobbies or social interests that take them outside of the home, thus increasing opportunities to be alone with the child for the abuse. Alternatively, they could isolate the non-abusing parents from friends and family to prevent any communication to others about possible suspicion of abuse. Also, some intrafamilial offenders may encourage drug or alcohol use by the parent so that they appear not credible if they were to raise concerns or report a child's disclosure.

Given the ongoing access, it has been suggested the intrafamilial offenders may continue familial grooming over long periods of time in order to engage in further abusive incidents (Eher & Ross, 2006). McAlinden (2012) proposed the bulk of the intrafamilial grooming would not take place at the onset of the abuse as it would in extrafamilial cases but rather would be used to prevent disclosure after the abuse and facilitate future abusive acts. Due to this later-stage sexual grooming, the child may feel confused as to whether the behaviors were abusive, feel fearful of telling as it may hurt others or the perpetrator themselves, and worry that they may not be believed; they may also experience guilt or a sense of responsibly for what happened.

7.4 Community Grooming

Community grooming is used to further surpass the "gatekeepers" of children so a person seeking to commit a sexual offense can find and access victims. The process of community grooming is present in items related to *gaining access and isolation* and *trust development* within the SGM (Winters et al., 2020); see Fig. 7.3.

The adult will aim to seamlessly integrate into the society, including becoming close to people who have contact with children and frequenting locations where children spend time in the community (Craven et al., 2006). For example, the individual may volunteer in youth-serving organizations, become a member of the church, or assist the community on tasks or jobs that are undesirable in order to make themselves indispensable (Leberg, 1997). In some cases, the adult may pose

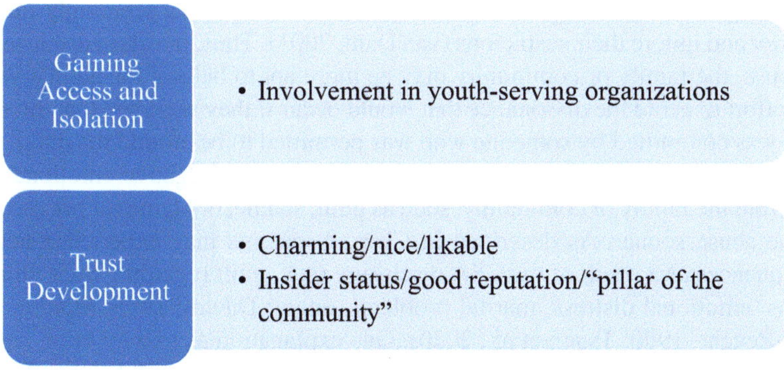

Fig. 7.3 SGM items relevant to community grooming

as a fellow parent to earn the trust of other parents. Regarding trust development tactics, Van Dam (2001) proposed that community grooming may include presenting as charming, trustworthy, dependable, and helpful, as well as include working toward gaining insider status and a good reputation. As Hare and Hart (1993) described, these adults skillfully "read the community like a book" so they can assess and subsequently fill the needs of their surroundings. For those who do seek to gain the insider status in the community before abusing a child, the sexual grooming is thought to be a long-term process (Sanford, 1982) that involves premeditation of how their efforts are going to result in rewarding situations in which the abuse can easily occur (Craven et al., 2006). Moreover, the use of community grooming is believed to serve as a protective barrier if the victim discloses, as the community may choose to support the adult whom they view as a pillar of the community.

7.5 Impact of Familial and Community Grooming on Disclosure

One of the motivations behind familial and community grooming is to ensure the abusive behavior will not be disclosed or discovered. In fact, it has been suggested that even if a victim does disclose, their account may not be believed if there was successful grooming of the family or community as citizens may deem the adult as more believable (Craven et al., 2006). One of the potential explanations for this is the purported role that *cognitive dissonance* plays in familial and community grooming (Craven et al., 2006; McAlinden, 2012; van Dam, 2001). Cognitive dissonance is the idea that when a person's thoughts and behaviors are incongruent, the person will make an effort to adjust these thoughts to be consistent with their actions. In the case of familial or community grooming, if there are any instinctive concerns about the person's trustworthiness or motivations after the family and community have welcomed and accepted the person, these individuals may change their thoughts or reasoning to be in line with the individual's seemingly innocent behavior and ignore their suspicions (van Dam, 2001). Thus, if a child discloses sexual abuse, the family or community may be more apt to believe the adult's version in an effort to avoid the dissonance that would occur if they accepted that the sexual abuse was committed by someone who was permitted to be around the child.

In instances that disclosure is believed, there may be negative emotional reactions from the family or community, such as guilt, shame, or blame for not recognizing the abuse sooner. As described in Chap. 4, parents may experience negative consequences as a result of the CSA disclosure (e.g., guilt regarding their failure as parents, emotional distress, marital problems, anger; Davies, 1995; Manion et al., 1996; Regehr, 1990; Tsang et al., 2020). One explanation as to why these negative emotional reactions may be heighted in the cases involving familial and community grooming is the *hindsight bias*. Empirical research has shown that there is a hindsight bias in cases of sexual grooming, in that people tend to overestimate the likelihood they would have predicted a person would sexually abuse children after learning about substantiated abuse (Winters & Jeglic, 2016). Yet data has shown that people are poor at recognizing sexual grooming behaviors as possibly deviant in the absence of outcome information about the CSA (Winters & Jeglic, 2017). This overestimation by individuals believing the abuse could have been prevented may lead to blaming the victim's family or community for not recognizing the seemingly obvious red flags before the CSA occurred.

7.6 Prevention

While prevention is described more broadly in Chap. 14, there are several preventive efforts specific to familial and community grooming worth noting. The CDC utilizes a socio-ecological model for the prevention of sexual violence using the acronym STOP SV (see Fig. 7.4). The strategies associated with T, O, and P as described are most applicable to familial and community grooming. Below, there are several broad recommendations applicable to these stages.

First, parents and communities should be provided with psychoeducation about CSA and sexual grooming in general (e.g., CSA is most often committed by someone known to the child, including those within the family system) but also more specifically about the grooming tactics that might be used to infiltrate a family and community. As one participant in Elliot et al.'s (1995) study noted, "parents are so naive—they're worried about strangers and should be worried about their brother-in-law. They just don't realize how devious we can be. I used to abuse children in the same room with their parents and they couldn't see it or didn't seem to know it was happening" (p. 590). Interestingly, an experimental study by Steedman et al. (in submission) showed that parents are not better able to recognize sexual grooming behaviors compared to nonparents. Thus, individuals must be educated on the myths about people who commit sexual offenses and their victims and how some individuals may seek to strategically develop relationships with families and communities in

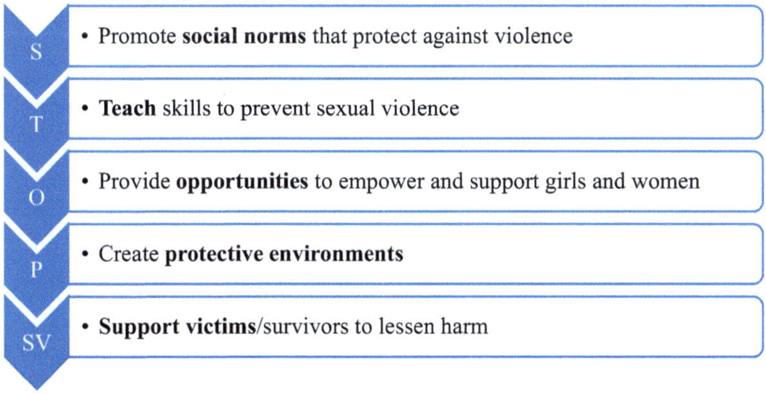

Fig. 7.4 CDC prevention of sexual violence: STOP SV

order to access and abuse children (McAlinden, 2006). Importantly, there is a notable dilemma that there are many individuals who will have genuine intentions regarding their relationship with children and may, in fact, be a positive or supportive figure in a child's life. Therefore, education efforts should acknowledge this reality as well and provide parents with information on when it is appropriate to raise concern (e.g., high frequency or severity of behaviors with children). Second, parents should also educate their children on what constitutes appropriate or inappropriate interactions with adults in their life. They should be informed about types of conversations and physical touch that is acceptable from both those within and outside of the family unit. The children should know they can relay any concerns to the caregiver and will not be punished for anything they report. Lastly, both caregivers and the community at large should be vigilant about the behaviors of adults in children's lives. Related to this, individuals should be informed of resources that can be sought out if they observe any potentially unusual or suspicious behavior with children (e.g., contacting law enforcement, anonymous crime tip lines, contacting child protective services).

7.7 Conclusion

In sum, it is evident that the family and community hold a significant role in CSA, contributing both to the risk and protection of children. Sexual grooming may not solely be used on the child, but it may also be used on the family or community. Through these familial and community grooming strategies, the adult develops a trusting relationship with the gatekeepers to children and, over time, gain easy access to potential victims. Moreover, it has been suggested the use of these behaviors may result in low rates of discovery and disclosure by victims, or disbelief if a victim does disclose the CSA. Additional research is needed on the construct of familial and community grooming, including the development of a standardized definition, as well as more research on the prevalence of these behaviors, the specific types of tactics that may be used, and how these behaviors can be more easily recognized in order to prevent CSA.

References

Assink, M., van der Put, C. E., Meeuwsen, M. W. C. M., de Jong, N. M., Oort, F. J., Stams, G. J. J. M., & Hoeve, M. (2019). Risk factors for child sexual abuse victimization: A meta-analytic review. *Psychological Bulletin, 145*(5), 459–459. https://doi.org/10.1037/bul0000188

Bagley, C., & Ramsey, R. (1986). Sexual abuse in childhood: Psycho-social outcomes and implications for social work practice. *Journal of Social Work and Human Sexuality, 4*, 33–47.

Belsky, J. (1980). Child maltreatment: An ecological integration. *American Psychologist, 35*, 320–335. https://doi.org/10.1037/0003-066X.35.4.320

Bennett, N., & O'Donohue, W. (2014). The construct of grooming in child sexual abuse: Conceptual and measurement issues. *Journal of Child Sexual Abuse: Research, Treatment, & Program Innovations for Victims, Survivors, & Offenders, 23*(8), 957–976. https://doi.org/10.1080/10538712.2014.960632

Berliner, L., & Conte, J. R. (1990). The process of victimization: The victims' perspective. *Child Abuse & Neglect, 14*(1), 29–40. https://doi.org/10.1016/0145-2134(90)90078-8

Black, D. A., Heyman, R. E., & Smith Slep, A. M. (2001). Risk factors for child sexual abuse. *Aggression and Violent Behavior, 6*(2), 203–229. https://doi.org/10.1016/S1359-1789(00)00023-9

Bronfenbrenner, U. (1979). *The ecology of human development*. Harvard University Press.

Centers for Disease Control and Prevention [CDC]. (2021). *Risk and protective factors*. https://www.cdc.gov/violenceprevention/childabuseandneglect/riskprotectivefactors.html

Child Welfare Information Gateway. (2004). *Risk and protective factors for child abuse and neglect*. https://www.childwelfare.gov/pubpdfs/riskprotectivefactors.pdf

Cohen, L. E., & Felson, M. (1979). Social change and crime rate trends: A routine activity approach. *American Sociological Review, 44*, 588–608. https://doi.org/10.2307/2094589

Conte, J. R., Wolf, S., & Smith, T. (1989). What sexual offenders tell us about prevention strategies. *Child Abuse & Neglect, 13*(2), 293–301. https://doi.org/10.1016/0145-2134(89)90016-1

Craven, S., Brown, S., & Gilchrist, E. (2006). Sexual grooming of children: Review of literature and theoretical considerations. *Journal of Sexual Aggression, 12*(3), 287–299. https://doi.org/10.1080/13552600601069414

Davies, M. G. (1995). Parental distress and ability to cope following disclosure of extra-familial sexual abuse. *Child Abuse & Neglect, 19*(4), 399–399.

Eher, R., & Ross, T. (2006). Reconsidering risk for reoffense in intrafamilial child molesters: New aspects on clinical and criminological issues. *Sexual Offender Treatment, 1*(2). http://www.sexual-offender-treatment.org/39.html

Elliott, M., Browne, K., & Kilcoyne, J. (1995). Child sexual abuse prevention: What offenders tell us. *Child Abuse & Neglect, 19*(5), 579–579.

Finkelhor, D. (1984). *Child sexual abuse: New theory and research*. Free Press/Collier Macmillan.

Fischer, D. G., & McDonald, W. L. (1998). Characteristics of intrafamilial and extrafamilial child sexual abuse. *Child Abuse & Neglect, 22*(9), 915–929.

Gruber, K. J., & Jones, R. J. (1983). Identifying determinants of risk of sexual victimization of youth: A multivariate approach. *Child Abuse & Neglect, 7*(1), 17–24. https://doi.org/10.1016/0145-2134(83)90025-X

Hare, R. D., & Hart, S. D. (1993). Psychopathy, mental disorder, and crime. In S. Hodgins (Ed.), *Mental disorder and crime* (pp. 104–115). Sage.

Herman, J. L., & Hirschman, L. (1981). *Father-daughter incest*. Harvard University Press.
Katz, C., & Barnetz, Z. (2016). Children's narratives of alleged child sexual abuse offender behaviors and the manipulation process. *Psychology of Violence, 6*(2), 223–232. https://doi.org/10.1037/a0039023
Leberg, E. (1997). *Understanding child molesters: Taking charge*. Sage.
Manion, I. G., McIntyre, J., Firestone, P., Ligezinska, M., Ensom, R., & Wells, G. (1996). Secondary traumatization in parents following the disclosure of extrafamilial child sexual abuse: Initial effects. *Child Abuse & Neglect, 20*(11), 1095–1109. https://doi.org/10.1016/0145-2134(96)00098-1
McAlinden, A. M. (2006). Setting 'em up': Personal, familial and institutional grooming in the sexual abuse of children. *Social & Legal Studies, 15*(3), 339–362. https://doi.org/10.1177/0964663906066613
McAlinden, A. M. (2012). *'Grooming' and the sexual abuse of children: Institutional, Internet and familial dimensions*. Oxford University Press.
National Criminal Intelligence Service (NCIS). (2003). *United Kingdom threat assessment of serious and organised crime*.
Olson, L. N., Daggs, J. L., Ellevold, B. L., & Rogers, T. K. K. (2007). Entrapping the innocent: Toward a theory of child sexual predators' luring communication. *Communication Theory, 17*, 231–251. https://doi.org/10.1111/j.1468-2885.2007.00294.x
Regehr, C. (1990). Parental responses to extrafamilial child sexual assault. *Child Abuse & Neglect, 14*(1), 113–120. https://doi.org/10.1016/0145-2134(90)90086-9
Salter, A. C. (1995). *Transforming trauma: A guide to understanding and treating adult survivors of child sexual abuse*. Sage.
Salter, A. (2003). *Predators, pedophiles, rapists, and other sex offenders: Who they are, how they operate, and how we can protect ourselves and our children*. Basic Books.
Sanderson, C. (2004). The grooming of children. In *The seduction of children: Empowering parents and teachers to protect children from sexual abuse* (pp. 165–190). Jessica Kinsley Publishers.
Sanford, L. T. (1982). *The silent children: A parent's guide to the prevention of child sexual abuse*. McGraw-Hill.
Sas, L. D., & Cunningham, A. H. (1995). *Tipping the balance to tell the secret: The public discovery of child sexual abuse*. London Family Court Clinic.
Sedlak, A. J., Mettenburg, J., Basena, M., Petta, I., McPherson, K., Greene, A., & Li, S. (2010). *Fourth National Incidence Study of child abuse and neglect (NIS–4): Report to Congress, executive summary*. U.S. Department of Health and Human Services, Administration for Children and Families.
Seto, M. C., Babchishin, K. M., Pullman, L. E., & McPhail, I. V. (2015). The puzzle of intrafamilial child sexual abuse: A meta-analysis comparing intrafamilial and extrafamilial offenders with child victims. *Clinical Psychology Review, 39*, 42–57. https://doi.org/10.1016/j.cpr.2015.04.001
Steedman, L., Jeglic, E., & Winters, G. (in submission). *Examining parental abilities to recognize sexual grooming behaviors of child sexual abusers*.
Tsang, V. M., Verlinden, E., van Duin, E. M., Twisk, J. W., Brilleslijper-Kater, S. N., Gigengack, M. R., Verhoeff, A. P., & Lindauer, R. J. (2020). The Amsterdam sexual abuse case: What scars did it leave? Long-term course of psychological problems for children who have been sexually abused at a very young age, and their parents. *Child Psychiatry & Human Development, 1–12*. https://doi.org/10.1007/s10578-020-01067-5
van Dam, C. (2001). *Identifying child molesters: Preventing child sexual abuse by recognizing the patterns of the offenders*. Haworth Maltreatment and Trauma Press/The Haworth Press.
Whittle, H., Hamilton-Giachritsis, C., Beech, A., & Collings, G. (2013). A review of young people's vulnerabilities to online grooming. *Aggression and Violent Behavior, 18*(1), 135–146. https://doi.org/10.1016/j.avb.2012.11.008

Winters, G. M., & Jeglic, E. L. (2016). I knew it all along: The sexual grooming behaviors of child molesters and the hindsight bias. *Journal of Child Sexual Abuse, 25*(1), 20–36. https://doi.org/10.1080/10538712.2015.1108945

Winters, G. M., & Jeglic, E. L. (2017). Stages of sexual grooming: Recognizing potentially predatory behaviors of child molesters. *Deviant Behavior, 38*(6), 724–733. https://doi.org/10.1080/01639625.2016.1197656

Winters, G. M., Kaylor, L. E., & Jeglic, E. L. (2017). Sexual offenders contacting children online: An examination of transcripts of sexual grooming. *Journal of Sexual Aggression, 23*(1), 62–76. https://doi.org/10.1080/13552600.2016.1271146

Winters, G. M., Jeglic, E. L., & Kaylor, L. E. (2020). Validation of the sexual grooming model of child sexual abusers. *Journal of Child Sexual Abuse: Research, Treatment, & Program Innovations for Victims, Survivors, & Offenders*. https://doi.org/10.1080/10538712.2020.1801935

Chapter 8
Institutions and Sexual Grooming

In the 1990s and 2000s, the public became aware of child sexual abuse (CSA) occurring within institutional settings. The abuse, which in many cases had been going on for decades, was pervasive in scope. It appears that no institutions are immune, as cases have occurred and continue to surface in schools, religious organizations, care homes, foster care, sporting organizations, volunteer organizations, and other youth-serving organizations such as the Boy Scouts of America and the Young Men's Christian Association (YMCA). Research examining sexual abuse within the Catholic Church both in Germany and the United States (US) found that approximately 4% of all Catholic priests were alleged to have perpetrated CSA (Dressing et al., 2021; John Jay College of Criminal Justice, 2004, 2006). In the US, it is estimated that over 12,000 boys had been abused by 7800 scoutmasters in the Boy Scouts of America between 1944 and 2006 (Dockterman, 2019). Inquiries in Canada revealed that one in five indigenous children who were placed in residential schools experienced CSA (Naumetz, 2009). Similarly, inquiries in the United Kingdom showed CSA occurring in children's homes, residential special schools, and boarding schools (Gallagher, 2000). While in Australia, the Royal Commission into Institutional Responses to CSA (2017) found that tens of thousands of children were sexually abused across a variety of different institutional contexts (e.g., education, recreation, sporting, and religious and/or cultural activity). Overall, it has been estimated that (depending upon the institution and the method of assessment employed) anywhere between 0.1% and 10% of children and youth placed in youth-serving organizations experienced CSA (Turner & Briken, 2015).

Gallagher (2000) defined institutional abuse as:

> The sexual abuse of a child (under 18 years of age) by an adult who works with him or her. The perpetrator may be employed in a paid or voluntary capacity; in the public, voluntary or private sector; in a residential or non-residential setting; and may work either directly with children or be in an ancillary role. (p. 797)

© The Author(s), under exclusive license to Springer Nature Switzerland AG 2022

G. M. Winters, E. L. Jeglic, *Sexual Grooming*,
https://doi.org/10.1007/978-3-031-07222-2_8

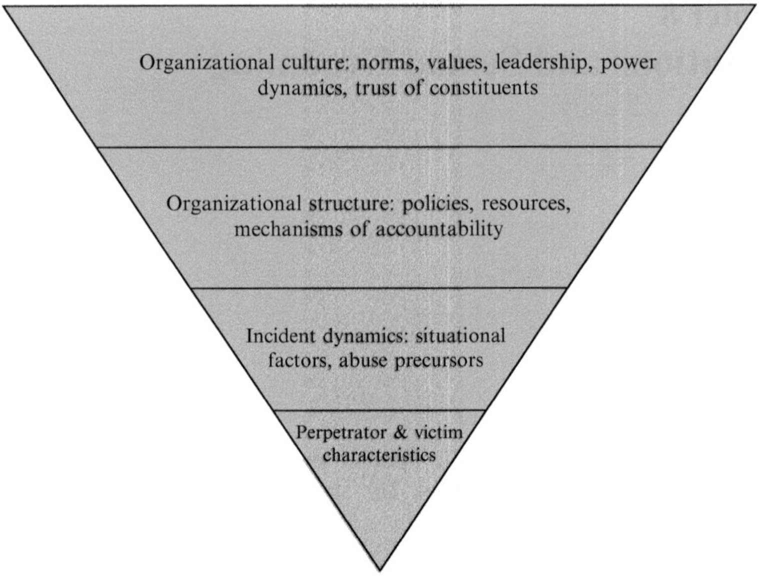
Organizational culture: norms, values, leadership, power dynamics, trust of constituents
Organizational structure: policies, resources, mechanisms of accountability
Incident dynamics: situational factors, abuse precursors
Perpetrator & victim characteristics

Fig. 8.1 Hierarchy of factors associated with CSA within institutions (Harris & Terry, 2019)

After many of these high-profile cases of institutional abuse were revealed, Sullivan and Beech (2002) described what they coined "professional perpetrators"—those individuals who use the organizations in which they work or volunteer to target and sexually abuse children. It is believed that these individuals seek out professions and organizations that cater to children specifically with the intention of abusing a child (Sullivan & Beech, 2004). Harris and Terry (2019) proposed a hierarchy of factors (see Fig. 8.1) which contribute to CSA within organizations. The bottom two levels represent the micro or individual level factors that contribute to CSA within institutions, while the top two levels represent the macro or organizational level factors.

In many of these cases, the perpetrators not only used sexual grooming techniques to abuse the children but also groomed institutions themselves so that they would not be detected (McAlinden, 2006). As such, this chapter will review what is known about those who perpetrate institutional CSA, explore the construct of institutional grooming, and examine how grooming strategies may be employed differently across settings (e.g., religious organizations, youth-serving organizations like the Boy Scouts of America, educational institutions, and sporting organizations).

8.1 Characteristics of Professional Perpetrators

While it has been known for some time that children could be abused by those who were not related to them (extrafamilial offenders; CSA-E), it was only when the widespread abuse of children within institutions was uncovered that researchers began studying the characteristics of those who perpetrated abuse within the context of working with children either in their employment or volunteer position (CSA-W). While the majority of the existing research on CSA-W to date has focused on the characteristics of clergy samples (John Jay College of Criminal Justice, 2004; Mercado et al., 2008; Perillo et al., 2008; Terry et al., 2008), more recent studies have examined characteristics of those who perpetrate abuse in the context of employment and volunteer work more generally, including educators, child care workers, coaches, and foster parents (i.e., CSA-Ws), and compared them to the characteristics of extrafamilial (CSA-E) and intrafamilial abusers (CSA-I). The findings of five of the main studies that have made these comparisons are summarized below in Table 8.1.

Table 8.1 Findings from studies examining the characteristics of CSA-W

Study (authors, date)	Comparison groups	Main findings for CSA-W
Sullivan et al. (2011)	CSA-I CSA-E	Less likely to have previous nonsexual or sexual convictions
		More likely to have offended against boys or have both boy and girl victims
		More likely to have post pubescent victims
		More likely to have more than 20 victims
		More sexual pre-occupation and overidentification with children
		Lower distorted attitudes about CSA
Sullivan and Beech (2004)	Non-CSA-W perpetrators (grouped both CSA-I and CSA-E)	More likely to be older and more intelligent
		Majority (90%) knew of their sexual interest in children before age 21
		More than half (57%) chose their profession in part to have access to minors
Falkenbach et al. (2017)	CSA-I CSA-E	More likely to be better educated and have higher income
		Less likely to be married
		Fewer nonsexual convictions.
		More likely to abuse male, post-pubescent children
Turner et al. (2016)	CSA-I CSA-E	Fewer antisocial tendencies.
		More likely to recidivate with a sexual offense
		Had more protective factors as measured by the Structured Assessment of Protective Factors (SAPROF)
		Had many indicators for pedophilic sexual interests
Turner et al. (2014)	CSA-I CSA-E	Lowest scores on the Psychopathy Checklist Revised
		Highest prevalence of pedophilic disorder diagnosis
		Highest frequency of male victims
		Highest total scores on Screening Scale for Pedophilic Interests

The studies highlighted in Table 8.1 suggest that CSA-W offenders differ significantly from CSA-E and CSA-I perpetrators and thus may constitute a separate typology of their own (Falkenbach et al., 2017; Sullivan & Beech, 2004; Sullivan et al., 2011; Turner et al., 2014, 2016). CSA-W offenders are more likely than either CSA-I and CSA-E offenders to be educated and unmarried, have pedophilic interests, have multiple victims, and offend against adolescent males, while they are less likely to have a criminal history of any kind and exhibit less psychopathic and antisocial traits. Taken together, these findings suggest that CSA-W offenders should not be characterized as CSA-I or CSA-E offenders. Further, Turner and Briken (2015) suggest that even within the CSA-W category there may be different subgroupings by profession (i.e., clergy, educator), but this has yet to be empirically studied. What makes CSA-W offenders particularly dangerous is that they often present to institutional employers, parents, and children as educated and socially stable, which may result in their behaviors not arousing suspicion. Also, they are less likely to have a criminal history, and thus, their deviance would not be detected using employment screening and background checks. Consequently, CSA-W perpetrators may be perceived as safe and trustworthy, so they are able gain the confidence of the institutions within which they are employed (Falkenbach et al., 2017).

8.2 Institutional Grooming

While the perpetrator may use their employment or volunteer position within a child-serving organization to gain access to children as part of the child sexual grooming process, to do so they must also gain the trust of the organization or institution so that the abuse can occur without detection—this process has been called *institutional grooming*. The term institutional grooming was first introduced into the literature by McAlinden in 2006. She used the term to describe the "special features of the institutional environment to facilitate abuse and prevent disclosure by children and other professionals. These particular dynamics include features such as opportunity, anonymity, secrecy and power" (McAlinden, 2006, p. 353).

According to McAlinden (2012), there are five main characteristics of the institutional environment that perpetrators utilize in the institutional sexual grooming process as depicted in Fig. 8.2: trust, opportunity, anonymity, secrecy, and power.

1. *Trust*. McAlinden likens institutional trust of the perpetrator to the trusting relationship they build with the potential victim, their family, and the community. The individual who seeks to engage in the sexual grooming of children manipulates the organization to gain a position of trust such that they now represents the organization to the child, their family, and the community, thus gaining access to minors. Their position of trust within the organization further reinforces their appearance of respectability, which is key as the grooming begins so that any behaviors that may arouse suspicion will be explained away, and they avoid detection.

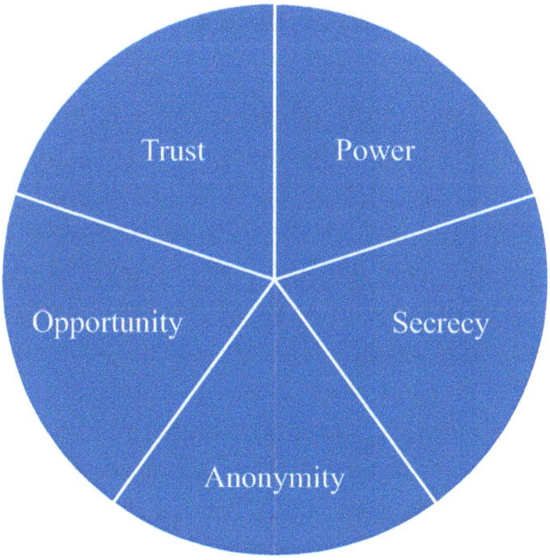

Fig. 8.2 Characteristics of institutional to environments that make them susceptible to sexual grooming

2. *Opportunity*. Those who wish to abuse children take advantage of opportunities to manipulate organizations. This can be due to a weak or hierarchical organizational culture in which those in positions of authority can abuse their power unchecked (McAlinden, 2012). Further, those who want to abuse minors will seek out and take advantage of organizations that either lack policies and procedures to prevent CSA or who fail to enforce them (Arnold & Jeglic, n.d.).
3. *Anonymity*. As grooming is considered a deceptive process, the individual who perpetrates sexual abuse within an institutional context can achieve anonymity as they can take on a new persona reflective of their institutional role, thus concealing their deviant intentions (McAlinden, 2012). For example, despite his deviant sexual interests as evidenced by his possession of child sexual exploitation material, Larry Nassar was able to represent USA gymnastics and hide his deviance through his medical work with the organization (Verhoeven, 2020).
4. *Secrecy*. According to McAlinden (2010), results of child abuse inquiries show that childcare institutions tend to be "self-protective, secretive and closed by nature" (p. 30). It is this secrecy that has allowed those who offend within institutional contexts to continue their abuse. For example, it was revealed that priests who were accused of sexual abuse within the Catholic Church were moved from one parish to another, thereby allowing the abuse to continue (Armbruster, 2021).
5. *Power*. McAlinden (2012) highlights that individuals in institutional roles that give them unchecked power can help to create a system in which abuse fails to be disclosed. This can be because they control the organizational culture, or there are no clear reporting lines such that even if abuse is suspected, there is no one but the abuser to report it to.

McAlinden (2012) states that it is these features of vulnerable organizations which permit the potentially abusive individual to "manipulate perceptions, create opportunities, and prevent suspicion" (p. 164).

8.2.1 Impact of Institutional Sexual Grooming

Institutional sexual abuse has lasting negative impacts not only on the victims of CSA (see Chap. 4 on the long-term consequences of CSA and sexual grooming) but also on communities and the institution itself. While there is the obvious financial liability incurred by the institutions for their failure to protect children, there is also damage to their public reputation and the public's trust in these organizations, as well as vicarious trauma to those who work within the organizations. Following the revelation of CSA within the Catholic Church, not only did survivors report a negative impact on their belief in God, church involvement, and spiritual practices, but peers, families, and communities also experienced a loss of trust and a sense of betrayal which has negatively impacted subsequent generations (Blakemore et al., 2017; Goode et al., 2003; Herbert et al., 2020; Kline et al., 2008; Rossetti, 1995). Blakemore et al. (2017) reviewed the research examining the impact of institutional CSA, and in addition to the negative consequences to the victim themselves. They highlighted the trauma experienced by colleagues of the perpetrator and other workers within the institutions following the revelations of abuse, especially if there was an institutional cover-up or the allegations were mishandled.

8.3 Child Sexual Abuse Across Institutional Settings

8.3.1 Religious Organizations

Following the Spotlight Investigation of abuse in the Catholic Church by the *Boston Globe* in 2002, the public became aware of the rampant CSA within the US Catholic Church (Rezendes, 2002). Between 1950 and 2002, allegations of sexual abuse were levied against 4% (n = 4392) of all active priests within the US Catholic Church (John Jay College of Criminal Justice, 2004, 2006; Terry et al., 2008). Similar scandals were reported in Canada, the United Kingdom, the Netherlands, Belgium, and Australia (Barnardos, 2010; Death, 2015). A recent study from Germany also found that 4.4% of clergy were alleged to have abused minors (Dressing et al., 2021). While the majority of attention has been focused on the Catholic Church, CSA scandals have also rocked the United Methodist Church (Strangeways-Booth, 2015), the Anglican Church, (Parkinson et al., 2012), the Mormon Church (Gerdes et al., 1996), and the Orthodox Jewish Community (Katzenstein & Fontes, 2017), among others.

It has long been speculated that clergy used sexual grooming strategies to enact CSA, which may account for the low rates of reporting (Spraitz & Bowen, 2020). However, it has only been recently that these strategies have been explored empirically. For example, evidence of sexual grooming was found in 17 out of 18 cases of alleged priest sexual abuse in one Benedictine Abbey in Minnesota (Mignon et al., 2017) and in 16 out of 17 priests with allegations of sexual abuse in a midwestern diocese (Burmeister et al., 2019). Spraitz et al. (2018, 2019) reviewed records from two samples of allegedly abusive priests in the US Midwest and developed a taxonomy of eight identified grooming behaviors of priests who engaged in CSA (see Chap. 3 for a more detailed description). Additionally, using data from the John Jay College study on CSA in the Catholic Church, Tallon and Terry (2008) found that sexual grooming tactics (i.e., threats, use of enticements, and socializing with family members) were allegedly used by some Catholic Church clergy (7–31%). More recently, Winters et al. (2022) examined sexual grooming behaviors among Catholic Church clergy using the John Jay College data and found that Catholic clergy used a variety of sexual grooming tactics and behaviors as described by the SGM (Table 8.2).

While many of the sexual grooming behaviors identified in these studies were similar to both the stages and behaviors described in the SGM, there is some evidence that there may be characteristics of grooming which may be unique to clergy or religious communities/figures. For example, religious figures may be less likely to choose vulnerable victims as they have easy access to minors. They may also possess the implicit trust and respect of children, families, and communities through their role within the religious institution (Raine & Kent, 2019; Spraitz & Bowen, 2020; Tishelman & Fontes, 2017). Consequently, within religious institutions there may be less emphasis by the perpetrator on the initial stages of the sexual grooming (i.e., choosing a vulnerable victim, and gaining access to the child). Indeed, Winters et al. (2022) found that in their large sample of Catholic clergy alleged to have perpetrated CSA, the clerics did not disproportionately target minors from single-parent households, and two-thirds of the clergy met their victims through their role in the church.

It has also been speculated that priests use their role as representatives of God (i.e., *in persona Christi*) or other religious figures to spiritually manipulate or cause reverential fear and religious duress among victims to prevent them from disclosing the abuse (Benkert & Doyle, 2009). Spraitz and Bowen (2020) found that more than half (57%) of the priests in their sample used reverential fear and religious duress as a possible mechanism to prevent disclosure. Interestingly, in another study they found that with the exception of one cleric, the use of reverential fear was not necessarily used explicitly or purposefully by the abusive clergy (Spraitz & Bowen, 2019). This is also in line with the Winters et al. (2022), who found that few (15%) of the clergy used threats to prevent disclosure, and of those who did, 28% could be characterized as spiritual manipulation. Given the established low rates of reporting of clergy sexual abuse (Terry, 2011) and the findings that priests used few post-abuse maintenance behaviors (Winters et al., 2022), this suggests that there may be something innate about the priest and their role that may prevent disclosure. While most of the research on clergy sexual grooming has focused on Christian religions, there is some evidence coming out of reports within the Jewish Orthodox community that abusers rely on the child's naivete (i.e., children are not taught sexual education or even language to describe sex, and sex and sexuality are considered a taboo topic) and other insular cultural values to prevent detection or reporting (Katzenstein & Fontes, 2017).

Table 8.2 Frequencies of priest grooming behaviors from Winters et al. (2022)

SGM stage	Behavior/tactic	*N* (%)
Victim selection	Living situation at the time of the alleged abuse	
	Both biological parents	5905 (78.6)
	Single parent	924 (12.3)
	Foster/orphanage	188 (2.5)
	Boarding school	172 (2.3)
	Church residence	120 (1.6)
	Other immediate family member	96 (1.3)
	Other unspecified residence	109 (1.5)
Gaining access and isolation	Location where alleged victim met cleric	
	Church-related location/event	8234 (83.8)
	School/youth activity	1578 (17.6)
	Victim's residence or family event	714 (7.9)
	Other location	746 (8.3)
	Cleric's primary duty when he met the alleged victim	
	Church-related duty	8234 (83.8)
	School or youth-based activity	1065 (10.8)
	Other role	523 (5.3)
	Cleric socialized with the family of the alleged victim(s)	
	Yes	2638 (49.8)
	If yes, ways in which they socialized	
	Victim's family residence	2033 (79.8)
	Church-related event	1227 (48.2)
	Vacations or social activities	439 (17.2)
	Other situations	146 (5.7)
	Where the alleged abuse occurred	
	Church-related location	5654 (71.8)
	At the home of the victim	1142 (14.5)
	At school	942 (12.0)
	In a car	899 (11.4)
	Outings (e.g., camp, park, pool)	790 (10.0)
	Other (e.g., hospital, other residence)	702 (8.9)
	In hotel room	677 (8.6)

(continued)

Table 8.2 (continued)

SGM stage	**Behavior/tactic**	*N* (%)
Trust development	Gifts were given to the alleged victim	
	Yes	837 (18.2)
	Enticements were given to the alleged victim	
	Yes	1650 (34.2)
	If yes, type of enticements*	
	Reward/privilege	1369 (74.4)
	Drugs/alcohol	712 (38.7)
	Other unspecified	281 (15.3)
	If yes, type of reward/privilege	
	Allowed to stay overnight	559 (40.8)
	Sports-related enticement	449 (32.8)
	Given money	377 (27.5)
	Access to pornography	151 (11.0)
	Allowed to drive a car	148 (10.8)
	Allowed to stay up late	130 (9.5)
	Special church activities	89 (6.5)
	Travel	67 (4.9)
	Food	33 (2.4)
	Toys or other gifts	7 (0.5)
Desensitization to physical contact and sexual touch	Desensitize to touch/increase sexual touching	4170 (65.3)
	Watch child undressing	1622 (25.4)
	Exposing naked body	1129 (17.7)
	Talk about sexual things	1105 (17.3)
	Seemingly innocent/nonsexual contact	593 (9.3)
	Showing pornography	278 (4.4)
Post-abuse maintenance	Threat	
	Yes	839 (14.6)
	If yes, type of threat:	
	Verbal threat of harm to the victim	243 (29.8)
	Spiritual manipulation	228 (27.9)
	Physical threat with weapon	139 (17.0)
	Threatened public exposure of victim's behavior to family or others	89 (10.9)
		42 (5.1)
	Verbal threat (that harm will come to the cleric	38 (4.7)
	Threatened family of victim	31 (3.8)
	Other threat	6 (.7)

8.3.2 Boy Scouts of America

CSA within the Boy Scouts of America (BSA) organization was first reported in a five-part series in the *Washington Times* in 1991. At the time, journalist Patrick Boyle unearthed records showing that between the years 1971 and 1989, 416 male employees were banned for sexual misconduct involving 1151 minors (Tallon & Terry, 2013). While this amount of abuse seemed incalculable, it was but the tip of the iceberg. As more lawsuits against the BSA were filed, the BSA filed for Chap. 11 bankruptcy in February of 2020 so that they could compensate the survivors, as a judge set a November 2020 deadline for survivors to file claims (Kelly, 2020). At the end of the deadline, 95,000 individuals had filed claims, and in July 2021, the BSA organization agreed to pay 850 million dollars to 84,000 claimants (Bella & Harkins, 2021) which was subsequently rejected. Overall, researchers have estimated that between 1960 and 1990 approximately 3.4% of all scoutmasters sexually abused children (Shon & Tewksbury, 2021).

Using 171 publicly available case files from the BSA, Shon and Tewksbury (2021) created three typologies of perpetrators for male-on-male CSA using a fishing analogy. They described 56% of the sample used an "angling-type" method to perpetrate the CSA. This method appears to correspond to cases involving sexual grooming where the perpetrators performed at least two to three steps (e.g., hugging, kissing, back rubs) before touching the child's penis. They describe the early behaviors in this process involving casual hugs and moving toward more obvious sexual contact such as fondling. Shon and Tewksbury (2021) describe these early grooming behaviors as "baiting" or "testing out" the child by gradually increasing the sexual contact so that the child was not able to discern the abuse until it got too serious. They further describe the "spearfishing" approach, in which the perpetrator would fondle the child while he is sleeping or otherwise occupied so he is not aware; this was present in about 28% of cases. The final strategy, "handpicking," involved undressing boys and touching them under the guise of some sort of medical exam or initiation ritual and was described in 15% of the cases (Shon and Tewksbury, 2021). While these data suggest that scoutmasters also employed some grooming strategies (e.g., desensitization to touch), more research is needed to better understand the tactics used.

8.3.3 Educational Institutions

Sexual abuse within educational institutions has also received significant media attention, although the scope of the problem remains relatively elusive (Abboud et al., 2020). Data suggest that most institutional CSA occurs in schools rather than religious organizations or other caretaking settings (Falkenbach et al., 2017). One of the largest studies of educational sexual misconduct was conducted by Charol Shakeshaft in 2004 at the behest of the US Department of Education. After reviewing the extant literature in the field, she found that the reported prevalence of educator misconduct in the literature ranged anywhere from 3.7% to 50.3%. For instance, Wishnietsky (1991) surveyed 140 school superintendents and 300 high school seniors in North Carolina and found that 14% of the students reported having engaged in sexual intercourse with a teacher, while 18% of males and 82% of females reported experiencing sexual harassment by an educator. However, there were methodological and sampling limitations of previous research, and Shakeshaft (2004) concluded that the best prevalence estimate should be based upon a secondary review American Association of University Women (AAUW). They surveyed a nationally representative sample of over 2000 students from grades eight through 11 and found that nearly 9.6% of students experienced educator sexual misconduct at some point during their school career (Shakeshaft, 2003). It should be noted that "sexual misconduct" was broadly defined as sexual comments, sexual rumors, forced kissing, being watched or spied upon, or being cornered or touched inappropriately. More recently, educator misconduct data from 1997 to 2017 involving K-12 educators was obtained from media reports, disciplinary decisions of educator misconduct, and published case law (Canadian Centre for Child Protection Inc. [CCCP], 2019). Overall, they found 750 cases of CSA involving 1272 student victims in the twenty-year period. Also, Jeglic and colleagues (2022) retrospectively queried 6632 college students about their experiences of educator misconduct from K-12. They found that overall, 11.7% ($n = 779$) of students reported some type of educator misconduct with the vast majority reporting experiencing sexual comments ($n = 711$; 10.9%), while many fewer reported receiving sexual images/photographs ($n = 39$; 0.6%), physical contact ($n = 57$; 0.9%), kissing ($n = 32$; 0.5%), or intercourse/oral sex ($n = 9$; 0.1%).

When looking at the characteristics of those who perpetrate CSA within educational settings, the largest number are teachers, followed by coaches, substitute teachers, bus drivers, teacher's aides, other school employees, security guards, principals, and counselors (AAUW, 2004; CCCP, 2019; Gallagher, 2000; Jeglic et al., 2022; Solis & Benedek, 2012). The majority of abusive educators are male (57–96%; CCCP, 2019; Jaffe et al., 2013; Mototsune, 2015; Moulden et al., 2010); however, it is speculated that CSA perpetrated by women is not uncommon, with estimates ranging anywhere between 4% and 43% and more conservative estimates ranging between 5% and 10% (Bunting, 2005; Darling, 2013; Gannon & Cortoni, 2010; Shakeshaft, 2004). Victims are most commonly girls, although men tend to target younger victims while women target boys aged 13 and older (Abboud et al., 2020; Ratliff & Watson, 2014).

It is believed that educators who engage in CSA use sexual grooming behaviors and tactics to perpetrate the abuse. For example, in their dataset, the CCCP (2019) found that sexual grooming strategies were commonly used by both male (80%, $n = 220$) and female (20%, $n = 55$) educators. While the precise behaviors were not identified the CCCP defined sexual grooming as "a conscious, deliberate, and carefully orchestrated approach used by the offender" (Knoll, 2010, p. 374), which involves manipulating the perceptions of children and adults around children to gain their trust and cooperation. It is also used to normalize inappropriate behavior through desensitization, to reduce the likelihood that a child will disclose, and to reduce the likelihood that a child will be believed if they do tell" (p. 54–55). Additionally, Darling et al. (2018) found that majority (77%) of females who perpetrated CSA within the context of their employment (most of whom were educators) utilized sexual grooming behaviors (e.g., sexual texts, encouraging the minor to visit the adult's home). Jeglic and colleagues (2022) also found that depending upon the nature of the contact, between 9% and 28% reported grooming behaviors such as receiving gifts, exchanging texts/emails, or receiving special attention from the educator.

In accordance with the SGM (Winters et al., 2020), perpetrators within the educational setting have been found to target more vulnerable children such as those who have been marginalized and have less supervision, or those with behavioral problems. Such students are often more susceptible to the sexual grooming tactics but are also less likely to be believed should they come forward about the abuse (West et al., 2010). Access to the minors is innate to the perpetrator's position within the institution, and perpetrators are often well-liked by students, trusted by parents, and have received accolades and rewards from their institutions (Abboud et al., 2020; McGrath, 1994; Shakeshaft, 2003). To isolate the child, teachers may offer special help, tutoring, or mentoring (Darling et al., 2018) and then may gain their trust by giving them special attention, praise, and gifts (Darling et al., 2018; Knoll, 2010; Moulden et al., 2010). More recently, text messaging and direct messaging has been found to be implicated in desensitizing minors to sexual content, as conversations become flirtatious and include sexual content and jokes (Henschel & Grant, 2019; Solis & Benedek, 2012). To maintain the abuse and prevent detection, some educators make threats about poor grades or the loss of the relationship. Older teens may come to believe that they are in a romantic relationship with the educator and that the sexual contact is consensual, thus decreasing the likelihood that they will make a report (Burgess et al., 2010; Deering & Mellor, 2011; Herbert, 1985; Mellor & Deering, 2010; Shakeshaft & Cohan, 1994).

8.3.4 Sporting Organizations

As described in Chap. 1, the Jerry Sandusky Pennsylvania State University CSA scandal brought to light CSA within sporting organizations. Sadly, major CSA scandals have been found in most sporting organizations including but not limited to gymnastics, swimming, ice skating, hockey, cheerleading, and soccer. For example, Larry Nassar gave restricted food and candy to gymnasts and would touch them inappropriately during back therapy (Verhoeven, 2020).

To date, only one study has attempted to assess the prevalence of CSA within sports, and they found that 14% of sport-involved youth reported sexual harassment and abuse (Vertommen et al., 2016). Sexual violence was more frequently reported by girls (17.2%) compared to boys (10.2%), although it is believed that males may be underreporting the abuse, or it may not be perceived by others as CSA (Vertommen et al., 2016). Sporting institutions are unique in that in many cases when children advance in the ranks of their chosen sport, they spend a significant amount of time outside the home and under the care and supervision of coaches. Indeed, there is evidence from qualitative studies that elite athletes are at greater risk for CSA (Bjørnseth & Szabo, 2018). Further, as sporting often requires physical touch, coaches, and other staff (e.g., physical therapists, doctors, trainers) may be able to engage in abuse under the guise of treatment, as was seen in the case of Dr. Larry Nassar. In most cases of abuse, it is the male coach that is the perpetrator (Bjørnseth & Szabo, 2018), although in an online survey conducted by Vertommen et al. (2017) in 45% of the cases, the perpetrator was another athlete, most often a peer of the same age.

Bjørnseth and Szabo (2018) describe sexual grooming as a key component of CSA within sports although it remains understudied. Many of the behaviors reported in case studies may also be described within the context of the SGM (see Chap. 1 description of the Jerry Sandusky case). Sexual grooming within sports may be more difficult to detect due to the intimate nature of many of the interactions. For example, any child who participates in elite sports will spend a considerable amount of time (and depending upon whether it is a team or individual sport) alone with an adult. The coach or other representative will have the full trust and consent of the child and family as that is required in order for the child to succeed and advance. Boundary violations, such as driving a child in a private vehicle back and forth to practice, may be considered more acceptable given the time commitment involved and viewed as a favor to the parents/guardians. As noted earlier, touch is commonplace, especially in individual sports where coaches and medical professionals often must manipulate the child's body to show them proper positioning or care for physical injuries. Further, in many sports (e.g., ice skating, gymnastics, swimming), the child is wearing minimal clothing, and changing and showering together is also not uncommon. Given the power held by the perpetrators within the sporting organization, disclosure of abuse may impact the victims' future prospects within the sport. Bjørnseth and Szabo (2018) highlighted several potential barriers to reporting, including the appraisal of the behavior as sexual abuse, fear of consequences, feelings of guilt and shame, and the impact of the disclosure on their sporting career.

In an effort to address the sexual violence occurring within sport, the US Olympic and Paralympic Committees introduced SafeSport in 2012 following the authorization of the *Protecting Young Victims from Sexual Abuse and Safe Sport Authorization Act of 2017* (S. 534). The US Center for SafeSport provides training, education to participants, families, and staff, as well as handling reports of abuse within sport (Harris & Terry, 2019).

8.4 Conclusion

Many youth-serving organizations have been impacted by CSA scandals. There is evidence that these institutions are sought out by a specific subsection of extrafamilial child abusers, called professional perpetrators. These individuals seek out the vulnerabilities within the institution itself in order to gain access to minors and carry out the abuse without detection. While it appears that many of the same stages and behaviors as those identified in the SGM are used in cases of institutional CSA, there also appear to be key differences, specifically related to the stages involving victim selection, gaining access, trust development, and post-abuse maintenance that may be unique to each type of institution. Given that most of this research has been conducted using archival records, interviews based on the SGM with survivors of institutional sexual abuse could help better understand the behaviors and tactics employed in the sexual grooming process and whether these behaviors differ by type of institution. The recent widespread disclosures of institutional CSA have significantly impacted policies and prevention measures used within child-serving organizations. While we still do not have data to make determinations, the increased awareness of institutional CSA and vigilance appears may be helpful at preventing future cases of CSA.

References

Abboud, M. J., Wu, G., Pedneault, A., Stohr, M. K., & Hemmens, C. (2020). Educator sexual misconduct: A statutory analysis. *Criminal Justice Policy Review, 31*(1), 133–153. https://doi.org/10.1177/0887403418806564

American Association of University Women. Educational Foundation. (2004). *Harassment-free hallways: How to stop sexual harassment in school*. American Association of University Women Educational Foundation.

Armbruster, A. (2021). On the undisclosed transfer of abusive Catholic priests: A field theoretical analysis of the sexual repression within the Catholic Church and the use of legitimate language. *Critical Research on Religion*. https://doi.org/10.1177/20503032211015282

Arnold, S., & Jeglic, E. L. (n.d.). *Stereotypes and unconscious bias in institutional child abuse: A hidden risk*. (in submission).

Barnardos. (2010). *Saving childhood Ryan: Fighting for children together*. http://www.barnardos.ie/assets/files/Advocacy/SAVING%20CHILDHOOD%20RYAN%20final%20report%20_2_.pdf

Bella, T., & Harkins, G. (2021, July 2). Boy Scouts of America settles for $850 million with more than 84,000 sexual abuse victims. *The Washington Post*. https://www.washingtonpost.com/dc-md-va/2021/07/02/boy-scouts-settlement-abuse-victims/

Benkert, M., & Doyle, T. P. (2009). Clericalism, religious duress and its psychological impact on victims of clergy sexual abuse. *Pastoral Psychology, 58*(3), 223–238. https://doi.org/10.1007/s11089-008-0188-0

Bjørnseth, I., & Szabo, A. (2018). Sexual violence against children in sports and exercise: A systematic literature review. *Journal of Child Sexual Abuse, 27*(4), 365–385. https://doi.org/10.1080/10538712.2018.1477222

Blakemore, T., Herbert, J. L., Arney, F., & Parkinson, S. (2017). The impacts of institutional child sexual abuse: A rapid review of the evidence. *Child Abuse & Neglect, 74*, 35–48. https://doi.org/10.1016/j.chiabu.2017.08.006

Bunting, L. (2005). *Females who sexually offend against children: Responses of the child protection and criminal justice systems*. NSPCC.

Burgess, A. W., Welner, M., & Willis, D. G. (2010). Educator sexual abuse: Two case reports. *Journal of Child Sexual Abuse, 19*(4), 387–402. https://doi.org/10.1080/10538712.2010.495045

Burmeister, N., Earle, S., & Spraitz, J. D. (2019). *Continued examination of sexual grooming by clergy: An analysis of one Wisconsin archdiocese.* https://minds.wisconsin.edu/bitstream/handle/1793/79889/BurmeisterSpr19.pdf?sequence=1&isAllowed=y

Canadian Centre for Child Protection Inc. (2019). The prevalence of sexual abuse by K-12 school personnel in Canada, 1997–2017. *Journal of Child Sexual Abuse, 28*(1), 46–66. https://doi.org/10.1080/10538712.2018.1477218

Darling, A. J. (2013). "Notes on a scandal": Why do females engage in abuse of trust behaviours? *International Journal of Criminology and Sociology.* https://doi.org/10.6000/1929-4409.2013.02.47

Darling, A. J., Hackett, S., & Jamie, K. (2018). Female sex offenders who abuse children whilst working in organisational contexts: Offending, conviction and sentencing. *The Journal of Sexual Aggression, 24*(2), 196–214. https://doi.org/10.1080/13552600.2018.1476601

Death, J. (2015). Bad apples, bad barrel: Exploring institutional responses to child sexual abuse by catholic clergy in Australia. *International Journal for Crime, Justice and Social Democracy, 4*(2), 94–110. https://doi.org/10.5204/ijcjsd.v4i2.229

Deering, R., & Mellor, D. (2011). An exploratory qualitative study of the self-reported impact of female- perpetrated childhood sexual abuse. *Journal of Child Sexual Abuse, 20*(1), 58–76. https://doi.org/10.1080/10538712.2011.539964

Dockterman, E. (2019). These men say the boy scouts' sex abuse problem is worse than anyone knew. *Time Magazine.* https://time.com/longform/boy-scouts-sex-abuse/

Dressing, H., Dölling, D., Hermann, D., Kruse, A., Schmitt, E., Bannenberg, B., Whittaker, K., Hoell, A., Voss, E., & Salize, H. J. (2021). Child sexual abuse by Catholic priests, deacons, and male members of religious orders in the authority of the German Bishops' Conference 1946–2014. *Sexual Abuse, 33*(3), 274–294. https://doi.org/10.1177/1079063219893371

Falkenbach, D., Foehse, A., Jeglic, E. L., Calkins, C., & Raymaekers, L. (2017). Sexual abuse within employment settings – A comparison of work-related, intra- and extra-familial child molesters. *Sexual Abuse: A Journal of Research and Treatment, 31(5), 524–542.* https://doi.org/10.1177/1079063217708202

Gallagher, B. (2000). The extent and nature of known cases of institutional child sexual abuse. *British Journal of Social Work, 30*, 795–817. https://doi.org/10.1093/bjsw/30.6.795

Gannon, T. A., & Cortoni, F. (Eds.). (2010). *Female sexual offenders: Theory, assessment and treatment.* Wiley-Blackwell.

Gerdes, K. E., Beck, M. N., Cowan-Hancock, S., & Wilkinson-Sparks, T. (1996). Adult survivors of childhood sexual abuse: The case of Mormon women. *Affilia, 11*(1), 39–60. https://doi.org/10.1177/088610999601100104

Goode, H., McGee, H. M., & OBoyle, C. A. (2003). *Time to listen: Confronting child sexual abuse by Catholic clergy in Ireland.* Liffey Press.

Harris, A. J., & Terry, K. J. (2019). Child sexual abuse in organizational settings: A research framework to advance policy and practice. *Sexual Abuse, 31*(6), 635–642. https://doi.org/10.1177/1079063219858144

Henschel, M. M., & Grant, B. J. (2019). Exposing school employee sexual abuse and misconduct: Shedding light on a sensitive issue. *Journal of Child Sexual Abuse, 28*(1), 26–45. https://doi.org/10.1080/10538712.2018.1483459

Herbert, M. (1985). What principals should know about child abuse. *Principal, 65*(2), 9–14.

Herbert, J. L., Bromfield, L., Arney, F., & Blakemore, T. (2020). Impacts of institutional child sexual abuse: What we have learned from research and the Royal Commission into Institutional Response to Child Sexual Abuse private sessions. In *Child sexual abuse* (pp. 221–240). Academic.

Jaffe, P., Straatman, A. L., Harris, B., Georges, A., Vink, K., & Reif, K. (2013). Emerging trends in teacher sexual misconduct in Ontario 2007–2012. *Education & Law Journal, 23*(1), 19.

Jeglic, E. L., Calkins, C., Kaylor, L., Margeotes, K., Doychak, K., Blasko, B., Chesin, M., & Panza, N. (2022). The nature and scope of educator misconduct in K 12. *Sexual Abuse*, Doi: 10790632221096421.

John Jay College. (2004). *The nature and scope of sexual abuse of minors by Catholic priests and deacons in the United States, 1950–2000*. USCCB.

John Jay College. (2006). *The nature and scope of sexual abuse of minors by Catholic priests and deacons in the United States – Supplemental data analysis*. USCCB.

Katzenstein, D., & Fontes, L. A. (2017). Twice silenced: The underreporting of child sexual abuse in orthodox Jewish communities. *Journal of Child Sexual Abuse, 26*(6), 752–767. https://doi.org/10.1080/10538712.2017.1336505

Kelly, C. (2020, May 26). Deadline set for abuse survivors to file claims in Boy Scouts bankruptcy. *USA TODAY.* https://www.usatoday.com/story/news/investigations/2020/05/26/boy-scouts-bankruptcy-deadline-abuse-survivor-claims-set-november/5229497002

Kline, P. M., McMackin, R., & Lezotte, E. (2008). The impact of the clergy abuse scandal on parish communities. *Journal of Child Sexual Abuse, 17*(3-4), 290–300. https://doi.org/10.1080/10538710802329817

Knoll, J. (2010). Teacher sexual misconduct: Grooming patterns and female offenders. *Journal of Child Sexual Abuse, 19*(4), 371–386. https://doi.org/10.1080/10538712.2010.495047

McAlinden, A. M. (2006). Setting 'em up': Personal, familial and institutional grooming in the sexual abuse of children. *Social & Legal Studies, 15*(3), 339–362. https://doi.org/10.1177/0964663906066613

McAlinden, A. M. (2010). Vetting sexual offenders: State over-extension, the punishment deficit and the failure to manage risk. *Social & Legal Studies, 19*(1), 25–48. https://doi.org/10.1177/0964663909346197

McAlinden, A. M. (2012). *'Grooming' and the sexual abuse of children: Institutional.* Oxford University Press.

McGrath, M. J. (1994). The psychodynamics of school sexual abuse investigations: An attorney's inside look. *School Administrator, 51*(9), 28–34.

Mellor, D., & Deering, R. (2010). Professional response and attitudes toward female-perpetrated child sexual abuse: A study of psychologists, psychiatrists, probationary psychologists and child protection workers. *Psychology, Crime & Law, 16*(5), 415–438. https://doi.org/10.1080/10683160902776850

Mercado, C. C., Tallon, J. A., & Terry, K. J. (2008). Persistent sexual abusers in the Catholic Church: An examination of characteristics and offenses patters. *Criminal Justice and Behavior, 35*, 629–642.

Mignon, A., Spraitz, J. D., & Langer, A. (2017). *Continued development of a taxonomy of clergy sexual grooming: Results from one Benedictine Abbey*. https://minds.wisconsin.edu/bitstream/handle/1793/77538/MignonSpr17.pdf?sequence=1

Mototsune, T. (2015). Ontario College of Teachers cases of teacher sexual misconduct. *Electronic Thesis and Dissertation Repository*, 2840. https://ir.lib.uwo.ca/etd/2840

Moulden, H. M., Firestone, P., Kingston, D. A., & Wexler, A. F. (2010). A description of sexual offending committed by Canadian teachers. *Journal of Child Sexual Abuse, 19*(4), 403–418. https://doi.org/10.1080/10538712.2010.495046

Naumetz, T. (2009). One in five students suffered sexual abuse at residential schools, figures indicate. *The Globe and Mail*. https://www.theglobeandmail.com/news/national/one-in-five-students-suffered-sexual-abuse-at-residential-schools-figures-indicate/article20440061/

Parkinson, P. N., Oates, R. K., & Jayakody, A. A. (2012). Child sexual abuse in the Anglican Church of Australia. *Journal of Child Sexual Abuse, 21*(5), 553–570. https://doi.org/10.1080/10538712.2012.689424

Perillo, A. D., Mercado, C. C., & Terry, K. J. (2008). Repeat offending, victim gender, and extent of victim relationship in Catholic Church sexual abusers. *Criminal Justice and Behavior, 35*, 600–614. https://doi.org/10.1177/0093854808314368

Raine, S., & Kent, S. A. (2019). The grooming of children for sexual abuse in religious settings: Unique characteristics and select case studies. *Aggression and Violent Behavior, 48*, 180–189. https://doi.org/10.1016/j.avb.2019.08.017

Ratliff, L., & Watson, J. (2014). A descriptive analysis of public school educators arrested for sex offenses. *Journal of Child Sexual Abuse, 23*(2), 217–228. https://doi.org/10.1080/10538712.2014.870275

Rezendes, M. (2002, January 6). Church allowed abuse by priest for years. *Boston Globe*. https://www.bostonglobe.com/news/special-reports/2002/01/06/church-allowed-abuse-priest-for-years/cSHfGkTIrAT25qKGvBuDNM/story.html

Rossetti, S. J. (1995). The impact of child sexual abuse on attitudes toward God and the Catholic Church. *Child Abuse & Neglect, 19*(12), 1469–1481. https://doi.org/10.1016/0145-2134(95)00100-1

Royal Commission into Institutional Responses to Child Sexual Abuse. (2017). *Final report. Nature and cause*. https://www.childabuseroyalcommission.gov.au/nature-and-cause

Shakeshaft, C. (2003). Educator sexual abuse. *Hofstra Horizons*, 10–13. https://www.hofstra.edu/pdf/orsp_shakeshaft_spring03.pdf

Shakeshaft, C. (2004). *Educator sexual abuse: A synthesis of existing literature*. U.S. Department of Education, Office of the Under Secretary. http://www.ed.gov/rschstat/research/pubs/misconductreview

Shakeshaft, C., & Cohan, A. (1994). *In Loco Parentis: Sexual abuse of students in schools. What administrators should know.* https://files.eric.ed.gov/fulltext/ED372511.pdf

Shon, L., & Tewksbury, R. (2021). Constructing a typology of male-on-male child molestation: A qualitative analysis of victims' narratives within the Boy Scouts of America. *Journal of Sexual Aggression, 27*(3), 338–352. https://doi.org/10.1080/13552600.2020.1805519

Solis, O. L., & Benedek, E. P. (2012). Female sexual offenders in the educational system: A brief overview. *Bulletin of the Menninger Clinic, 76*(2), 172–188. https://doi.org/10.1521/bumc.2012.76.2.172

Spraitz, J. D., & Bowen, K. N. (2019). Examination of a nascent taxonomy of priest sexual grooming. *Sexual Abuse, 31*(6), 707–728. https://doi.org/10.1177/1079063218809095

Spraitz, J. D., & Bowen, K. N. (2020). Religious duress and reverential fear in clergy sexual abuse cases: Examination of victims' reports and recommendations for change. *Criminal Justice Policy Review*. https://doi.org/10.1177/0887403420921232

Spraitz, J. D., Bowen, K. N., & Strange, L. (2018). Proposing a behavioral taxonomy of priest sexual grooming. *International Journal for Crime, Justice and Social Democracy, 7*(1), 30–43. https://doi.org/10.5204/ijcjsd.v&i1.387

Strangeways-Booth, A. (2015, May 23). *Methodist church apologies for abuse spanning decades. BBC*. https://www.bbc.com/news/uk-32909444

Sullivan, J., & Beech, A. (2002). Professional perpetrators: Sex offenders who use their employment to target and sexually abuse the children with whom they work. *Child Abuse Review: Journal of the British Association for the Study and Prevention of Child Abuse and Neglect, 11*(3), 153–167. https://doi.org/10.1002/car.737

Sullivan, J., & Beech, A. (2004). A comparative study of demographic data relating to intra- and extra-familial child sexual abusers and professional perpetrators. *Journal of Sexual Aggression, 10*(1), 39–50. https://doi.org/10.1080/13552600410001667788

Sullivan, J., Beech, A. R., Craig, L. A., & Gannon, T. A. (2011). Comparing intra-familial and extra-familial child sexual abusers with professionals who have sexually abused children with whom they work. *International Offender Therapy and Comparative Criminology, 55*(1), 56–74. https://doi.org/10.1177/0306624X09359194

Tallon, J. A., & Terry, K. J. (2008). Analyzing paraphilic activity, specialization, and generalization in priests who sexually abused minors. *Criminal Justice and Behavior, 35*(5), 615–628. https://doi.org/10.1177/0093854808314374

Tallon, J., & Terry, K. J. (2013). *Child sexual abuse: A review of the literature*. https://www.bishop-accountability.org/reports/2004_02_27_JohnJay/LitReview/2004_06_Literature_Review_Complete_Optimized.pdf

Terry, K. J. (2011). *The causes and context of sexual abuse of minors in the Catholic Church in the United States, 1950–2002*. U.S. Conference of Catholic Bishops.

Terry, K. J., Mercado, C. C., & Perillo, A. (2008). Priests who abuse and were abused: Understanding victimization in the Catholic Church. *Victims & Offenders, 3*, 412–422. https://doi.org/10.1080/15564880802338559

Tishelman, A. C., & Fontes, L. A. (2017). Religion in child sexual abuse forensic interviews. *Child Abuse & Neglect, 63*, 120–130. https://doi.org/10.1016/j.chiabu.2016.11.025

Turner, D., & Briken, P. (2015). Child sexual abusers working with children – Characteristics and risk factors. *Sexual Offender Treatment, 10*(1).

Turner, D., Rettenberger, M., Lohmann, L., Eher, R., & Briken, P. (2014). Pedophilic sexual interests and psychopathy in child sexual abusers who work with children. *Child Abuse & Neglect, 38*, 326–335. https://doi.org/10.1016/j.chiabu.2013.07.019

Turner, D., Rettenberger, M., Yoon, D., Klein, V., Eher, R., & Briken, P. (2016). Risk assessment in child sexual abusers working with children. *Sexual Abuse: A Journal of Research and Treatment*, 1–25. https://doi.org/10.1177/1079063214564390

Verhoeven, B. (2020, June 24). 'Athlete A': 9 most shocking details from Larry Nassar sexual abuse documentary. *The Wrap*. https://www.thewrap.com/athlete-a-shocking-details-larry-nassar-sexual-abuse-documentary/

Vertommen, T., Schipper-van Veldhoven, N., Wouters, K., Kampen, J. K., Brackenridge, C. H., Rhind, D. J., Neels, K., & Van Den Eede, F. (2016). Interpersonal violence against children in sport in the Netherlands and Belgium. *Child Abuse & Neglect, 51*, 223–236. https://doi.org/10.1016/j.chiabu.2015.10.006

Vertommen, T., Kampen, J., Schipper-van Veldhoven, N., Wouters, K., Uzieblo, K., & Van Den Eede, F. (2017). Profiling perpetrators of interpersonal violence against children in sport based on a victim survey. *Child Abuse & Neglect, 63*, 172–182. https://doi.org/10.1016/j.chiabu.2016.11.029

West, S. G., Hatters-Friedman, S., & Knoll, J. L., IV. (2010). Lessons to learn: Female educators who sexually abuse their students. *Psychiatric Times, 27*(8), 9. https://link.gale.com/apps/doc/A233502884/AONE?u=anon~e3063fe3&sid=googleScholar&xid=4ac89994

Winters, G. M., Jeglic, E. L., & Kaylor, L. E. (2020). Validation of the sexual grooming model of child sexual abusers. *Journal of Child Sexual Abuse, 29*(7), 855–875. https://doi.org/10.1080/10538712.2020.1801935

Winters, G. M., Jeglic, E. L., & Terry, K. J. (2022). The prevalence of sexual grooming behaviors in a large sample of clergy. *Sexual Abuse: A Journal of Research and Treatment*. https://doi.org/10.1177/10790632211070803

Wishnietsky, D. H. (1991). Reported and unreported teacher-student sexual harassment. *The Journal of Educational Research, 84*(3), 164–170. https://doi.org/10.1080/00220671.1991.10886010

Chapter 9
Women and Sexual Grooming

Sexual offending is typically thought to be a male-perpetrated crime (Jeglic & Calkins, 2018). While the majority of individuals who commit sexual offenses are indeed male, there is evidence that a sizeable proportion of sex offending is in fact perpetrated by women. Official records suggest that women are responsible for only 2.2% of all sex crimes (Cortoni et al., 2017), with most of those crimes being perpetrated against children. However, a recent meta-analysis of child sexual abuse (CSA) from 12 countries showed that the self-reported prevalence of female-perpetrated sexual abuse is up to six times higher (approximately 11.6%) than that reported to authorities. Further, there were gender differences in reported victimization rates, with 40% of men reporting that they were sexually abused during childhood by a woman compared to only 4% of women (Cortoni et al., 2017). Given that very few of these women who sexually abuse children actually come into contact with the criminal justice system, relatively little is known about them and their offense process. There is some preliminary evidence that at least some women use sexual grooming strategies to perpetrate the abuse, but much of that conjecture comes from case studies and media reports (Kaylor et al., 2021). This chapter will review what is known about women who sexually offend and review some common typologies of this population that have been proposed in the literature. Next, we will use case examples to discuss how a subset of women who engage in CSA may utilize sexual grooming in the perpetration of the crime and present some preliminary data about female sexual grooming behaviors as reported by victims. The chapter will conclude with female-specific prevention and treatment recommendations.

© The Author(s), under exclusive license to Springer Nature Switzerland AG 2022

G. M. Winters, E. L. Jeglic, *Sexual Grooming*,
https://doi.org/10.1007/978-3-031-07222-2_9

9.1 Characteristics of Females Who Commit Sex Crimes

While the number of women who are incarcerated globally for committing sex crimes is very low (approximately 2% of all those convicted of a sexual offense; Cortoni et al., 2017) compared to men, the limited research on these women has provided a "typical profile" of women who sexually offend. Women who perpetrate sex crimes tend to be young (between 20 and 32 years of age) and White and have a history of severe abuse including domestic violence (see Gannon et al., 2008; Wijkman et al., 2011). They have been found to experience elevated levels of post-traumatic stress disorder symptoms, suicidal thoughts, substance abuse problems, low self-esteem and self-worth, poor coping skills, emotional instability, depressive symptoms, the inability to form healthy adult relationships, and personality disorders (Darling et al., 2018; Freeman & Sandler, 2008; Johansson-Love & Fremouw, 2009; Mathews et al., 1997; Oliver, 2007; West et al., 2010).

While most of the research on women who commit sexual abuse comes from samples in the United States (US) and Canada, Wijkman et al. (2010) examined the characteristics of 111 females who committed crimes in the Netherlands—which represents the entire population of women known to the criminal justice system between 1994 and 2005. They found that almost one-third of their sample had experienced sexual abuse in childhood (31%) and almost two thirds (59%) experienced mental health problems.

In a study conducted in Ireland, Bourke et al. (2014) used self-report data from a study of adults' experiences of CSA to look at the characteristics of the perpetrators. What makes this study unique was that many of the cases were never reported to authorities (6% of those abused by males and none of those abused by females were reported to the police). They found that 6% of their sample reported CSA perpetrated by a woman. The large majority of those reporting female-perpetrated sexual abuse were male (85%), between the ages of 9 and 14 (40%) or 15 and 17 (40%) at the time of abuse. Unlike some of the other studies that focused only on adults who commit sexual abuse, in this study, 32% of the individuals who perpetrated the abuse were under the age of 16, 45% were 16 to 25, while only 23% were over 26 years of age. Most reported that no force was used (92%) and/or no penetration took place (79%). Importantly, most victims did not disclose the abuse to others (60%), and no one reported to the police.

As will be discussed in the typology section below, some women sexually offend on their own (solo), while others offend in concert with a male perpetrator (co-offender). Ten Bensel et al. (2019) studied females convicted of sexual offenses over an 18-year period in the state of Arkansas (n = 223), comparing offender, victim, and offense characteristics of solo and co-offenders. Of their sample, two-thirds (64.6%) were solo offenders. Several themes emerged from the data. They found that overall, solo offenders were more likely to be employed, single, and younger, have multiple prior arrests, and have been charged with a sexual offense as compared to co-offenders. Solo offenders were also less likely to be mothers of the victims but instead hold an authoritative position over the minor such as teacher or caregiver. In terms of the crime, solo offenders were more likely to have engaged in consensual acts (age of consent was 14 years in Arkansas at the time of the study; however, the authors note that "although consent was considered in the charging decision, the act itself still remained illegal due to victim's age, or the offender's position held over the victim," p. 4071) and less likely to use force. Crimes perpetrated by solo offenders were less likely to occur in their residence. The victims of solo offenders were much more likely to be male, nonrelatives, and older than those of co-offenders. Wijkman et al. (2010) also examined differences between solo and co-offenders in their sample and similarly found that solo offenders were more likely to have male, unrelated victims. They also found that co-offenders were more likely to be diagnosed with a personality disorder than solo offenders.

9.1.1 Typologies of Sexually Abusive Women

In an effort to better understand the motivations for offending, offending pathways, and to help the development of targeted interventions, sexual researchers have proposed typologies of women who sexually offend.

One of the original categorizations of women who committed sex crimes was created by Mathews et al. (1989) who developed three typologies of women who sexually abuse children. These typologies were based upon interviews with 16 women who received treatment as part of their nonprofit agency that provides community corrections and treatment for women and their children in Minneapolis, Minnesota. They used a holistic-inductive approach to categorize the women into three categories as depicted in Fig. 9.1 below:

Syed and Williams (1996) expanded upon Mathews and colleagues' typologies using case studies of 19 females who were incarcerated in the Correctional

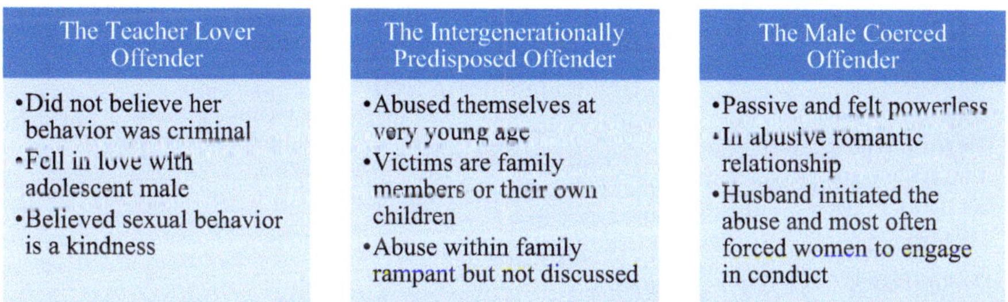

Fig. 9.1 Mathews et al. (1989) typology of female sex offenders

Services of Canada following conviction for a sex crime (mostly for crimes against minors). They found that in their sample, only about half of the women could be classified according to the Mathews et al. (1989) typology. They found that while many of the women committed the sex offenses with a male companion, they did not appear to be coerced, and as such, they proposed a *male-accompanied* typology to be separate from the *male-coerced* typology. They further proposed breaking down the male-accompanied typology into familial and nonfamilial. Finally, given the violence they saw in some of the cases, they proposed an *angry-impulsive* category.

Subsequently, Vandiver and Kercher (2004) used a much larger sample of females who committed sexual offenses against both children and adults ($N = 471$) and conducted a cluster analysis to develop an empirically derived typology of females who were convicted of sex crimes. Their analysis yielded six types of females who commit sex crimes as depicted below in Fig. 9.2.

In 2007, Sandler and Freeman replicated Vandiver and Kercher's (2004) study using a sample of all the females on the sex offender registry in New York state ($N = 390$), which represented 2% of all the registered sex offenders in the state (male and female). Their cluster analysis also yielded six typologies, some of which

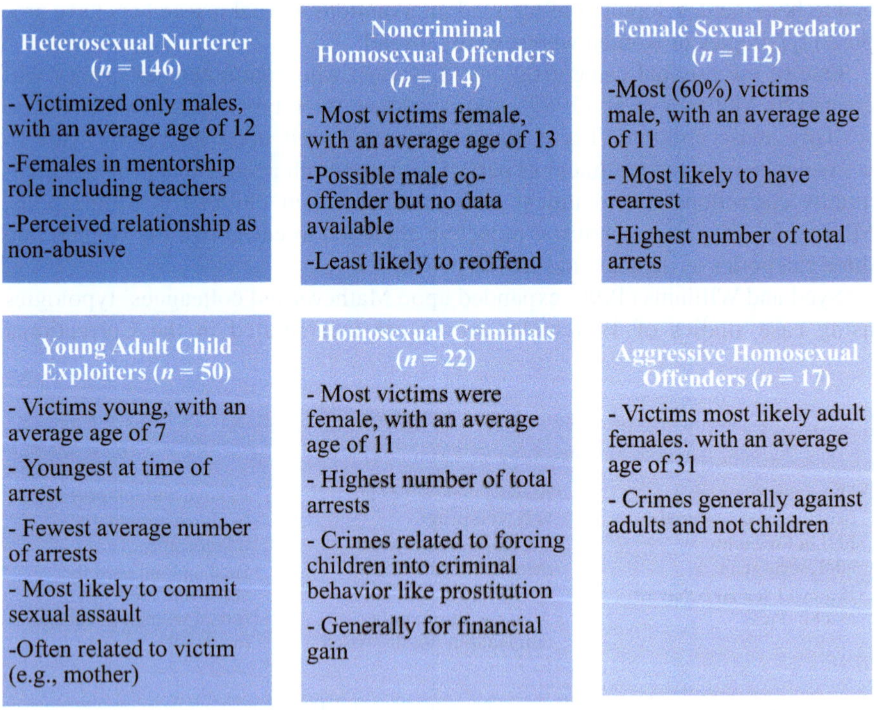

Fig. 9.2 Vandiver and Kercher (2004) six typologies of female sex offenders

overlapped with Vandiver and Kercher's typologies and some which yielded different characteristics. Overall, they found evidence for six types of women who sexually abuse as listed below.

1. *Criminally limited hebephiles* (*n* = 158) – This type is similar to Vandiver and Kercher's *heterosexual nurturers* and is comprised of older women (*M* = 32.6 years), with early adolescent victims (*M* = 13.8 years), the majority of whom were male (70%) with low recidivism rates (9%).
2. *Criminally prone hebephiles* (*n* = 105) – This type was very similar to the *criminally limited hebephile* except they had a more extensive criminal history and higher rearrest rates (53%).
3. *Young adult child molesters* (*n* = 27) – This type is similar to Vandiver and Kercher's *young adult child exploiters*. This type had the youngest offender age (*M* = 28.2 years) and the youngest victim age (*M* = 4.1 years). They were almost equally likely to have male and female victims.
4. *High-risk chronic offenders* (*n* = 25) – This group had the highest average number of total arrests (*M* = 15.4) and recidivism (76%). This group was most likely to target young (*M* = 5.4 years) female victims and had the most non-White offenders (38%).
5. *Older non-habitual offenders* (*n* = 20) – This group had the oldest offender age (*M* = 51.1 years) with an average victim age of 12.2 years and little to no criminal history or reoffending (0%).
6. *Homosexual child molesters* (*n* = 11) – This type was also older (*M* = 44.2 years) but offended against young females (91%; *M* = 5.3 years). They had few past convictions and low rearrest rates (18%).

While these typologies are helpful for synthesizing information, in terms of profiling women who sexually offend against children, there is variation across studies and samples, and the typologies are based and developed upon women who have been either convicted or incarcerated for sex crimes; therefore, they may not resemble those who were not detected by the justice system. In terms of prevention and intervention, it is important to determine the behaviors and tactics used to perpetrate the abuse to develop prevention and intervention strategies to prevent abuse.

9.2 Sexual Grooming by Females Who Commit Sex Crimes

While the academic literature on sexual grooming in general is sparse to begin with, the research on female sexual grooming is almost nonexistent. The limited research to date has been based on the theoretical literature or case studies (e.g., Darling et al., 2018; Johansson-Love & Fremouw, 2009; Kaylor et al., 2021). However, in a recent study examining sexual grooming as reported by victims of CSA based on the Sexual Grooming Model (SGM; Winters et al., 2020), we found that of the 115 respondents, 12 (10.4%) reported that they experienced CSA perpetrated by a woman (Winters et al., in submission). Further analyses showed that almost all of the victims (11 out of the 12 or 92%) reported that the woman who committed the abuse used at least one of the sexual grooming behaviors as described in the SGM, with an average of 15.8 (range = 0–26) behaviors reported (see Table 9.1; Winters et al., in submission). Moreover, we found that over two-thirds of the victims endorsed that the woman used at least one behavior from each of the five SGM stages. The behaviors and tactics in the desensitization to sexual content and touch stage were the most frequently endorsed (10 out of the 12 victims), and the most common sexual grooming behavior reported was for the females to expose their naked body to the victim in 83% of the cases. What was unique about the females in our study was that many were minors themselves when the abuse occurred. While we know that about one-third of those who perpetrate CSA are juveniles (i.e., under the age of 18 at the time of the abuse; Finkelhor et al., 2009), of which between 7 and 15% are estimated to be female (Finkelhor et al., 2009; Tsopelas et al., 2011), there is little known about the behaviors and tactics employed by female youth who commit sex crimes. However, our findings did show that adolescent females who perpetrate CSA are engaging in sexual grooming behaviors that are like those reportedly used by males (Winters et al., in submission).

Recently, our group (see Kaylor et al., 2021) put forth a theoretical model of sexual grooming for female-perpetrated sexual abuse based upon the SGM that may apply to those women who fall into the *teacher-lover typology* (i.e., adult women who use sexual grooming strategies to engage in what they believe to be romantic relationships with minor teenage boys) and those who fall within the *sex trafficker typology* (i.e., women who use sexual grooming to entrap victims into the sex trafficking) as described below.

9.2.1 Teacher/Lover

Recent government inquiries in Canada, the United Kingdom (UK), and Australia, among others, have highlighted the rampant CSA that has taken place for decades within institutional settings including schools (see Chap. 8 for review). While most of those who were accused and prosecuted within educational settings were men, there is some evidence that some female teachers were also sexually abusing their students (Christensen & Darling, 2020). According to Shakeshaft (2004), who conducted a review of the research on educator misconduct in the US, rates of female-perpetrated abuse within educational settings ranged anywhere from 4% (Gallagher, 2000) to 43% (Cameron et al., 1986). More recently, Ratliff and Watson (2014) examined the publicly available records of educator arrests for sexual misconduct between 2007 and 2011 in nine southeastern US states. They found that of those arrested, 112 (26%) were women, with the majority ($n = 99$; 88%) offending against middle and high school students, in line with the teacher-lover typology.

As described earlier, women categorized within the teacher-lover typology may use sexual grooming strategies, such as their position of power and access to students, to perpetrate the abuse (Robertiello & Terry, 2007; Vandiver & Walker, 2002).

Table 9.1 SGS-V item endorsement

SGS-V item	*n* (%)
Victim selection	
I was lonely and/or isolated.	7 (58.3)
I was compliant and/or trusting of adults.	5 (41.7)
I lacked confidence and/or had low self-esteem.	5 (41.7)
I felt unwanted or unloved by others.	4 (33.3)
I was not close to my parents and/or they were not resources for me.	2 (16.7)
I lacked adult supervision.	2 (16.7)
I had a single mother and/or was in need of a "father figure."	2 (16.7)
I was a troubled child/teen.	1 (8.3)
I was a needy child/teen.	0 (0.0)
Other reason not listed	4 (33.3)
Gaining access and isolation	
They did activities alone with me without other adults.	5 (41.7)
They separated or isolated me from friends, other kids, and/or family.	4 (33.3)
They manipulated my family to gain access to me.	3 (25.0)
They took me on overnight stays or outings.	3 (25.0)
They were involved in youth-serving organizations.	1 (8.3)
Other reason not listed	1 (8.3)
Trust development	
They were affectionate and loving toward me.	7 (58.3)
They gave me compliments.	7 (58.3)
They spent a lot of time with me and/or communicated with me often.	7 (58.3)
They were charming, nice, and/or likeable.	6 (50.0)
They gave me a lot of attention.	6 (50.0)
They showed favoritism toward me and/or formed a special relationship with me.	6 (50.0)
They engaged in childlike activities with me.	5 (41.7)
They had insider status and a good reputation and/or were considered a "pillar of the community."	2 (16.7)
They gave me rewards and/or privileges.	2 (16.7)
They provided me with drugs and/or alcohol.	1 (8.3)
Other reason not listed	1 (8.3)
Desensitization to sexual content and physical contact	
They exposed their naked body to me.	10 (83.3)
They used inappropriate sexual language and/or told dirty jokes.	8 (66.7)
They used seemingly innocent and/or nonsexual touching.	7 (58.3)
They gradually increased the amount of sexual touching over time.	7 (58.3)
They showed me pornography photographs or videos.	6 (50.0)
They used accidental touching and/or distracted me while touching me.	5 (41.7)
They asked questions about my sexual experiences and/or relationships.	5 (41.7)
They talked about sexual things they had done.	5 (41.7)
They watched me undressing.	5 (41.7)

(continued)

Table 9.1 (continued)

SGS-V item	*n* (%)
They educated me about sexual behavior.	5 (41.7)
Other reason not listed	1 (8.3)
Post-abuse maintenance	
They told me not to tell anyone what happened.	7 (58.3)
They convinced me it was acceptable and/or normal behavior.	7 (58.3)
They told me they loved me and/or that I was special.	6 (50.0)
They encouraged secrets.	5 (41.7)
They made me feel responsible for the abuse.	2 (16.7)
They misstated the moral standards regarding touch.	4 (33.3)
They gave me rewards and bribes or allowed me to avoid punishment.	2 (16.7)
They threatened abandonment, rejection, or my family breaking up.	0 (0.0)
Other reason not listed	2 (16.7)

Note: Taken from Winters et al. (in submission)

In a recent review of cases of charged and/or prosecuted female-perpetrated sexual abuse within the UK between 2000 and 2016, Darling et al. (2018) found that the majority of the 71 cases (n = 43; 61%) were educators and that sexual grooming behaviors were evident in two-thirds of the cases, including sexualized contact via text (45%), meeting outside the organization (34%), allowing or encouraging visits to the teacher's house (31%), talking via cell phone (62%), and online/social media contact (42%). More specifically, the data suggested that women developed close relationships with often vulnerable victims and sent flirtatious text messages before the abuse occurred.

As shown in Fig. 9.3 below, Kaylor et al. (2021) proposed that the teacher-lover may select victims who are vulnerable due to their emotional/psychological needs or home situation, which may decrease the risk of detection and/or disclosure (Darling et al., 2018; Knoll, 2010; Plummer, 2018; Shakeshaft, 2004; West et al., 2010). In their role as educators, the potential perpetrator has easy access to victims and often has the support of guardians to spend time alone with victims as they are believed to be a positive influence (Darling et al., 2018; Knoll, 2010; Winters et al., 2020). Once access is established, the educator can use a variety of techniques to gain the trust of the potential victim and community, such as capitalizing on their reputation and/or a teenage boy's fantasy of a sexual relationship with a teacher, as well as using rewards, attention, and praise to solidify the relationship (Christensen, 2018; Knoll, 2010; Lanning & Dietz, 2014; Marshall et al., 2015; Plummer, 2018; West et al., 2010).

According to the SGM, the next step in the grooming process involves desensitizing the minor to sexual content and physical contact such as accidental touch, increased physical contact (e.g., hugs, sending/receiving flirty or suggestive/nude texts), or misrepresenting sexual contact as part of a consensual relationship (Christensen & Darling, 2020; Darling et al., 2018; Knoll, 2010). Once the abuse has transpired, the woman may engage in post-abuse maintenance behaviors to

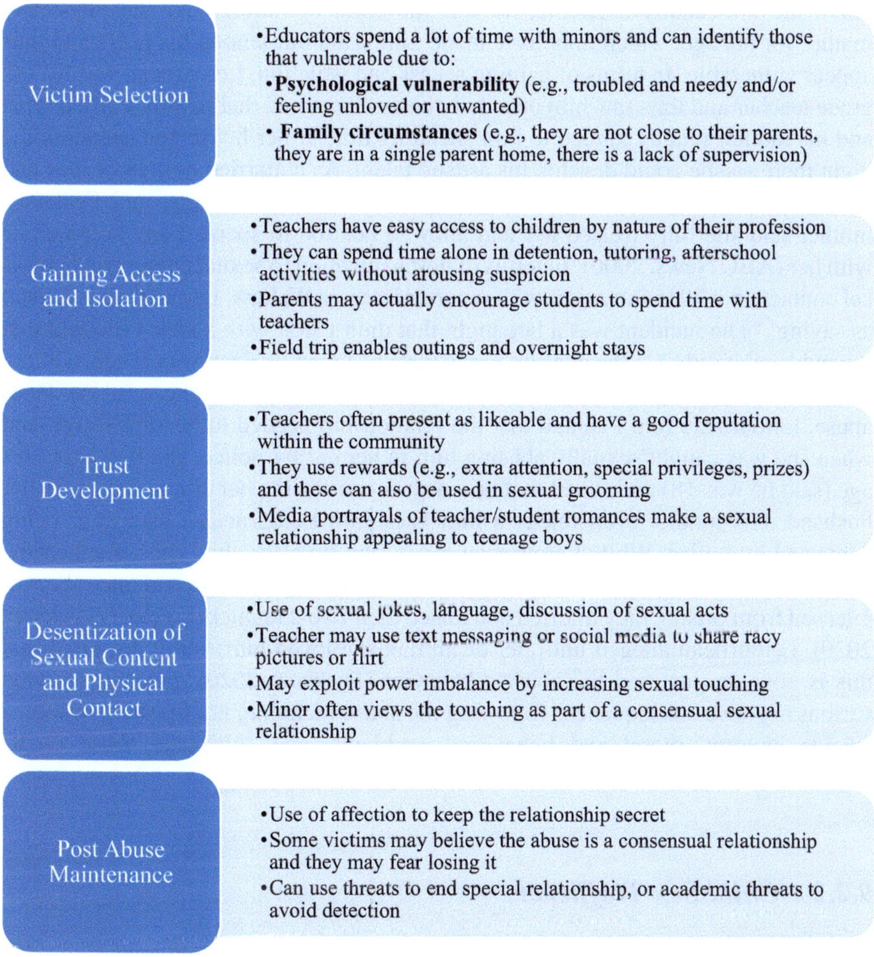

Fig. 9.3 The teacher-lover profile of grooming behavior among females who perpetrate the abuse

continue the abusive relationship without detection such as showing affection, threatening to terminate the relationship if it disclosed, making academic threats, or making the minor feel as they were complicit in the abuse (Lang & Frenzel, 1988; West et al., 2010). The behaviors as delineated in the SGM are presented below, followed by a description of sexual grooming behaviors depicted through a case study of Mary Kay Letourneau.

Case Example: Mary Kay Letourneau

An example of a teacher that used sexual grooming was Mary Kay Letourneau—perhaps the most famous "female sex offender." In 1996, she was a married primary school teacher and mother of four. She began what she later called "a love affair" with her then 12 year-old student Vili Fualaau (Dickson, 2020). While details of his youth are not readily available, he was the child of immigrants and physically mature for his age, which may have made him stand out among his peers and thus appear vulnerable. In terms of gaining access and isolation, Letourneau was his 6th grade teacher and thus saw him on a daily basis. She noted that he was a gifted artist and his mother readily agreed to him spending time at her house and spending the night there so she could develop his artistic talent. As a married mother of four and a teacher, Letourneau had good standing within the community, and Fualaau's mother said she fully trusted her and allowed her son to spend many hours alone with her (ABC News, 2006). In terms of desensitization to sexual content and physical contact, in a 2015 interview with reporter Barbara Walters, Letourneau is quoted as saying: "The incident was a late night that didn't stop with a kiss. I thought that it would and it didn't." She goes on to say that she loved Fualaau very much, adding, "and I kind of thought, 'Why can't it ever just be a kiss?'" (Walters, 2015). Post-abuse, Letourneau told Fualaau that the relationship needed to be kept secret, and when she was caught sexually abusing him in her car by police, she lied about his age (said he was 18) and stated that he was just comforting her after a fight with her husband. His mother even released him back into Letourneau's care after being contacted by police. While Letourneau served jail time for child rape, she became pregnant twice with Fualaau's children while he was still a minor, and once she was released from prison, they married and raised their two daughters together (Dickson, 2020). Letourneau alleged until her death that she loved him, and it appeared that this is how she justified the abusive behavior (Dickson, 2020). Fualaau reported various negative consequences following the abuse including not finishing school, a suicide attempt, mood and behavioral problems, and substance abuse (ABC News, 2006).

9.2.2 Child Sex Trafficker

While the stereotype of an individual who engages in sex trafficking is a man, globally, it is estimated that up to 38% of those who engage in trafficking are women (UNDOC, 2014). While there are various routes for women to engage in sex trafficking behavior, a recent analysis found many of the women engaged in trafficking voluntarily as part of a partnership with a male (be it a business arrangement, a romantic arrangement, or part of the family business). Further, they may have many roles including ringleader, enforcer, and recruiter. In one study of US traffickers, Veldhuizen-Ochodnicanova and Jeglic (2021) found that half of the women in the sample were the ringleaders of the operation while another 40% had some role in the recruitment of new victims. It is often within this recruitment role that females engaged in sex trafficking may use grooming behaviors to lure victims into the sex trade (Siegel & de Blank, 2010). According to Kaylor et al. (2021), women who engage in the recruitment of victims for trafficking meet two potential profiles of females who sexually abuse: (1) If they engage in the recruitment of victims at the behest of a male partner, they may fall into the *male-accompanied* type (Mathews et al., 1989), while (2) others who are ringleaders and who are driven by economic gains or antisocial traits may fit the *homosexual criminal* (i.e., sex trafficker) type (Spruce, 2018).

As described in Chap. 10, Winters and colleagues (2021a, b) proposed that those who traffic minors for sexual purposes, in general (both male and female), may utilize sexual grooming behaviors as described in the SGM to entrap victims into the sex trafficking trade. Kaylor et al. (2021) further outlined how females who recruit victims and can be described as the sex trafficking type of females who commit sexual offenses may use sexual grooming behaviors (see Fig. 9.4). In the victim selection phase, the women may select minors vulnerable due to environmental circumstances; for example, the minors may be homeless or runaways, be involved in the criminal justice or child welfare system, as well as psychologically vulnerable due to low self-esteem, substance abuse, mental health problems, or abusive home situations (FBI, 2020; Hampton & Lieggi, 2017; Litam, 2017; Reid, 2016; Varma et al., 2015). Once a potential target has been identified, the woman may work to gain access to the minor through social media and places where at-risk youth congregate, such as shopping malls, foster care facilities, homeless shelters, and juvenile detention facilities and isolate them by changing their identity, engaging in constant monitoring, and working to separate them from guardians and peers (Reid, 2016; Roe-Sepowitz, 2019). Next, they may build trust with minors by acting as a caring mother/sister figure, making promises of a safer and better life, providing material luxuries or lifestyle stability, and providing often-missing kindness, attention, and compliments (Hampton & Lieggi, 2017; Litam, 2017; Reid, 2016; Roe-Sepowitz, 2019; Williamson & Prior, 2009). In preparation for ensuing work as a trafficked individual, the woman may desensitize the minor to sexual content and physical touch by exposing them to pornography, taking sexually suggestive photographs, and having male accomplices "break them in," sometimes under the guise of a romantic relationship (Dank et al., 2014; Reid, 2016). Once the minor has begun being trafficked, the woman will engage in various post-abuse strategies and tactics to avoid disclosure so that the youth can continue to be trafficked, including psychological manipulation, threats of being arrested or put back on the street if they disclose, physical and sexual abuse, or making them feel culpable for being trafficked (Roe-Sepowitz, 2019; Veldhuizen-Ochodnicanova & Jeglic, 2021). The hypothesized tactics used by the females engaged in sex trafficking are presented below, followed by a case description describing the sexual grooming behaviors used by a convicted female trafficker—Ghislaine Maxwell.

Case Study: Ghislaine Maxwell

Ghislaine Maxwell, a consort of convicted sex trafficker Jeffrey Epstein, has herself been convicted of sex trafficking minors and young women. She was also convicted of conspiracy to entice a minor to travel to engage in illegal sex acts, conspiracy to transport a minor with the intent to engage in criminal sexual activity, transporting a minor with the intent to engage in criminal sexual activity, and conspiracy to commit sex trafficking of minors (Garsd & Romo, 2021). Some of the allegations made by victims suggest that Maxwell engaged in sexual grooming techniques to entrap

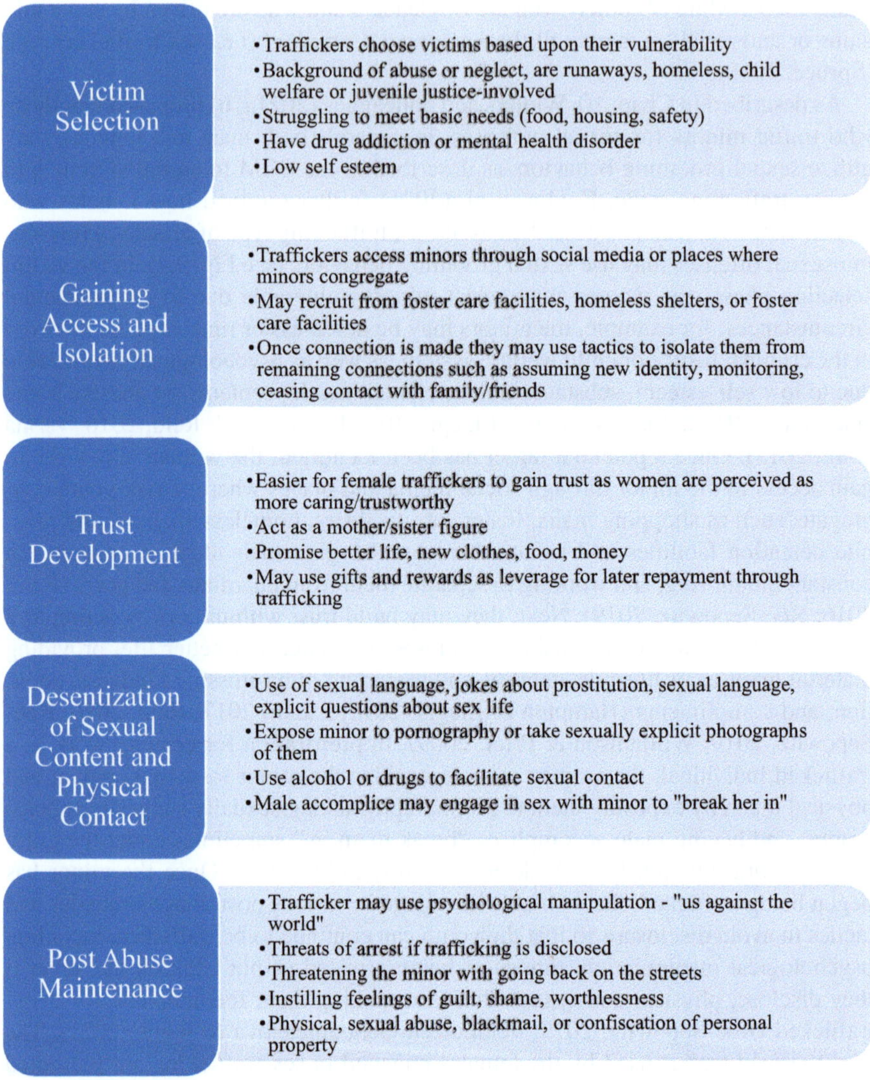

Fig. 9.4 The female sex trafficker profile of grooming behavior among females who perpetrate the abuse

the minors into Epstein's trafficking operation (Dockterman, 2021). It was known that Epstein preferred minors (between the ages of 13 and 17), and many of Epstein's victims came from disadvantaged or abusive homes or foster care and consequently were more vulnerable to the allure of the "jet-setting lifestyle" (Dastagir, 2019). Epstein was also said to have a specific "type" and selected teens who had a certain appearance. While many allege that Maxwell recruited girls for Epstein, court documents suggest that she targeted minors and young women who were more naive and trusting (Dastagir, 2019). In terms of gaining access and isolating the victims, it was said that Maxwell frequented massage spas and massage schools to recruit trainees. She would also have minor victims recruit other vulnerable minors for large cash payments and a jet-setting lifestyle (Hurtado, 2021). One victim reported that she was taken to Epstein's ranch in New Mexico to attend a program with other students who were interested in learning about studying abroad; however, when she arrived, it was only Maxwell and Epstein who were present (Hurtado, 2021). To gain her trust, Maxwell would ask about the victim's family and other aspects of her life to build rapport. It was also claimed that she gave the minors gifts of lingerie and hundreds of dollars in cash for conducting naked massages. Another victim described Maxwell as "an older sister" type who bought her expensive clothing during shopping sprees and engaged in witty conversation with her (Dockterman, 2021). In terms of desensitizing the minors to sexual content and physical contact, Maxwell talked about sexual topics around the girls in the massage room when the minor was naked (Hurtado, 2021). It was also alleged that Maxwell would give the minors massages herself, and during the massage, she would take down the sheet, so their breasts were exposed. Another victim reported that Maxwell taught her to give foot massages as Epstein enjoyed foot rubs (Dockterman, 2021). The three of them also watched a movie with themes of sexuality and pedophilia. Minors were also recruited to give Epstein massages for large sums of money that then became sexual in nature. Once the minors were abused, Maxwell was alleged to have paid them large sums of money for their "services" and asked them to find other minors for massages. This may have caused feelings of confusion as they may have perceived that they went willingly and feel guilt and shame for their actions, thus preventing disclosure and allowing the abuse to continue (Aradillas, 2019).

9.3 Female-Specific Prevention and Treatment

Given that many people are not aware or may not believe that women can engage in sexual violence, prevention initiatives specifically targeting this subgroup may be particularly warranted. As noted earlier, societal biases and stereotypes may enable females who engage in sexual offending to go undetected, while social stigma and confusion may prevent reporting (Cortoni et al., 2017; Darling et al., 2018). Thus, most existing child abuse prevention materials generally exclude the mention of women who commit sexual abuse. Given the evidence that female-perpetrated sexual abuse is more prevalent than was originally believed and there is some evidence that women use some of the same sexual grooming behaviors as men, all training materials and resources must be updated to reflect this information. For example, children and guardians should be made aware that women can perpetrate sexual abuse, and they should be taught how to recognize and report inappropriate touch or red flag behaviors exhibited by a woman. For instance, our research suggested that a common tactic used by sexually abusive female adolescents was to show the victim their naked body.

Educational institutions and youth-serving organizations in which women have mentoring roles should also be aware of the *teacher-lover typology* and the sexual grooming tactics that women in such roles may engage in. While most youth-serving institutions and organizations now have protocols to prevent the sexual abuse of children, these are largely based on the prototype of a male offender. However, due to biases and stereotypes of women as caring and nurturing, female grooming behaviors within institutions are more likely to go undetected (Arnold & Jeglic, 2021; Kienast et al., 2015; Reid & Jones, 2011). As such, explicit trainings identifying sexual grooming behaviors that may be more likely to be exhibited by women should be highlighted and addressed.

Similarly, organizations that work with at-risk youth should be familiar with the grooming techniques that may be used by women that fall into the *sex trafficker typology*. These behaviors and tactics should be included in educational materials and trainings. Further, caregivers, those in the service industry, medical providers, and the community at large should be knowledgeable of how female sex trafficking recruiters can befriend vulnerable teens and young women with the promise of a better life or material goods in order to develop better prevention and intervention programs.

Law enforcement and those who may be most likely to detect CSA, such as educators and medical professionals, should also be aware of how biases and stereotypes about females may impact their ability to detect, report, and prosecute female-perpetrated sexual abuse. For example, women are more likely to bring children to the doctor (Henry J. Kaiser Family Foundation, 2018) and stay in the room during medical evaluations, which is typically the time that doctors probe and examine for signs of abuse. If the female who committed the abuse is in the room, the child may be less likely to disclose the abuse. As such, medical professionals should perhaps ask the guardian to step out and a nurse to step in so that they may ask such questions without the female present.

Knowledge about female-perpetrated abuse patterns and behaviors may also be important for the treatment of both the victim of the abuse and the female who committed the abuse. In self-report surveys, up to 40% of men report that their abuser was a woman, and none of them had reported the abuse to authorities (Cortoni et al., 2017). Men who have experienced sexual abuse by a woman report the same or even more negative consequences of sexual abuse than those victimized by a man. This can be due in part to the perceived stigma, including feelings of shame or fear that either they will not be believed or that their manliness would be questioned if they reported (Sable et al., 2006). Addressing the myths surrounding female-perpetrated CSA and how women may also use sexual grooming tactics in the commission of the abuse may help diminish the feelings of stigma and shame and consequently reduce some of the negative consequences of the abuse.

Finally, understanding of female offending patterns is important for targeted treatment. Many treatment programs for individuals with sexual offenses address the perpetrators' abusive behaviors and risk factors using self-management strategies and relapse prevention plans (Moster et al., 2008). Understanding the behaviors and tactics employed by females who perpetrate CSA may help to identify high-risk situations, and as such, effective coping strategies can be taught and applied in an effort to reduce reoffending.

9.4 Conclusion

While we know that females do perpetrate sexual abuse, the sexual grooming literature as it pertains to females remains largely theoretical and underdeveloped. There are many stereotypes and biases that prevent female sexual abuse from being reported and detected, limiting the number of women who come in contact with the criminal justice system and thus can be studied. While it appears likely that at least some types of females who commit sexual abuse use grooming techniques, especially those in mentorship/teaching roles and those who engage in sex trafficking, much research still needs to be done. This will likely start by using case studies of women who committed the abuse and victim reports until more data can be gathered. In the meantime, prevention initiatives, especially within educational facilities and organizations that work with at-risk youth, should be aware of sexual grooming tactics and strategies that may be employed by women.

References

ABC News. (2006, January 7). *Mom testifies in teacher sex case.* https://abcnews.go.com/US/story?id=91755&page=1

Aradillas, E. (2019, August 28). More than 12 of Jeffrey Epstein's alleged victims speak out in court: 'The pain will never go away'. *People.* https://people.com/crime/jeffrey-epstein-accusers-speak-out-in-courtroom/

Arnold, S., & Jeglic, E. L. (2021). *Stereotypes and unconscious bias in institutional child abuse: A hidden risk.* Manuscript submitted for publication.

Bourke, A., Doherty, S., McBride, O., Morgan, K., & McGee, H. (2014). Female perpetrators of child sexual abuse: characteristics of the offender and victim. *Psychology, Crime & Law, 20*(8), 769–780. https://doi.org/10.1080/1068316X.2013.860456

Cameron, P., Proctor, K., Coburn, W., Jr., Forde, N., Larson, H., & Cameron, K. (1986). Child molestation and homosexuality. *Psychological Reports, 58*, 327–337. https://doi.org/10.2466/pr0.1986.58.1.327

Christensen, L. S. (2018). The new portrayal of female child sexual offenders in the print media: A qualitative content analysis. *Sexuality & Culture, 22*(1), 176–189. https://doi.org/10.1007/s12119-017-9459-1

Christensen, L. S., & Darling, A. J. (2020). Sexual abuse by educators: A comparison between male and female teachers who sexually abuse students. *Journal of Sexual Aggression, 26*(1), 23–35. https://doi.org/10.1080/13552600.2019.1616119

Cortoni, F., Babchishin, K. M., & Rat, C. (2017). The proportion of sexual offenders who are female is higher than thought: A meta-analysis. *Criminal Justice and Behavior, 44*(2), 145–162. https://doi.org/10.1177/0093854816658923

Dank, M. L., Khan, B., Downey, P. M., Kotonias, C., Mayer, D., Owens, C., Pacifici, L., & Yu, L. (2014). *Estimating the size and structure of the underground commercial sex economy in eight major US cities*. The Urban Institute.

Darling, A. J., Hackett, S., & Jamie, K. (2018). Female sex offenders who abuse children whilst working in organisational contexts: offending, conviction and sentencing. *Journal of Sexual Aggression, 24*(2), 196–214. https://doi.org/10.1080/13552600.2018.1476601

Dastagir, A. E. (2019, July 9). Jeffrey Epstein's alleged sex trafficking targets: 'The more vulnerable the better,' investigator says. *USA Today*. https://www.usatoday.com/story/news/nation/2019/07/09/how-jeffrey-epstein-allegedly-chose-his-sex-trafficking-victims/1683420001/

Dickson, E.J. (2020). How the media turned child rape into a 'tryst' for Mary Kay Letourneau. *Rolling Stone*. https://www.rollingstone.com/culture/culture-features/mary-kay-letourneau-vili-fualauu-relationship-media-child-rape-tryst-1025466/

Dockterman, E. (2021, December 2). Ghislaine maxwell's trial centers on allegations of 'grooming' young girls. Here's what that means. *Time*. https://time.com/6125081/ghislaine-maxwell-grooming-trial/

FBI. (2020). *Internet Crime Complaint Center: Human Traffickers Continue to Use Popular Online Platforms to Recruit Victims*. https://www.ic3.gov/Media/Y2020/PSA200316

Finkelhor, D., Ormrod, R., & Chaffin, M. (2009). Juveniles who commit sex offenses against minors. *Juvenile Justice Bulletin*. https://www.ojp.gov/pdffiles1/ojjdp/227763.pdf

Freeman, N. J., & Sandler, J. C. (2008). Female and male sex offenders: A comparison of recidivism patterns and risk factors. *Journal of Interpersonal Violence, 23*(10), 1394–1413. https://doi.org/10.1177/0886260508314304

Gallagher, B. (2000). The extent and nature of known cases of institutional child sexual abuse. *British Journal of Social Work, 30*, 795–817. https://doi.org/10.1093/bjsw/30.6.795

Gannon, T. A., Rose, M. R., & Ward, T. (2008). A descriptive model of the offense process for female sexual offenders. *Sexual Abuse, 20*(3), 352–374. https://doi.org/10.1177/1079063208322495

Garsd, J., & Romo, V. (2021, December 29). Ghislaine Maxwell found guilty of helping Jeffrey Epstein sexually abuse girls. *NPR*. https://www.npr.org/2021/12/29/1066219689/ghislaine-maxwell-verdict-trial-jeffrey-epstein

Hampton, M. D., & Lieggi, M. (2017). Commercial sexual exploitation of youth in the United States: A qualitative systematic review. *Trauma, Violence, & Abuse, 21*, 57–70. https://doi.org/10.1177/1524838017742168

Henry J. Kaiser Family Foundation. (2018). *Women, work, and family health: Key findings from the 2017 Kaiser Women's Health Survey*. https://files.kff.org/attachment/Issue-Brief-Women-Work-and-Family-Health-Key-Findings-from-the-2017-Kaiser-Womens-Health-Survey

Hurtado, P. (2021, November 12). Epstein scapegoat or sexual abuser: The trial of Ghislaine Maxwell. *Bloomberg*. https://www.bloomberg.com/features/ghislaine-maxwell-jeffrey-epstein-trial-2021/

Jeglic, E. L., & Calkins, C. (2018). *Protecting your child from sexual abuse: What you need to know to keep your kids safe*. Skyhorse.

Johansson-Love, J., & Fremouw, W. (2009). Female sex offenders: A controlled comparison of offender and victim/crime characteristics. *Journal of Family Violence, 24*(6), 367–376. https://doi.org/10.1007/s10896-009-9236-5

Kaylor, L. E., Winters, G. M., & Jeglic, E. L. (2021). Exploring sexual grooming in female perpetrated child sexual abuse. *Journal of Child Sexual Abuse*, 1–19.

Kienast, J., Lakner, M., Neulet, A., Kangaspunta, K., & Szalai, A. (2015). *The role of female offenders in sex trafficking organizations*. In ACUNS Vienna Annual Conference 2015 Lessons Learned from the Millennium Development Goals and Perspectives for the Post-2015 Development Agenda. https://acuns.org/wp-content/uploads/2014/11/vienna-vision.pdf#page=136

Knoll, J. (2010). Teacher sexual misconduct: Grooming patterns and female offenders. *Journal of Child Sexual Abuse: Research, Treatment, & Program Innovations for Victims, Survivors, & Offenders, 19*(4), 371–386. https://doi.org/10.1080/10538712.2010.495047

Lang, R., & Frenzel, R. (1988). How sex offenders lure children. *Annals of Sex Research, 1*, 303–317. https://doi.org/10.1007/BF00852802

Lanning, K. V., & Dietz, P. (2014). Acquaintance molestation and youth-serving organizations. *Journal of Interpersonal Violence, 29*(15), 2815–2838. https://doi.org/10.1177/0886260514532360

Litam, S. D. A. (2017). Human sex trafficking in America: What counselors need to know. *Professional Counselor, 7*, 45–61. https://doi.org/10.15241/SDAL.7.1.45
Marshall, W. L., Smallbone, S., & Marshall, L. E. (2015). A critique of current child molester subcategories: A proposal for an alternative approach. *Psychology, Crime & Law, 21*(3), 205–218. https://doi.org/10.1080/1068316X.2014.925724
Mathews, R., Hunter, J. A., & Vuz, J. (1997). Juvenile female sexual offenders: Clinical characteristics and treatment issues. *Sexual Abuse: A Journal of Research and Treatment, 9*(3), 187–199. https://doi.org/10.1007/BF02675064
Mathews, R., Matthews, J. K., & Speltz, K. (1989). *Female sexual offenders: An exploratory study*. Safer Society Press.
Moster, A., Wnuk, D. W., & Jeglic, E. L. (2008). Cognitive behavioral therapy interventions with sex offenders. *Journal of Correctional Health Care, 14*(2), 109–121. https://doi.org/10.1177/1078345807313874
Oliver, B. E. (2007). Preventing female-perpetrated sexual abuse. *Trauma, Violence, & Abuse, 8*(1), 19–32. https://doi.org/10.1177/1524838006296747
Plummer, M. (2018). Lived experiences of grooming among Australian male survivors of child sexual abuse. *Journal of Interpersonal Violence, 33*(1), 37–63. https://doi.org/10.1177/0886260517732539
Ratliff, L., & Watson, J. (2014). A descriptive analysis of public school educators arrested for sex offenses. *Journal of Child Sexual Abuse, 23*(2), 217–228. https://doi.org/10.1080/10538712.2014.870275
Reid, J. A. (2016). Entrapment and enmeshment schemes used by sex traffickers. *Sexual Abuse, 28*, 491–511. https://doi.org/10.1177/1079063214544334
Reid, J. A., & Jones, S. (2011). Exploited vulnerability: Legal and psychological perspectives on child sex trafficking victims. *Victims & Offenders, 6*(2), 207–231. https://doi.org/10.1080/15564886.2011.557327
Robertiello, G., & Terry, K. J. (2007). Can we profile sex offenders? A review of sex offender typologies. *Aggression and Violent Behavior, 12*, 508–518. https://doi.org/10.1016/j.avb.2007.02.010
Roe-Sepowitz, D. (2019). A six-year analysis of sex traffickers of minors: exploring characteristics and sex trafficking patterns. *Journal of Human Behavior in the Social Environment, 29*, 608–629. https://doi.org/10.1080/10911359.2019.1575315
Sable, M. R., Danis, F., Mauzy, D. L., & Gallagher, S. K. (2006). Barriers to reporting sexual assault for women and men: Perspectives of college students. *Journal of American College Health, 55*(3), 157–162. https://doi.org/10.3200/JACH.55.3.157-162
Sandler, J. C., & Freeman, N. J. (2007). Typology of female sex offenders: A test of Vandiver and Kercher. *Sexual Abuse, 19*(2), 73–89. https://doi.org/10.1177/107906320701900201
Shakeshaft, C. (2004). *Educator sexual misconduct: A synthesis of existing literature (U.S. Department of Education Document No. 2004-09)*. U.S. Department of Education.
Siegel, D., & De Blank, S. (2010). Women who traffic women: the role of women in human trafficking networks–Dutch cases. *Global Crime, 11*(4), 436–447. https://doi.org/10.1080/17440572.2010.519528
Spruce, H. (2018, November 6). *Methods of Human Trafficking: #AntiSlaveryDay*. The Hub. https://www.highspeedtraining.co.uk/hub/methods-of-human-trafficking/
Syed, F., & Williams, S. (1996). *Case studies of female sex offenders in the Correctional Service of Canada*. Ottawa, Canada: Correctional Service Canada.
Ten Bensel, T., Gibbs, B., & Burkey, C. R. (2019). Female sex offenders: Is there a difference between solo and co-offenders? *Journal of Interpersonal Violence, 34*(19), 4061–4084. https://doi.org/10.1177/0886260516674202
Tsopelas, C., Spyridoula, T., & Athanasios, D. (2011). Review on female sexual offenders: Findings about profile and personality. *International Journal of Law and Psychiatry, 34*(2), 122–126. https://doi.org/10.1016/j.ijlp.2011.02.006
UNDOC. (2014). *Global report on trafficking in persons 2014*. UNDOC.

Vandiver, D. M., & Kercher, G. (2004). Offender and victim characteristics of registered female sexual offenders in Texas: A proposed typology of female sexual offenders. *Sexual Abuse: A Journal of Research and Treatment, 16*(2), 121–137. https://doi.org/10.1177/107906320401600203

Vandiver, D. M., & Walker, J. T. (2002). Female sex offenders: An overview and analysis of 40 cases. *Criminal Justice Review, 27*(2), 284–300. https://doi.org/10.1177/073401680202700205

Varma, S., Gillespie, S., McCracken, C., & Greenbaum, V. J. (2015). Characteristics of child commercial sexual exploitation and sex trafficking victims presenting for medical care in the United States. *Child Abuse & Neglect, 44*, 98–105. https://doi.org/10.1016/j.chiabu.2015.04.004

Veldhuizen-Ochodnicanova, E., & Jeglic, E. L. (2021). Of madams, mothers and mistresses: Conceptualising the female sex trafficker in the United States. *International Journal of Law, Crime and Justice, 64*(e100455). https://doi.org/10.1016/j.ijlcj.2020.100455

Walters, B. (2015). *Mary Kay Letourneau Fualaau, Vili Fualaau open up in 'American Scandal'.* https://abcnews.go.com/GMA/video/mary-kay-letourneau-fualaau-vili-fualaau-interivew-couple-30224200

West, S. G., Hatters-Friedman, S., & Knoll, J. L., IV. (2010). Lessons to learn: Female educators who sexually abuse their students. *Psychiatric Times, 27*(8), 9. https://link.gale.com/apps/doc/A233502884/AONE?u=anon~e3063fe3&sid=googleScholar&xid=4ac89994

Wijkman, M., Bijleveld, C., & Hendriks, J. (2010). Women don't do such things! Characteristics of female sex offenders and offender types. *Sexual Abuse, 22*(2), 135–156. https://doi.org/10.1177/1079063210363826

Williamson, C., & Prior, M. (2009). Domestic minor sex trafficking: A network of underground players in the Midwest. *Journal of Child and Adolescent Trauma, 2*(1), 46–61. https://doi.org/10.1080/19361520802702191

Winters, G. M., Jeglic, E. L., & Kaylor, L. E. (2020). Validation of the sexual grooming model of child sexual abusers. *Journal of Child Sexual Abuse: Research, Treatment, & Program Innovations for Victims, Survivors, & Offenders*. https://doi.org/10.1080/10538712.2020.1801935

Winters, G. M., Jeglic, E. L., & Kaylor, L. (2021a). *Victims' perspectives of sexual grooming behaviors of females who commit child sexual abuse*. Manuscript submitted for Publication.

Winters, G., Schaaf, S., Grydehoj, R., Allan, C., Lin, A., & Jeglic, E. (2021b). The sexual grooming model of child sex trafficking. *Victims & Offenders*. https://doi.org/10.1080/15564886.2021.1926031

Chapter 10
Sex Trafficking and Sexual Grooming

Child sex trafficking has become a global problem that impacts over one million children (International Labour Organization, 2017), which has prompted researchers to examine the tactics used by sex traffickers to lure victims into these sexually exploitative situations. These recruitment and maintenance strategies of victims have been compared to those utilized in cases of intimate partner violence, hostage situations, and cults (Reid et al., 2013). In some cases, authors have suggested that this process is akin to the sexual grooming process of individuals who commit child sexual abuse (Brayley et al., 2011; Reid, 2016; Winters et al., 2021). For example, Brayley et al. (2011) explained that there was increased awareness in the United Kingdom (UK) regarding sexual grooming of minors, but they stressed that the application of this construct to cases of child sex trafficking remained "a knowledge black hole" (p. 134). Indeed, many of the behaviors utilized in cases of child sex trafficking mirror those of the sexual grooming behaviors a person seeking to commit child sexual abuse may use in the offense process (Winters et al., 2021). However, there remains little crossover between the scholarship on sexual offending and sex trafficking despite the apparent similarities between the strategies and tactics used to perpetrate the crimes. For example, instead of utilizing the term "grooming," the sex trafficking literature has adopted a range of vocabulary to reflect the process by which a victim is selected, recruited, and controlled. These include terminology to describe the victim selection and access stages of grooming, such as "recruitment" (Dank et al., 2014; Kennedy et al., 2007), "persuasion" (Dank et al., 2015), "find" (Brayley et al., 2011), or "entrapment" (Reid, 2016), as well as terms related to the core sexual grooming process, such as "coercive control" (Raphael et al., 2010), "management of work relationship" (Dank et al., 2014), "enmeshment" (Reid, 2016), or "methods of control" (Roe-Sepowitz, 2019). This chapter aims to bridge the distance between the child sexual grooming and child sex trafficking literature in order to develop a shared understanding and lexicon of the overlapping strategies, behaviors, and tactics that are used both in child sexual abuse (CSA) and sex trafficking.

© The Author(s), under exclusive license to Springer Nature Switzerland AG 2022

G. M. Winters, E. L. Jeglic, *Sexual Grooming*,
https://doi.org/10.1007/978-3-031-07222-2_10

10.1 Overview of Child Sex Trafficking

Sex trafficking refers to the "the recruitment, harboring, transportation, provision, or obtaining of a person for the purpose of a commercial sex act," with severe forms occurring when "a commercial sex act is induced by force, fraud, or coercion, or in which the person induced to perform such act has not attained 18 years of age" (Office on Violence Against Women, 2000, p. 1470). This is considered to be one of the fastest growing global criminal enterprises worldwide (International Labour Organization, 2012). The forced sexual labor of minors is of particular concern given the serious consequences it may have on the victims (e.g., physical, psychological, and social well-being; Adelson, 2009; Miller-Perrin & Wurtele, 2017; Rafferty, 2008; Silverman et al., 2009). Consistent with CSA in general, the sex trafficking definition acknowledges that sex trafficking of a minor is illegal given that a minor is unable to consent to such activity.

In 2016, it was estimated that over one million minors were in forced sexual labor across the globe (International Labour Organization, 2017), including documented cases in all 50 states in the United States (US; Clawson et al., 2009). Importantly, while it is well established that child sex trafficking is a prevalent problem, the actual rates may far surpass current estimates (The Crimes Against Children Research Centre, 2008). This is likely attributable to a number of reasons. The existing research is limited as it is based on known and documented cases of sex trafficking (i.e., self-identified victims and offenders identified through law enforcement, independent agencies, or social services), and there is no central database or uniform report to track these cases (Duger, 2015; Gerassi, 2015; McClain & Garrity, 2011). Moreover, there are victims' internal barriers to reporting, including that they may not identify as a victim or may decline to report out of fear or shame (Bales & Lize, 2007; Goodey, 2008; Hodge & Lietz, 2007; Jones et al., 2007; Logan et al., 2009); thus, the research is unable to account for those who do not come forward. As a result, the Crimes Against Children Research Centre (2008) stress that the available prevalence rates may underestimate the full scope of child sex trafficking.

10.1.1 The Individuals Who Commit Sex Trafficking and Their Victims

In order to better understand the behaviors used in the sex trafficking process, it is important to understand those involved in trafficking youth—both those who commit the sex trafficking and their victims. Prior research on sex traffickers ("pimps") have grouped them into three categories: (1) the "gorilla pimp" (i.e., uses coercion and violence to control victims), (2) the "finesse/Romeo pimp" (i.e., uses affection, charm, and romance to manipulate victims), and (3) the "business/CEO pimp" (i.e., uses promises of a glamorous career and legitimate income; Godoy et al., 2016;

Hammond & McGlone, 2014; Harris, 2012; Marcus et al., 2014). Sex traffickers may operate independently or within an organized group context (i.e., "third-party" sex trafficking). Roe-Sepowitz (2019) found the majority of sex traffickers worked within these group contexts, and one in five reported being a member of a gang. For those operating independently, some target family, peers, or romantic partners to recruit individuals into sex trafficking (Godoy et al., 2016; Marcus et al., 2014; Miller-Perrin & Wurtele, 2017; Polaris Project, 2013; Sprang & Cole, 2018).

The sex traffickers tend to be male (Godoy et al., 2016; Roe-Sepowitz, 2019; Veldhuizen et al., 2020), but there are cases of females who are used to recruit others or facilitate the sexual exploitation (Miccio-Fonseca, 2017; Raphael et al., 2010; Roe-Sepowitz, 2019). Indeed, Roe-Sepowitz (2019) found that 24% of sex traffickers were female in 2015, which was an increase from 13% in 2010. These female traffickers have been grouped into two categories: (1) those who operate under the direction of their traffickers (e.g., to recruit victims; Anderson et al., 2014; Roe-Sepowitz, 2019) and (2) caregivers or guardians who exploit their own children (Mitchell et al., 2010; Roe-Sepowitz, 2019; Sprang & Cole, 2018).

Data has shown that most victims are recruited into the sex trafficking industry before the age of 18 (Swaner et al., 2016), with the average age being 12–15 years (Clawson et al., 2009; Franchino-Olsen, 2019; Roe-Sepowitz, 2019). Females represent the majority of those who are sex trafficked (between 60 and 94%; Banks & Kyckelhahn, 2011; Swaner et al., 2016), but males may be trafficked as well. Minor victims from all races, ethnicities, and socioeconomic statuses have been documented within the illegal sex trade (Litam, 2017; McClain & Garrity, 2011). Furthermore, the majority of child sex trafficking cases in the US are citizens or permanent legal residents (Banks & Kyckelhahn, 2011; Franchino-Olsen, 2019; McClain & Garrity, 2011).

10.2 Models of Sex Trafficking

Within the child sex trafficking literature, several authors have proposed models to conceptualize the process of recruitment and maintenance of the minors. As will be elucidated in the sections below, these conceptualizations vary significantly in the terminology used and the description of the tactics involved in the process. This results in inconsistencies across the literature, which promotes confusion regarding what exactly the recruitment and management process entails. Nonetheless, it is important to understand prior conceptualizations in order to highlight similarities among the tactics used by sex traffickers and how they may map onto the child sexual grooming literature (see Table 10.1 for a description of the various models).

In 2007, Kennedy et al. identified various "routes" of recruitment used by sex traffickers through interviews with 22 informants (e.g., former victims, parents of victims, VICE police officers, outreach workers, nurses, and social service providers), as well as interviews with 44 victims of sex trafficking. The qualitative findings

Table 10.1 Models of child sex trafficking tactics

Authors	Stages/tactics	Description
Kennedy et al. (2007)	*Routes of recruitment*	Violence
		Love
		Debt
		Drugs
		"Gorilla" technique
		Position of authority
Raphael et al. (2010)	*Violence*	Punching
		Hair pulled
		Pinched
		Spanked
		Kicked
		Kidnapped
		Ripped clothes
		Something thrown
		Threatened rape
		Forced sex
	Coercive control	Money taken by pimp
		Threats of being kicked out of home
		Drugs provided to encourage addiction
		Withholding drugs by pimp
		Claims of indebtedness with food, clothing, and gifts
		Threats to end romantic relationship
		Threats of harm
		Verbal abuse
Brayley et al. (2011)	*Find*	Searching for a new girl
		Receiving a request for a girl
	Groom	Flattery
		Building trust
		Normalizing sexual activity
		Isolation
		Disorientation
		Intimidation
	Abuse	Invite girl to socialize
		Pick up/arrange meeting
		Enter abuse location
		Isolate girl
		Abuse
		Release girl

(continued)

Table 10.1 (continued)

Authors	Stages/tactics	Description
Dank et al. (2015)	*Recruitment/persuasion tactics*	Romance or sexual relationship
		Mutual dependency
		Monetizing sex
		Associated lifestyle
		Reputation
	Management of work relationship	Rules
		Punishment (force/coercion)
		Competition between "employees"
Reid (2016)	*Entrapment schemes*	Flattery or romance
		Become ally/build trust
		Normalize sex
		Isolate
		Abduct and drug
		"Bait and switch"
		Target intellectually disabled youth
		Persuaded by "boyfriend/gang"
	Enmeshment schemes	Shame/blackmail
		Obligation
		Make complicit in crime
		Pregnancy/child
		Isolate
		Financial control
		Intimidate
		Hope, connection, and faux family
Roe-Sepowitz (2019)	*Recruitment tactics*	Targeting vulnerable victims
		Promises of money and wealth
		Glamorize prostitution
		Offer a place to stay
		Use friendship
		Use romantic relationship
		Physical violence
		Sexual violence
		Provide drugs and alcohol
	Methods of control	Physical violence
		Sexual violence
		Psychological abuse
		Provide drugs
		Use of firearm to intimidate

suggested that the majority of sex traffickers used violence as a controlling technique, along with five additional frequently used techniques, including:

1. Love (e.g., having an emotional attachment or romantic relationship with the pimp)
2. Debt (i.e., given gifts, money, clothing, or drugs, then later demand payment)
3. Drugs (i.e., exploiting victims' drug use)
4. The "gorilla" technique (i.e., use of only force and violence)
5. Position of authority (i.e., using the position of power over the victim, such as cases in which family members recruit relatives in sex trade)

Raphael et al. (2010) created a model that focused on the violence and coercive control used by sex traffickers. Using a snowball sample, the authors interviewed 71 women (ages 16–25) who were engaged in prostitution in Chicago about their experiences during recruitment, as well as at the present time (i.e., the time of the interview). Through quantitative and qualitative analyses, the authors found that 21% experienced violence during recruitment, while 75% reported current violence against them. There was a range of violent behaviors reported, such as punching, hair pulling, pinching, spanking, kicking, kidnapping, ripping clothes, being thrown down, something was thrown, threatening rape, or forcing sex. The authors also investigated nonviolent coercion and control (based on definitions within the intimate partner violence literature), including the creation of vulnerabilities and indebtedness, exploiting existing vulnerabilities, manipulation, and threats. Approximately half of the sample reported coercion used during recruitment (49%) and at the time of the interview (59%). The most common tactics were verbal abuse and having money taken by the pimp. Other tactics included threats of being kicked out of the home, being provided with or withholding drugs, claims of debt, threats to end a romantic relationship, and threats of harm.

Brayley et al. (2011) are among the few sex trafficking researchers that utilized the term "grooming" to describe the recruitment/maintenance strategies employed by sex traffickers. They used data (e.g., interviews, case summaries, phone records, charge lists) from child sex trafficking cases in the UK that included 25 offenders and 36 victims to develop a "crime script" by grouping similar actions that ultimately lead to the commission of the abuse against the sex-trafficked minor. There were three overarching stages involved, including *find*, *groom*, and *abuse*. The *find* stage refers to how the sex traffickers locate and target potential victims, such as through use of psychological manipulation, approaching a high number of potential targets, or various "unsophisticated" attempts (e.g., giving the minor attention, flirting, bantering). During the *groom* stage, Brayley et al. (2011) indicated there was a range of the type, degree, duration, and frequency of grooming tactics used. Broadly, these grooming tactics fell into six categories:

1. Flattery (e.g., complimenting, flirting, professing love)
2. Building trust (e.g., being a friend or boyfriend, offering to help solve problems, giving food or cigarettes, protecting the girl from other men)

3. Normalizing sexual activity (e.g., sexual jokes, asking about sexual experiences or preferences, talking about sex, exposure to pornography)
4. Isolation (e.g., insulting relatives or friends, taking the victim to unfamiliar locations, separating them from friends, locking or blocking exits)
5. Disorientation (e.g., giving alcohol or drugs, spiking drinks, switching between nice and mean, speaking a different language)
6. Intimidation (e.g., threats to harm the girl or her family, physical violence, insulting the minor)

Lastly, during the *abuse* phase, there is a linear progression that occurs: invite the minor to socialize, pick up/arrange the meeting, enter abuse location, isolation, abuse, and release the minor.

Dank et al. (2015) investigated the commercial sex industry in eight US cities (San Diego, Seattle, Dallas, Denver, Washington DC, Kansas City, Atlanta, and Miami) using a mixed methods approach. For the qualitative data, they conducted interviews with sex traffickers and sex workers involved in court diversion. They organized their conceptualization of sex trafficking tactics into (1) *methods of recruitment/persuasion* and (2) *management of work relationships*. Broadly, Dank et al. (2015) described two recruitment strategies used by sex traffickers, including "finesse pimping" (i.e., recruit using "bait and switch" tactics) and "gorilla pimping" (i.e., use intimidation and coercion), based on the work of Williamson and Prior (2009). The sex traffickers in the sample described that finesse pimps may use violence as a means of controlling and persuading sex workers, but it is not intended as the primary tactic; indeed, only 15% of their sample used violence during the recruitment process. In terms of persuasion, the authors described that the sex traffickers used the following:

1. Romantic and sexual relationships (i.e., developing a romantic and physical relationship with the victim)
2. Mutual dependency (i.e., promoting the benefits of sex work and encouraging a shared lifestyle)
3. Monetizing sex (i.e., discouraging sex without compensation)
4. Associated lifestyle (i.e., verbally promising material comforts, displaying wealth and money)
5. Reputation (i.e., maintaining a reputation as a "good" pimp to attract sex workers)

Once a person is recruited into the sexually exploitative relationship, the sex trafficker may use management techniques to maintain the work relationship, such as establishing and enforcing rules (e.g., drug use, limitations with clientele, communication with other pimps, quotas), punishment via force or coercion, and competition between employees (e.g., promote competition and jealousy to maintain control and drive earnings).

Reid (2016) collected archival data from 2007 to 2012 of 43 child sex trafficking cases of girls (age 4–17 years) involving nonrelative traffickers, along with data from 10 semi-structured interviews conducted by social service providers. Through this qualitative data analysis, Reid proposed the behaviors utilized by sex traffickers can be understood through two overarching categories: *entrapment* (i.e., the initial recruitment strategies used by sex traffickers) and *enmeshment* (i.e., the long-term strategies used for ongoing exploitation). There were eight entrapment schemes identified in the data, including:

1. Flattery and romance (e.g., showing love and attention, taking the child on special dates or outings)
2. Becoming an ally/building trust (e.g., helping the child run away from home or avoid police, providing drugs or a place to stay)
3. Normalizing sex (e.g., talking about sexual topics, exposure to pornography, sex with the child)
4. Isolation (e.g., moving to another city/state, controlling cell or computer devices)
5. Giving drugs and abducting the child
6. "Bait and switch" (e.g., giving money or assistance, then later demanding repayment)
7. Selecting intellectually disabled youth
8. Persuading by boyfriend/gang member

Then in the case of longer-term exploitation, there may be additional enmeshment techniques used, such as:

1. Shame and blackmailing (e.g., threatening to share explicit photographs, telling the child they are not wanted)
2. Obligations (e.g., convincing the child they are better off and should remain loyal)
3. Making the child complicit in crimes (e.g., recruiting other children for sexual exploitation)
4. Impregnating the child
5. Isolating the child
6. Financial control
7. Intimidation
8. Providing hope, connection, and sense of family

Roe-Sepowitz (2019) examined 1,416 cases of sex trafficking of minors in the US from 2010 to 2015. The data was derived from an online search engine, electronic court documents, and online government agency press releases. Roe-Sepowitz described the tactics of sex traffickers in terms of *recruitment* and *methods of control*. The findings showed many sex traffickers engaged in recruitment (43% of the sample), and there was a range of tactics that may be used. Roe-Sepowitz identified that traffickers may seek out vulnerable victims (e.g., runaways), lure them with promises of money and wealth, glamorize prostitution, provide a place to stay, or use friendship or romantic relationships. In many cases, the sex trafficker used sexual assault or physical abuse in the recruitment process. Once the victim is recruited, the sex trafficker may use various methods of control including sexual, physical, or psychological abuse (e.g., threats). The physical violence may occur with a weapon or without, and some cases may involve torture. In other cases, the sex trafficker may use drugs to control the victim.

10.2.1 *Sexual Grooming Model of Child Sex Trafficking*

Importantly, while there have been numerous proposed models and tactics involved in the sex trafficking recruitment and maintenance process, there are notable limitations. The terminology across all the models, as well as the description of these stages or behaviors, varies significantly. This makes it difficult to draw consistent and thorough conclusions across the literature. Additionally, it has been suggested that sex trafficking behaviors may be similar to tactics used by other types of offenses, such as sexual offenses, intimate partner violence, kidnapping, and cults (Reid et al., 2013). Of relevance, there tends to be a lack of attention to how these recruitment and maintenance processes within sex trafficking may be akin to the sexual grooming tactics used in CSA cases. Indeed, these areas have seemingly remained independent from one another, with little overlap between the constructs and theories despite the parallel processes (e.g., the term "grooming" is rarely seen within sex trafficking despite the similarities). As Brayley et al. (2011) noted, there has been increased awareness about sexual grooming in CSA cases in the past decade, but the application to child sex trafficking remained "a knowledge black hole" (p. 134). It is necessary to more thoroughly explore how the construct of sexual grooming may apply to sex trafficking cases as it does to those within CSA as knowledge from these different areas may help inform one another.

Winters et al. (2021) argued that the variation within the field of sex trafficking, coupled with the largely unexplored parallels of sexual grooming as it applies to sex trafficking, warranted investigation. Thus, through a thorough review of the literature, they proposed overlaps between the "entrapment" tactics used by sex traffickers and child sexual grooming behaviors. They proposed a Sexual Grooming Model of Child Sex Trafficking (SGM-CST; Winters et al., 2021) based on the application of the sex trafficking literature to the SGM (Winters et al., 2020) of individuals who commit child sexual abuse. See Table 10.2 for a review of the sex trafficking stages/tactics that seemingly correspond to the broad stages or behaviors included in the SGM.

While the exact tactics used by those who commit child sexual abuse versus child sex trafficking may differ, Winters et al. (2021) suggests the recruitment and control strategies used by sex traffickers can be conceptualized in the five stages of the SGM as described below.

10.2.1.1 Victim Selection

The victim selection stage of the SGM includes targeting a minor based on perceived vulnerabilities, such as psychological/emotional, environmental, and familial instabilities, which has been documented in cases of child sex trafficking. Regarding psychological vulnerabilities, research has shown that sex traffickers may target children with low confidence, intellectual deficits, mental health issues, or drug problems (Dank et al., 2014; Hampton & Lieggi, 2017; Reid, 2016; Twill et al., 2010). Additionally, a child may be targeted based on external/

Table 10.2 The sex trafficking stages/tactics that correspond to the Sexual Grooming Model

SGM stage	Corresponding model stages
Victim selection	Brayley et al. (2011)—find
	Reid (2016)—target intellectually disabled youth
	Roe-Sepowitz (2019)—target vulnerable victim
Gaining access and isolation	Brayley et al. (2011)—groom (isolation)
	Reid (2016)—isolate
Trust development	Kennedy et al. (2007)—love, debt, drugs, and position of authority
	Raphael et al. (2010)—drugs and indebtedness
	Brayley et al. (2011)—groom (flattery, building trust)
	Dank et al. (2015)—romance relationship, mutual dependency, associated lifestyle, and reputation
	Reid (2016)—flattery or romance, build trust, drug, "bait and switch," and persuaded by boyfriend/gang
	Roe-Sepowitz (2019)—promise money and wealth, offer place to stay, use friendship or romantic relationship, and provide drugs/alcohol
Desensitization to sexual content and physical contact	Brayley et al. (2011)—groom (normalizing sexual activity)
	Dank et al. (2015)—sexual relationship
	Reid (2016)—normalize sex
Post-abuse maintenance	Raphael et al. (2010)—threats
	Brayley et al. (2011)—intimidation
	Reid (2016)—shame, intimidation, and hope/connection
	Roe-Sepowitz (2019)—psychological abuse

environmental factors such as an inhospitable home (e.g., subject to physical, sexual, or emotional abuse), unmet basic needs (e.g., neglect, lack of food or clothing), and maladaptive influences (e.g., deviant peers or relatives; Hampton & Lieggi, 2017). Indeed, research has supported the notion that the majority of sex trafficked minors experienced physical, sexual, verbal, and emotional abuse (Clawson et al., 2009; Dank et al., 2015; Hampton & Lieggi, 2017; Litam, 2017), with many reporting parental neglect, lack of supervision, or having experienced a shortage of food, clothes, or housing (Cecchet & Thoburn, 2014; Dank et al., 2015; Edinburgh et al., 2015; Hampton & Lieggi, 2017). In terms of bad influences, many trafficked minors were found to have been raised in homes where sex trafficking, crime, or drug use was present (Cobbina & Oselin, 2011; Curtis et al., 2008; Dank et al., 2015; Edinburgh et al., 2015; Hampton & Lieggi, 2017); thus, these children may have more exposure and susceptibility to the world of sex trafficking (McClain & Garrity, 2011).

10.2.1.2 Gaining Access and Isolation

Once the victim is selected, according to the SGM-CST, the sex trafficker will aim to gain access to the child and isolate them from others. Studies have shown that sex traffickers may manipulate their existing relationships with a minor (e.g., family member, friends, romantic partner, acquaintance) to recruit potential victims (Kiensat et al., 2014; Litam, 2017; Miccio-Fonseca, 2017; Williamson & Prior, 2009). In other cases, sex traffickers have searched for victims at vulnerable locations, such as shelters, detention centers, or foster care (Hampton & Lieggi, 2017; Litam, 2017; Roe-Sepowitz, 2019), and many specifically target runaways who may be in need of financial support and housing (Jordan et al., 2013). As noted previously, some cases of sex trafficking involved third parties during the access phase, including using trafficked females to approach and access other minors (e.g., Carpenter & Gates, 2016; Curtis et al., 2008; Dank et al., 2015; Kiensat et al., 2014). With regard to isolation tactics, sex traffickers may aim to emotionally isolate victims from relatives or peers (O'Connor & Healy, 2006) or physically isolate them (e.g., placing them in unfamiliar environments, surveillance; Brayley et al., 2011; Dank et al., 2014; Reid, 2016; Roe-Sepowitz, 2019).

10.2.1.3 Trust Development

The third stage of the SGM describes the process of developing trust with the victims, as is also seen in child sex trafficking. Indeed, studies have shown some of the more effective trafficking tactics revolve around establishing trustworthy relationships with targeted youth (Carpenter & Gates, 2016; Curtis et al., 2008; Kiensat et al., 2014). The sex trafficker may present themselves in a manner that is likable and caring, including feigning romantic interests, showing attention/affection, or appearing of high status or wealth (e.g., Brayley et al., 2011; Dank et al., 2014; Reid, 2016; Roe-Sepowitz, 2019); this may result in a sense of dependency or strong emotional bonds for the victim, especially those who are emotionally or psychologically vulnerable as described in the *victim selection* stage of the SGM. Reid (2016) described a "bait and switch" technique in which traffickers use this kindness (e.g., giving gifts, money, shelter, etc., for "free") as leverage later (e.g., demanding repayment). Moreover, other trust development tactics include glorifying sex work or being befriended by other sex workers and promising the victim they will obtain a prosperous life that includes money and material goods (Dank et al., 2015; Reid, 2016; Roe-Sepowitz, 2019).

10.2.1.4 Desensitization to Sexual Content and Physical Contact

Consistent with the SGM *desensitization* stage, sex trafficking literature has shown that the sex traffickers aim to desensitize the youth to sexual content and physical contact typically in such a way that it gradually escalates over time. Research has described a "breaking-in" phase where the sex trafficker uses increasingly sexual language, such as jokes about sex or prostitution, asks the youth about their sexual experiences or preferences, or shows them pornography (Reid, 2016). Sexual contact is also gradually increased, such as escalating sexual requests and behaviors (e.g., engaging in sexual contact with the new recruit and then encouraging friends to have sexual contact as well; Dank et al., 2014).

10.2.1.5 Post-abuse Maintenance

As with the SGM *post-abuse maintenance* phase, there are strategies a sex trafficker may use to promote future abuse and avoid disclosure/reporting. More so than in cases of child abuse, sex trafficking post-abuse maintenance often involves violence, blackmail, threats, and other overtly coercive tactics to exert continued control over victims (Anderson et al., 2014; Brayley et al., 2011; Cecchet & Thoburn, 2014; Dank et al., 2014; Reid, 2016; Roe-Sepowitz, 2019). For example, several studies showed severe forms of physical abuse (i.e., beatings, burns, physical torture), sexual abuse (e.g., rape), and neglect (i.e., deprivation of food, sleep, and shelter). Other studies have shown ongoing psychological manipulation is used, such as promoting competition between individuals who were trafficked (Dank et al., 2014; Reid, 2016), fostering feelings of connectedness (Reid, 2016), or making the victim feel ashamed, guilty, or worthless (Reid, 2016). A sense of fear might also be induced in that the person being trafficking might worry they were breaking the law and could be punished if they reported.

10.3 Conclusion

In sum, the child sex trafficking literature has been largely isolated from the CSA literature. Indeed, the sex trafficking field uses various terminologies in describing how sex traffickers find, recruit, and maintain their victims, many of which are analogous to the sexual grooming process. Winters et al. (2021) proposed the SGM-CST as a first step in conceptualizing the construct of sexual grooming in the realm of child sex trafficking. However, future research is needed to empirically investigate this model, such as examining real-world cases of victims or sex traffickers as it applies to this model. If empirically supported, this model may be helpful in preventing child sex trafficking by identifying early warning signs before someone is exploited or recognizing cases of exploitation sooner. For example, at-risk youth, caregivers, hospitality workers, health-care providers, and others could benefit from a further understanding of sex trafficker tactics. Law enforcement and courts may also utilize this knowledge as the information can be used to aid investigations (e.g., gathering evidence related to sexual grooming) or inform guilt or sentencing decisions. Moreover, clinicians working with victims could use this model to foster a better understanding of their experiences as a means of reducing guilt and shame, while sex traffickers can gain insight into these behaviors in treatment in order to establish relapse prevention plans. Ultimately, the sex offense and sex trafficking fields would likely benefit from more partnership and collaboration to promote a more thorough understanding of these distinct but similar populations.

References

Adelson, W. (2009). Child prostitute or victim of trafficking? *University of St. Thomas Law Journal, 6*(1), 96–128. https://ir.stthomas.edu/cgi/viewcontent.cgi?article=1178&context=ustlj

Anderson, P. M., Coyle, K. K., Johnson, A., & Denner, J. (2014). An exploratory study of adolescent pimping relationships. *The Journal of Primary Prevention, 35*, 113–117. https://doi.org/10.1007/s10935-014-0338-3

Bales, K., & Lize, S. (2007). Investigating human trafficking: Challenges, lessons learned, and best practices. *FBI Law Enforcement Bulletin, 76*(4), 24–32.

Banks, D., & Kyckelhahn, T. (2011). *Characteristics of suspected human trafficking incidents, 2008–2010*. Bureau of Justice Statistics. https://www.bjs.gov/content/pub/pdf/cshti0810.pdf

Brayley, H., Cockbain, E., & Laycock, G. (2011). The value of crime scripting: Deconstructing internal child sex trafficking. *Policing: A Journal of Policy and Practice, 5*, 132–143. https://doi.org/10.1093/POLICE/PAR024

Carpenter, A., & Gates, J. (2016). *The nature and extent of gang involvement in sex trafficking in San Diego County* (Final Report Grant No.: NIJ-2012-R2-CX-0028 USDOJ). U.S. Department of Justice. https://www.ncjrs.gov/pdffiles1/nij/grants/249857.pdf

Cecchet, S., & Thoburn, J. (2014). The psychological experience of child and adolescent sex trafficking in the United States: Trauma and resilience in survivors. *Psychological Trauma: Theory, Research, Practice, and Policy, 6*(5), 482–493. https://doi.org/10.1037/a0035763

Clawson, H. J., Dutch, N., Solomon, A., & Grace, L. G. (2009). *Human trafficking into and within the United States: A review of the literature*. Office of the Assistant Secretary for Planning and Evaluation. https://aspe.hhs.gov/report/human-trafficking-and-within-united-states-review-literature

Cobbina, J. E., & Oselin, S. S. (2011). It's not only for the money: An analysis of adolescent versus adult entry into street prostitution. *Sociological Inquiry, 81*(3), 310–332. https://doi.org/10.1111/j.1475-682X.2011.00375.x

Crimes Against Children Research Centre. (2008). *How many juveniles are involved in prostitution in the U.S.?* http://www.unh.edu/ccrc/prostitution/Juvenile_Prostitution_factsheet.pdf

Curtis, R., Terry, K., Dank, M., Dombrowski, K., Khan, B., Muslim, A., Labriola, M., & Rempel, M. (2008). *The commercial sexual exploitation of children in New York City*. Center for Court Innovation. https://www.courtinnovation.org/sites/default/files/CSEC_NYC_Executive_Summary.pdf

Dank, M. L., Khan, B., Downey, P. M., Kotonias, C., Mayer, D., Owens, C., Pacifici, L., & Yu, L. (2014). *Estimating the size and structure of the underground commercial sex economy in eight major US cities*. The Urban Institute. https://www.urban.org/research/publication/estimating-size-and-structure-underground-commercial-sex-economy-eight-major-us-cities/view/full_report

Dank, M., Yahner, J., Madden, K., Banuelos, I., Yu, L., Ritchie, M., & Conner, B. (2015). *Surviving the streets of New York: Experiences of LGBTQ youth, YMSM, and YWSW engaged in survival sex*. The Urban Institute. http://www.urban.org/research/publication/surviving-streets-new-york-experiences-lgbtq-youthymsm-and-ywsw-engaged-survival-sex

Duger, A. (2015). Focusing on prevention: The social and economic rights of children vulnerable to sex trafficking. *Health and Human Rights, 17*(1), 114–123. https://dash.harvard.edu/bitstream/handle/1/23586707/Duger.pdf?sequence=1

Edinburgh, L., Pape-Blabolil, J., Harpin, S. B., & Saewyc, E. (2015). Assessing exploitation experiences of girls and boys seen at a child advocacy center. *Child Abuse & Neglect, 46*, 47–59. https://doi.org/10.1016/j.chiabu.2015.04.016

Franchino-Olsen, H. (2019). Vulnerabilities relevant for commercial sexual exploitation of children/domestic minor sex trafficking: A systematic review of risk factors. *Trauma, Violence, & Abuse*, 1–13. https://doi.org/10.1177/1524838018821956

Gerassi, L. (2015). From exploitation to industry-definitions, risks, and consequences of domestic sexual exploitation and sex work among women and girls. *Journal of Human Behavior in the Social Environment, 25*(6), 591–605. https://doi.org/10.1080/10911359.2014.991055

Godoy, S., Sadwick, R., & Baca, K. (2016). *Shedding light on sex trafficking: Research, data, and technologies with the greatest impact*. UCLA Luskin Center for Innovation. https://innovation.luskin.ucla.edu/wp-content/uploads/2019/03/Shedding_Light_on_Sex_Trafficking.pdf

Goodey, J. (2008). Human trafficking: Sketchy data and policy responses. *Criminology & Criminal Justice, 8*(4), 421–442. https://doi.org/10.1177/1748895808096471

Hammond, G. C., & McGlone, M. (2014). Entry, progression, exit, and service provision for survivors of sex trafficking: Implications for effective interventions. *Global Social Welfare, 1*, 157–168. https://doi.org/10.1007/S40609-014-0010-0

Hampton, M. D., & Lieggi, M. (2017). Commercial sexual exploitation of youth in the United States: A qualitative systematic review. *Trauma, Violence, & Abuse, 21*(1), 57–70. https://doi.org/10.1177/1524838017742168

Harris, K. (2012). *The state of human trafficking in California*. State of California Department of Justice Office of the Attorney General. https://oag.ca.gov/sites/all/files/agweb/pdfs/ht/human-trafficking-2012.pdf

Hodge, D. R., & Lietz, C. A. (2007). The international sexual trafficking of women and children: A review of the literature. *Journal of Women and Social Work, 22*, 163–174. https://doi.org/10.1177/0886109907299055

International Labour Organization. (2012). *ILO global estimate of forced labour 2012: Results and methodology*. http://www.ilo.org/global/topics/forced-labour/publications/WCMS_182004/lang–en/index.htm

International Labour Organization. (2017). *Forced labour, modern slavery and human trafficking*. https://www.ilo.org/global/topics/forced-labour/lang%2D%2Den/index.htm

Jones, L., Engstrom, D. W., Hilliard, T., & Diaz, M. (2007). Globalization and human trafficking. *Journal of Sociology & Social Welfare, 34*, 107–122.

Jordan, J., Patel, B., & Rapp, L. (2013). Domestic minor sex trafficking: A social work perspective on misidentification, victims, buyers, traffickers, treatment, and reform of current practice. *Journal of Human Behavior in the Social Environment, 23*, 356–369. https://doi.org/10.1080/10911359.2013.764198

Kennedy, M. A., Klein, C., Bristowe, J., Cooper, B., & Yuille, J. (2007). Routes of recruitment: Pimps' techniques and other circumstances that lead to street prostitution. *Journal of Aggression, Maltreatment & Trauma, 15*(2), 1–19. https://doi.org/10.1300/J146v15n02_01

Kiensat, J., Lakner, M., & Neulet, A. (2014). *Role of female offenders in sex trafficking organizations*. Regional Academy on the United Nations (RAUN). http://www.ra-un.org/uploads/4/7/5/4/47544571/the_role_of_female_offenders_in_sex_trafficking_organizations.pdf

Litam, S. D. A. (2017). Human sex trafficking in America: What counselors need to know. *Professional Counselor, 7*, 45–61. https://doi.org/10.15241/SDAL.7.1.45

Logan, T. K., Walker, R., & Hunt, G. (2009). Understanding human trafficking in the United States. *Trauma, Violence, & Abuse, 10*, 3–30. https://doi.org/10.1177/1524838008327262

Marcus, A., Horning, A., Curtis, R., Sanson, J., & Thompson, E. (2014). Conflict and agency among sex workers and pimps: A closer look at domestic minor sex trafficking. *The ANNALS of the American Academy of Political and Social Science, 653*, 225–246. https://doi.org/10.1177/0002716214521993

McClain, N. M., & Garrity, S. E. (2011). Sex trafficking and the exploitation of adolescents. *Journal of Obstetric, Gynecology, & Neonatal Nursing, 40*, 243–252. https://doi.org/10.1111/j.1552-6909.2011.01221.x

Miccio-Fonseca, L. C. (2017). Juvenile female sex traffickers. *Aggression and Violent Behavior, 35*, 26–32. https://doi.org/10.1016/j.avb.2017.06.001

Miller-Perrin, C., & Wurtele, S. K. (2017). Sex trafficking and the commercial sexual exploitation of children. *Women & Therapy, 40*, 123–151. https://doi.org/10.1080/02703149.2016.1210963

Mitchell, K. J., Finkelhor, D., & Wolak, J. (2010). Conceptualizing juvenile prostitution as child maltreatment: Findings from the National Juvenile Prostitution Study. *Child Maltreatment, 15*, 18–36. https://doi.org/10.1177/1077559509349443

O'Connor, M., & Healy, G. (2006). *The links between prostitution and sex trafficking: A briefing handbook*. Coalition Against Trafficking in Women.

Office on Violence Against Women. (2000). *Victims of trafficking and violence prevention act of 2000*. United States Department of Justice.

Polaris Project. (2013). *Human trafficking trends in the United States: National human trafficking resource center 2007–2012*. https://polarisproject.org/wp-content/uploads/2019/09/Human-Trafficking-Trends-in-the-US-11-21-13.pdf

Rafferty, Y. (2008). The impact of trafficking on children: Psychological and social policy perspectives. *Child Development Perspectives, 2*, 13–18. https://doi.org/10.1111/j.1750-8606.2008.00035.x

Raphael, J., Reichert, J. A., & Powers, M. (2010). Pimp control and violence: Domestic sex trafficking of Chicago women and girls. *Women & Criminal Justice, 20*, 89–104. https://doi.org/10.1080/08974451003641065

Reid, J. A. (2016). Entrapment and enmeshment schemes used by sex traffickers. *Sexual Abuse, 28*, 491–511. https://doi.org/10.1177/1079063214544334

Reid, J. A., Haskell, R. A., Dillahunt-Aspillaga, C., & Thor, J. A. (2013). Trauma bonding and interpersonal violence. In T. Van Leeuwen & M. Brouwer (Eds.), *Psychology of trauma* (pp. 35–62). Nova Science Publishers.

Roe-Sepowitz, D. (2019). A six-year analysis of sex traffickers of minors: Exploring characteristics and sex trafficking patterns. *Journal of Human Behavior in the Social Environment, 29*, 608–629. https://doi.org/10.1080/10911359.2019.1575315

Silverman, J. G., Decker, M. R., McCauley, H. L., & Mack, K. P. (2009). *Sex, trafficking and STI/HIV in Southeast Asia: Connections between sexual exploitation, violence and sexual risk*. UNDP Regional Center. https://www.undp.org/content/dam/undp/library/hivaids/English/SexTrafficking.pdf

Sprang, G., & Cole, J. (2018). Familial sex trafficking of minors: Trafficking conditions, clinical presentation, and system involvement. *Journal of Family Violence, 33*, 185–195. https://doi.org/10.1007/s10896-018-9550-y

Swaner, R., Labriola, M., Rempel, M., Walker, A., & Spadafore, J. (2016). *Youth involvement in the sex trade: A national study*. Center for Court Innovation. https://www.ncjrs.gov/pdffiles1/ojjdp/grants/249952.pdf

Twill, S. E., Green, D. M., & Traylor, A. (2010). A descriptive study on sexually exploited children in residential treatment. *Child & Youth Care Forum, 39*, 187–199. https://doi.org/10.1007/s10566-010-9098-2

Veldhuizen, E., Jeglic, E. L., & Boskovic, I. (2020). Separate routes, similar crimes? Conceptualising differences between domestic and international sex traffickers in the United States. *International Journal of Law, Crime and Justice, 62*(100395). https://doi.org/10.1016/j.ijlcj.2020.100395

Williamson, C., & Prior, M. (2009). Domestic minor sex trafficking: A network of underground players in the Midwest. *Journal of Child and Adolescent Trauma, 2*(1), 46–61. https://doi.org/10.1080/19361520802702191

Winters, G., Jeglic, E., & Kaylor, L. (2020). Validation of the sexual grooming model of child sexual abusers. *Journal of Child Sexual Abuse, 29*(7), 855–875. https://doi.org/10.1080/10538712.2020.180193

Winters, G., Schaaf, S., Grydehoj, R., Allan, C., Lin, A., & Jeglic, E. (2021). The sexual grooming model of child sex trafficking. *Victims & Offenders*. https://doi.org/10.1080/15564886.2021.1926031

Chapter 11
Juveniles and Sexual Grooming

Starting in the 1980s, there was an increased focus on juveniles who engaged in sexually inappropriate and illegal behaviors (Chaffin et al., 2002). This was largely attributed to the 40-fold increase in juveniles placed in sexual offender treatment programs from 1982 to 1992 (Knopp et al., 1992). Indeed, data has shown that over one-third (35.6%) of sexual offenses against minors that were reported to law enforcement were committed by juveniles (Finkelhor et al., 2009). A cascade of federal funding, empirical articles, and policy and practice guidelines has since targeted issues related to juvenile sexual offenses, with the focus primarily being on examining the characteristics of these juveniles, treatment efforts, risk assessment, and reoffending rates (Becker, 1998). One area that has remained neglected in the juvenile sex offense literature is the use of sexual grooming tactics by youth, and it remains largely unclear whether youth may also employ sexual grooming strategies in the perpetration of sexual offenses. To this end, this chapter will provide an overview of juveniles who commit sexual offenses, followed by an examination of the empirical literature and theory related to juvenile sexual grooming.

11.1 Juveniles Who Commit Sexual Offenses Against Minors

There are potentially inappropriate sexual behaviors engaged in by youth that are considered relatively developmentally normative and ultimately not problematic (Association for Treatment of Sexual Abusers [ATSA], 2021). For instance, it is normal for children of a younger age or developmental level to be curious about sexual activity and not fully understand appropriate boundaries. In fact, between 42 and 73% of children engage in some sexual behavior before the age 13 (Kellogg, 2010; Larsson, 2002), including solitary (e.g., masturbation, viewing pornography) or mutual (e.g., kissing, cuddling, showing or touching genitals, inserting objects in genitals/rectum) sexual experiences. The behaviors that are not problematic are

© The Author(s), under exclusive license to Springer Nature Switzerland AG 2022

G. M. Winters, E. L. Jeglic, *Sexual Grooming*,
https://doi.org/10.1007/978-3-031-07222-2_11

generally infrequent, exploratory, voluntary, and spontaneous acts by younger children, either alone or with other children of similar size and age (Friedrich et al., 1992; National Center for Sexual Behavior of Youth, 2021). This might include looking at genitals, touching (without insertion or use of mouth), or masturbation (ATSA, 2021). Conversely, behaviors deemed problematic involve acts that are developmentally inappropriate, may cause harm or distress to the child/youth or others, are repetitive or excessive, or involve coercion, aggression, or force (National Center for Sexual Behavior of Youth, 2021). These atypical behaviors tend to involve children of different ages, sizes, and development levels (e.g., social, emotional). Importantly, some of these problematic behaviors may be illegal in nature, which can result in a minor being charged with a criminal sexual offense.

In general, juveniles who commit sexual offenses are a heterogenous group which is consistent with the adult sexual offense literature (Finkelhor et al., 2009); indeed, these juveniles have different characteristics, backgrounds, motivations, behaviors, and risk factors. There is evidence to suggest that youth who commit sexual offenses may have experienced child sexual abuse (CSA) or maltreatment, including physical abuse, neglect, or witnessing family violence (Kobayashi et al., 1995; Righthand & Welch, 2001; Ryan et al., 1996). Many have a history of family instability, psychiatric problems (e.g., conduct disorder, anxiety, attention deficit hyperactivity disorder), social skills deficits, academic and learning disabilities, or substance use (Center for Sex Offender Management [CSOM], 1999).

There are many motivations for juveniles who commit a sexual offense, such as sexual curiosity, antisocial tendencies, mental health issues, or impulsivity and poor judgment (Becker, 1998; CSOM, 1999; Chaffin, 2005; Hunter et al., 2003). The offenses can include noncontact or contact behaviors, such as creating and sharing pornography of minors, fondling over or under the clothes, gang or date rape, or engaging in oral, anal, or vaginal rape. Regarding details of the offenses, data has suggested that juvenile sexual offenses most often occur in the home (nearly 70%; Finkelhor et al., 2009); although in comparison to adults who commit sexual offenses against minors, juveniles with these types of offenses are more likely to commit them at school and in groups than adults. They are also more likely to have male and younger victims compared to their adult counterparts. See Table 11.1 for a description of the age and sex of juveniles who commit offenses, as well as their relationship to the victim.

Regarding reoffending, one study showed that most juveniles (85–95%) convicted of a sexual offense do not commit a subsequent sexual crime per official records (Finkelhor et al., 2009). Following a review of relevant literature, Lobanov-Rostovsky (2015) reported the sexual recidivism rate likely ranges between 7 and 13% following a 59-month follow-up period depending on the specific study. These rates are lower than those of adults, and the data suggests general recidivism is more likely than sexual recidivism for juveniles who commit a sexual offense.

Table 11.1 Age, sex, and relationship to victim based on Finkelhor et al.'s (2009) findings

Juvenile age	
Younger than 12 years	16%
12–14 years old	38%
15–17 years old	46%
Juvenile sex	
Male	93%
Female	7%
Victim relationship to juvenile	
Family	25%
Acquaintance	63%
Stranger	3%
Other	1%
Unknown	8%

11.1.1 Typologies

There have been numerous proposed typologies of juveniles who commit sexual offenses. Typically, these typologies aim to categorize the juveniles based on age of the victim, history of delinquent behavior, and personality traits.

There are several typologies that focus on the *age of the victim*. Hunter et al. (2000) studied 126 juveniles with sex offenses, including 62 who had offended against prepubescent children and 64 who offended against pubescent (peer) and postpubescent (adult) victims. Those with peer or adult victims, compared to juveniles with prepubescent victims, were more likely to offend against a stranger or acquaintance and offend against a female victim. They were also more likely to commit the offense in public, in a group, or in the context of other criminal activity, and they had more instances of aggression or use of a weapon during the offense. Overall, the group with peer or adult victims tended to have more antisocial and violent tendencies as compared to those who had child victims. In 2003, Hunter et al. found further evidence to support the distinction between these groups in a sample of 206 youth with sexual offenses, which was followed by subsequent research further demonstrating the differences (Daversa & Knight, 2007; Knight & Sims-Knight, 2004; Leroux et al., 2016; Zakireh et al., 2008). Table 11.2 summarizes the findings from the studies comparing juveniles with child versus peer or adult victims.

Of note, some researchers have suggested that the distinction based on victim age is too simplistic. Kemper and Kistner (2010) examined data from 296 male youth with sexual offenses committed to a residential facility. While their findings showed juveniles with peer victims tend to have female acquaintance victims and more general delinquency compared to those with child victims, they did not find

Table 11.2 Juveniles with prepubescent child victims versus juveniles with pubescent and postpubescent victims

Juveniles with prepubescent child victims	Juveniles with pubescent and postpubescent victims
• Greater psychosocial functioning deficits • Fewer aggressive sexual offenses • More likely to have victims who are a relative • More likely to have depression or anxiety • More likely to be submissive, dependent, and isolated • Less sexually experienced • More typical sexual interests • Less general delinquent behaviors	• More likely to use force, violence, and/or weapon • More likely to use of drugs or alcohol during the offense • More likely to have nonrelative victim • More likely to commit offense in the victim's or their own home • More likely to have prior arrests and severe behavioral problems • Less anxiety, depression, and self-esteem deficits • More likely to have a disturbed family situation, caregiver instability, and childhood victimization • More peer-aged friends • More sexual experience (e.g., consensual sex with same-aged peers) • More instances of borderline intellectual functioning • Greater hypersexuality and sexual deviance

Note. Findings summarized from Daversa and Knight (2007), Hunter and Figueredo (2000), Hunter et al. (2003), Joyal et al. (2016), Knight and Sims-Knight (2004), Leroux et al. (2016), and Zakireh et al. (2008)

significant associations between groups for other variables (e.g., social skills, child maltreatment). The authors suggest that victim age may be a proxy for other relevant variables associated with juvenile sexual offending (e.g., physical or emotional development of the victim, such as physical maturity, intellectual functioning, social skills, etc.) and that consideration of both the juvenile's and victim's age may be most useful. Moreover, Miner et al. (2010) studied 156 male youth convicted of a sexual offense and compared groups based on the age of the victim (those with child victims versus adult/peer victims). They found similarities between these groups regarding child maltreatment, antisocial tendencies, psychiatric issues, family history, and risk; the only factors that differentiated the group in the variables examined was hypersexuality and sociosexuality. Thus, they suggest that incorporating criminal history and personality factors in a typology may be beneficial.

Some typologies focus on *juvenile delinquency/crime type* in categorizing juveniles with sexual offenses. Butler and Seto (2002) examined a sample of 32 juveniles with sexual offenses, 48 juveniles who were criminally versatile, and 34 who had nonaggressive offenses. They categorized the juveniles who had sexual offenses as either "sex only" (i.e., they only had a sexual offense) or "sex plus" (i.e., they had a sexual offense and a nonsexual offense). Results showed significant differences between the groups in terms of social, behavioral, and risk variables; that is, the sex-only group had fewer current and childhood behavioral problems, more prosocial

Table 11.3 Juveniles with "sex-only" versus "sex plus" offenses

Sex only	Sex plus
• Fewer conduct problems • More prosocial attitudes • Atypical sexual interests • Deficits in romantic relationships • More likely to have child and male victims • Better current adjustment • Lower risk for delinquency	• Antisocial personality traits • Use drugs • More psychiatric issues • Greater deficits in social skills • More likely to cause physical injury to victim and use weapon • Familial psychiatric and substance abuse history • Living in a single-parent home • Physically abused

Note. Findings summarized from Butler and Seto (2002) and Pullman et al. (2014)

Table 11.4 Worling's (2001) personality-based typology

Antisocial/ impulsive	Unusual/isolated	Overcontrolled/reserved	Confident/ aggressive
• Rule violations and general delinquency • Anxious, unhappy, and rebellious	• Insecure, isolated, and emotionally troubled • Difficulty developing and maintaining healthy relationships	• Hold prosocial attitudes but are cautious in their interactions and keep their emotions inside	• Confident, self-focused, outgoing, aggressive, and sociable

attitudes, and lower risk compared to sex plus. A follow-up study by Pullman et al. (2014) further supported the distinction between these groups. The summary of findings for the two studies are presented in Table 11.3.

A third method of categorizing juvenile sexual offenders is based on *personality traits*. Worling (2001) proposed a personality-based typology based on findings from 112 male adolescents with sexual offenses, which includes four categories: antisocial/impulsive, unusual/isolated, overcontrolled/reserved, and confident/aggressive. See Table 11.4 for a description of the groups. The groups showed differences in terms of history of physical abuse, parental marital status, residence, and criminal charges but not for victim age and gender or history of sexual victimization. The results further demonstrated the antisocial/impulsive and unusual/isolated groups were the riskier groups as they were more likely to commit a future violent or nonviolent offense as compared to the other two groups (overcontrolled/reserved and confident/aggressive).

11.2 Sexual Grooming by Juveniles

To our knowledge, there has been little to no literature specifically addressing sexual grooming tactics that may be used by juveniles who commit sexual offenses. Similar to the adult literature, the research on juveniles with sexual offenses tends to focus on assessment and treatment of this population rather than pre-offense behaviors. According to the United States (US) Department of Justice (Thomas, 1992), differentiating whether a sexual act by a juvenile is a criminal offense can be informed by whether there was (1) a clear power differential between the victim and offender, (2) exploitation, (3) emotional or physical coercion, (4) abusive manipulation or control, and (5) threats of violence. These constructs (e.g., "exploitation," "emotional coercion," "manipulation," "control") seemingly describe the overarching purpose of and strategies for sexually grooming victims, yet the specific term "grooming" has largely been omitted from the literature. Nonetheless, the legal definition of what constitutes a sexual offense by a juvenile suggests that these pre-offense tactics may be used to facilitate the offense process. Thus, in the section below, we discuss what sexual grooming by juveniles may entail through exploration of related constructs, such as coercion, manipulation, and control used prior to the offense.

Winters et al. (n.d.) aimed to explore sexual grooming behaviors used by females, but, coincidentally, the results showed that in 8 of 12 instances of CSA, the females who perpetrated the crimes were juveniles themselves at the time of the offense. The findings showed that based upon victim report, all but one (92%) of the females (most of whom were juveniles) who committed a sexual offense used at least one sexual grooming behavior during the offense (based on the content-validated Sexual Grooming Model [SGM]; Winters et al., 2020). The authors also examined the percentage of victims who reported experiencing at least one behavior for each stage of the SGM, with the majority reporting at least one behavior: *victim selection* (83%), *gaining access and isolation* (67%), *trust development* (83%), *desensitization to sexual content and physical touch* (92%), and *post-abuse maintenance* (83%). Overall, out of the 42 possible sexual grooming behaviors in the SGM, the victims reported an average of 15.8 behaviors overall (range = 0–26), suggesting that sexual grooming was relatively commonly used by females who committed sexual offenses based on the self-report from the victims.

Hogan et al. (2020) presented data from cases of sexual abuse committed by children against other minors. The authors conducted a review of 106 forensic psychosocial evaluations of CSA committed by another minor from a treatment center for children and families involved with child protective services; 82% of the reports were evaluations of victims, and 18% were evaluations of the juvenile who committed the sexual behavior. The authors reported age of the juvenile who committed the offense in terms of those who were younger than 12 (n = 29; 27%) or older than 12 (n = 77; 66%). The files were coded for themes that reflected potential sexual grooming behaviors: manipulation, boundary violations, and inducements. The results showed that seven cases (6.6%) described positive emotional manipulation tactics (e.g., compliments, special attention), while negative emotional manipulation (e.g., name-calling, isolation, threats) was used in one-third of cases (n = 35; 33%). Boundary violations, such as gradually increasing touch or talking about sexual topics, were found in one-quarter of cases (n = 27; 25.5%). Lastly, inducements (e.g., gifts, special privileges) were used in 22% (n = 23) of the cases. The authors concluded that sexual grooming behaviors may be used by youth who commit child sexual offenses although it remains unclear if they are implemented the same way as adults who commit sexual abuse.

Although not described as "sexual grooming" per se, Leclerc et al. (2008) conducted a study on the "modus operandi" (MO) of adolescents who commit sexual offenses against children. Using the Modus Operandi Questionnaire (MOQ; Kaufman, 1994; see Chap. 13 for a description of the measure), they gathered self-report data from 103 adolescents (age 13–17) who had victims younger than age 12. They were interested in examining the following strategies: gaining trust (e.g., love, attention, and gifts; reported in 88% of cases), gaining cooperation (e.g., desensitizing the victim; reported in 85% of cases), gifts and privileges (reported in 44% of cases), maintaining silence (e.g., emotional blackmail; reported in 52% of cases), and violent behavior (reported in 20% of cases). The aim was to explore how situational factors (e.g., location of crime, victim-offender relationship, deviant sexual interests) were related to MO. The authors report the most frequently used strategies included providing love, attention, or gifts (88%) and desensitization to sexual contact (85%). The authors found that location had an important impact of which MO strategies were used; for example, the adolescents used gaining cooperation strategies in "less risky" locations (e.g., where someone is unlikely to interfere) and used emotional blackmail in their own home. When examining the relationship between the juvenile and victim, they found gift giving and privileges was more commonly used by those who had either intrafamilial or extrafamilial victims compared to juveniles who had both types of victims. The findings also showed that juveniles with deviant sexual interests were more likely to adopt MO strategies, and used more varied behaviors, compared to those who did not. Overall, the data suggested that juveniles may use sexual grooming-type strategies in the offense process, which may be differentially used depending on certain situational factors.

Other research has explored the strategies used by juveniles to manipulate or pressure a victim into sexual contact. A multi-wave longitudinal survey examining the impact of media on adolescents' behavior was conducted from 2006 through 2012, which included questions regarding self-reported sexual violence. Ybarra and Mitchell (2013) reported that 9% of the 1,058 youths (aged 10 to 15 at recruitment) in the sample endorsed having perpetrated sexual violence during their lifetime (i.e., coercive and forced sexual behavior). These behaviors included forced sexual contact (i.e., kissed, touched, or other sexual contact when the other individual did not consent; 8%), coercive sexual contact (i.e., pressuring someone to "give in" to sex when they did not want to; 3%), attempted rape (3%), and completed rape (2%). Relevant to sexual grooming, the youths were asked about the tactics used in the attempted or completed forced sex. The results showed the most common tactic was getting angry and making the person feel guilty (63%), followed by arguing or pressuring the person (32%) and the use of alcohol (15%). Few reported using threats (5%) or physical force (8%), which is consistent with findings from the sexual grooming literature. Approximately three in four of the victims were the romantic partner of the perpetrator, suggesting that these coercive behaviors are often used by those known to the victim.

There are a few hypotheses about juvenile sexual grooming that can be derived from the literature. The typologies of *juveniles who offend against peer and adult victims* possess particular traits and characteristics that suggests they may be more apt to use sexual grooming strategies. They are more likely to have nonrelative victims and, thus, may be likely to use *victim selection* or *gaining access and isolation* tactics. They also exhibit more antisocial tendencies and sexual deviance, which may result in increased use of manipulative tactics consistent with sexual grooming. Of note, however, this group is also more likely to be aggressive and use a weapon, which is not necessarily consistent with sexual grooming. Thus, it may be that a particular subgroup of this typology, those who are more psychologically and emotionally manipulative, that would utilize sexual grooming tactics. Another hypothesis is that the *confident/aggressive typology* of juveniles who commit sexual offenses may be more apt to use sexual grooming. This group is described as confident, self-focused, outgoing, and sociable as compared to the other groups who are less socially adept. Therefore, it may be that this group might use the interpersonal tactics consistent with sexual grooming in an offense process. Further research is needed to explore what types of juveniles may use sexual grooming tactics in their offense.

11.3 Conclusion

Research has shown that nearly one-third of sexual offenses are committed by juveniles, yet there is little research on the behaviors leading up to these offenses. Very few empirical studies have explored the tactics and strategies that a juvenile might use in preparation for committing a sexual offense, but of the little data we have, it suggests that juveniles may in fact use sexual grooming similar to their adult counterparts. In general, research is needed to identify whether, and to what extent, juveniles are using sexual grooming in the offense process. This may help inform not only treatment strategies for juveniles with sex offenses but also educate people on how to better identify strategies that might be used by juveniles before the offense occurs. Further research is also needed to explore whether there are particular types of juveniles who will use these behaviors, such as the juvenile typologies identified in prior literature (e.g., typologies based on age, crime type, etc.). This can shed light on whether there are particular subgroups of juveniles who commit sexual offenses who may be more likely to use sexual grooming and whether there are group differences on the types of behaviors utilized. Another proposed line of research is comparing the sexual grooming patterns of juveniles with those identified by adults who commit sexual offenses (as outlined in the SGM). It is possible that there may be distinct differences between what behaviors are used, the number of behaviors used, and the length of time spent sexual grooming; this can better inform treatment providers on unique treatment targets for juvenile versus adults who commit sexual offenses. Overall, while the research remains scarce, it is recommended that prevention and treatment efforts incorporate the construct of sexual grooming to ensure that any of these "red flag," preparatory behaviors are identified before the abuse. Additional vigilance to potentially inappropriate behaviors by youth can result in earlier intervention and potential prevention of the sexual abuse of a minor.

References

Association for Treatment of Sexual Abusers. (2021). *Fast facts about children who display problematic sexual behaviors.*. https://www.atsa.com/fast-facts-about-children-who-display-problematic-sexual-behaviors

Becker, J. V. (1998). What we know about the characteristics and treatment of adolescents who have committed sexual offenses. *Child Maltreatment, 3*, 317–329. https://doi.org/10.1177/1077559598003004004

Butler, S. M., & Seto, M. C. (2002). Distinguishing two types of adolescent sex offenders. *Journal of the American Academy of Child and Adolescent Psychiatry, 41*(1), 83–90. https://doi.org/10.1097/00004583-200201000-00015

Center for Sex Offender Management [CSOM]. (1999). *Understanding juvenile sexual offending behavior: Emerging research, treatment approaches and management practices*. Center for Effective Public Policy.

Chaffin, M. (2005). Can we develop evidence-based practice for adolescent sex offenders? In R. E. Longo & D. Prescott (Eds.), *Current perspectives. Working with sexually aggressive youth and youth with sexual behavior problems* (pp. 119–141). NEARI Press.

Chaffin, M., Letourneau, E., & Silovsky, J. F. (2002). Adults, adolescents, and children who sexually abuse children: A developmental perspective. In J. E. B. Myers, L. Berliner, J. Briere, C. T. Hendrix, C. Jenny, & T. A. Reid (Eds.), *The APSAC handbook on child maltreatment* (2nd ed., pp. 205–232). Sage.

Daversa, M. T., & Knight, R. A. (2007). A structural examination of the predictors of sexual coercion against children in adolescent sexual offenders. *Criminal Justice and Behavior, 34*(10), 1313–1333. https://doi.org/10.1177/0093854807302411

Finkelhor, D., Ormrod, R., & Chaffin, M. (2009). *Juveniles who commit sexual offenses*. Office of Justice Programs. https://www.ojp.gov/pdffiles1/ojjdp/227763.pdf

Friedrich, W. N., Grambsch, P., Broughton, D., Kuiper, J., & Beilke, R. L. (1992). Normative sexual behavior in children. *Journal of the American Academy of Child & Adolescent Psychiatry, 31*(2), 203. https://doi.org/10.1542/peds.101.4.e9

Hogan, C., Byrnes, K., & Zottoli, T. (2020). *Grooming behaviors in child-on-child sexual abuse cases*. Poster presented at the American Psychology-Law Society, New Orleans, Louisiana.

Hunter, J. A., & Figueredo, A. J. (2000). The influence of personality and history of sexual victimization in the prediction of juvenile perpetrated child molestation. *Behavior Modification, 24*(2), 241–263. https://doi.org/10.1177/0145445500242005

Hunter, J. A., Hazelwood, R. R., & Slesinger, D. (2000). Juvenile perpetrated sex crimes: Patterns of offending and predictors of violence. *Journal of Family Violence, 15*(1), 81–93. https://doi.org/10.1023/A:1007553504805

Hunter, J. A., Figueredo, A. J., Malamuth, N. M., & Becker, J. (2003). Juvenile sex offenders: Toward the development of a typology. *Sexual Abuse: A Journal of Research and Treatment, 15(1)*, 27–48. https://doi.org/10.1023/A:1020663723593

Joyal, C. C., Carpentier, J., & Martin, C. (2016). Discriminant factors for adolescent sexual offending: On the usefulness of considering both victim age and sibling incest. *Child Abuse & Neglect, 54*, 10–10. https://doi.org/10.1016/j.chiabu.2016.01.006

Kaufman, K. L. (1994). *Modus operandi questionnaire* (Rev ed.). Author (Children's Hospital).

Kellogg, N. D. (2010). Sexual behaviors in children: Evaluation and management. *American Family Physician, 82*(10), 1233–1238.

Kemper, T. S., & Kistner, J. A. (2010). An evaluation of classification criteria for juvenile sex offenders. *Sexual Abuse: A Journal of Research and Treatment, 22*(2), 172–190. https://doi.org/10.1177/1079063210366270

Knight, R. A., & Sims-Knight, J. E. (2004). Testing an etiological model for male juvenile sexual offending against females. *Journal of Child Sexual Abuse, 13*(3-4), 33–55. https://doi.org/10.1300/j070v13n03_03

Knopp, F. H., Freeman-Longo, R., & Stevenson, W. F. (1992). *Nationwide survey of juvenile and adult sex-offender treatment programs and models.* The Safer Society Press.

Kobayashi, J., Sales, B. D., Becker, J. V., Figueredo, A. J., & Kaplan, M. S. (1995). Perceived parental deviance, parent-child bonding, child abuse, and child sexual aggression. *Sexual Abuse: A Journal of Research and Treatment, 7*(1), 25–44. https://doi.org/10.1177/107906329500700105

Larsson, I. B. (2002). Sexual experiences in childhood: Young adults' recollections. *Archives of Sexual Behavior, 31*(3), 263–273. https://doi.org/10.1023/a:101525903931

Leclerc, B., Beauregard, E., & Proulx, J. (2008). Modus operandi and situational aspects in adolescent sexual offenses against children. *International Journal of Offender Therapy and Comparative Criminology, 52*(1), 46–61. https://doi.org/10.1177/0306624X07300271

Leroux, E. J., Pullman, L. E., Motayne, G., & Seto, M. C. (2016). Victim age and the generalist versus specialist distinction in adolescent sexual offending. *Sexual Abuse: A Journal of Research and Treatment, 28*(2), 79–95. https://doi.org/10.1177/1079063214535814

Lobanov-Rostovsky, C. (2015). *Adult sex offender management.* U.S. Department of Justice. https://smart.ojp.gov/sites/g/files/xyckuh231/files/media/document/adultsexoffendermanagement.pdf

Miner, M. H., Robinson, B. E., Knight, R. A., Berg, D., Swinburne Romine, R., & Netland, J. (2010). Understanding sexual perpetration against children: Effects of attachment style, interpersonal involvement, and hypersexuality. *Sexual Abuse, 22*(1), 58–77. https://doi.org/10.1177/1079063209353183

National Center for the Sexual Behavior of Youth. (2021). *Sexual behavior: Typical or problematic?*. https://ncsby.org/content/sexual-behavior-typical-or-problematic

National Center for the Sexual Behavior of Youth, Center for Sex Offender Management [CSOM], & U.S. Department of Justice, Office of Juvenile Justice and Delinquency Prevention. (2001). *Juveniles who have sexually offended; A review of the professional literature report.* http://www.ojjdp.ncjrs.org/

Pullman, L. E., Leroux, E. J., Motayne, G., & Seto, M. C. (2014). Examining the developmental trajectories of adolescent sexual offenders. *Child Abuse & Neglect, 38*(7), 1249–1249. https://doi.org/10.1016/j.chiabu.2014.03.003

Righthand, S., & Welch, C. (2001). *Juveniles who have sexually offended a review of the professional literature.* U.S. Department of Justice. https://www.ojp.gov/pdffiles1/ojjdp/184739.pdf

Ryan, G., Miyoshi, T. J., Metzner, J. L., Krugman, R. D., & Fryer, G. E. (1996). Trends in a national sample of sexually abusive youths. *Journal of the American Academy of Child and Adolescent Psychiatry, 35*(1), 17–17. https://doi.org/10.1097/00004583-199601000-00008

Thomas, D. W. (1992). *A special report on juvenile sex offenders.* U.S. Department of Justice. https://www.ojp.gov/pdffiles1/Digitization/141661NCJRS.pdf

Winters, G. M., Jeglic, E. L., & Kaylor, L. E. (2020). Validation of the sexual grooming model of child sexual abusers. *Journal of Child Sexual Abuse: Research, Treatment, & Program Innovations for Victims, Survivors, & Offenders.* https://doi.org/10.1080/10538712.2020.1801935

Winters, G., Jeglic, E., & Kaylor, L. (n.d.). *Victims' perspectives of sexual grooming behaviors of females who commit child sexual abuse.* (in submission).

Worling, J. R. (2001). Personality-based typology of adolescent male sexual offenders: Differences in recidivism rates, victim-selection characteristics, and personal victimization histories. *Sexual Abuse: A Journal of Research and Treatment, 13*(3), 149–166. https://doi.org/10.1023/A:1009518532101

Ybarra, M. L., & Mitchell, K. J. (2013). Prevalence rates of male and female sexual violence perpetrators in a national sample of adolescents. *Jama Pediatrics, 167*(12), 1125–1134. https://doi.org/10.1001/jamapediatrics.2013.2629

Zakireh, B., Ronis, S. T., & Knight, R. A. (2008). Individual beliefs, attitudes, and victimization histories of male juvenile sexual offenders. *Sexual Abuse: A Journal of Research and Treatment, 20*(3), 323–351. https://doi.org/10.1177/1079063208322424

Chapter 12
Adults and Sexual Grooming

The term sexual grooming has been used in the research literature to describe only the behaviors used by those who perpetrate sexual abuse against minors. While the majority of research has focused on child sexual abuse (CSA) perpetrated against younger children, more recent data suggests that sexual grooming strategies and tactics are also used in the perpetration of CSA among adolescents (Winters & Jeglic, 2021). However, in recent years, the term sexual grooming has also been used in popular media to describe sexually and emotionally abusive behaviors directed toward adults. For example, the actress Rachel Evan Wood alleged that her former husband, Brian Warner, known to most by his stage name Marilyn Manson, groomed her and sexually abused her for years (Grow & Newman, 2021). Also, *Zoey 101* star Alexa Nikolas alleged that her ex-husband Michael Milosh sexually groomed her for years (Blistein, 2021). To our knowledge, there is no empirical research on adult sexual grooming, and the only reference in the academic literature to adult sexual grooming is by Grant Sinnamon in 2017 wherein he proposed a model of adult sexual grooming. However, research has discovered parallel phenomena and processes that have been identified as contributing to the emotional, physical, and sexual abuse of adults, including sexual harassment, sexual coercion, coercive control, and "catfishing," that may all have bearing on adult sexual grooming. As such, this largely exploratory chapter will begin by examining what we know about adult abuse, a description of Sinnamon's Seven-Stage Model of Adult Sexual Grooming, a review of how adult sexual grooming has been defined in the popular media, and an examination of the literature on related constructs to understand how these behaviors may be indicative of adult sexual grooming. We will conclude with some proposals for future research to better understand whether the tactics and strategies used to perpetrate sexually abusive behaviors against adults constitute sexual grooming.

© The Author(s), under exclusive license to Springer Nature Switzerland AG 2022

G. M. Winters, E. L. Jeglic, *Sexual Grooming*,
https://doi.org/10.1007/978-3-031-07222-2_12

12.1 What We Know About Adult Sexual Abuse

Similar to CSA, adult sexual abuse is most often perpetrated by someone known to the victim. According to the Department of Justice 2010–2016 National Crime Victimization Survey (2017), only 19.5% of adult sexual assaults (rapes) are committed by a stranger, with the largest portion (39%) being perpetrated by an acquaintance, followed by a current or former intimate partner (33%). However, the majority of research focusing on the behaviors and tactics, or the modus operandi, used by those who perpetrate sex crimes against adults has typically focused on cases involving stranger rape or multiple detected sexual assaults and individuals who were convicted for the offense (see Beauregard et al., 2007). Yet most adult sexual assaults are not reported to authorities, or if they are, few are prosecuted with even fewer resulting in conviction (RAINN, n.d.). In 2019, only 34% of rape/sexual assault cases were formally reported to authorities (Morgan & Truman, 2020). Further, survivors of sexual violence are less likely to report, or are delayed in reporting, the crime to law enforcement if the perpetrator was known to them, especially if they were a family member (Jones et al., 2009; McCall-Hosenfeld et al., 2009; Monroe et al., 2005).

Those who perpetrate adult sexual assault have reported that they select those they offend against because they are vulnerable or "easy prey" (Stevens, 1994). This vulnerability may include a lack of guardianship or mental illness (Creighton & Jones, 2012; Rebocho & Goncalves, 2012). Alcohol use by both parties is also more common in the sexual abuse of adults than children (Kirk-Provencher et al., 2021). These common strategies may overlap with sexual grooming strategies such as *victim selection* (e.g., vulnerable victim), *gaining access and isolation* (e.g., lack of guardianship), and *trust development* (e.g., provision of alcohol).

12.2 Sinnamon's Seven-Stage Model of Adult Sexual Grooming

The only description in the literature of adult sexual grooming comes from a chapter written by Grant Sinnamon in 2017 in which he proposes his model of adult sexual grooming. Sinnamon states that his model, "while having some application in the description of child sexual grooming, has been developed to explain the specific character of predatory sexual behavior involving and targeting of vulnerable adults, the engagement in the preparatory processes characterized as grooming, and the instigation and maintenance of sexually exploitative and abusive relationships with adult victims by sexual predators" (p. 460). While it is not clear how Sinnamon derived his model, he indicated that the adult grooming literature is hampered by low reporting rates by victims. He also points out, importantly, that the study of adult sexual grooming can be challenging as the victims are adults, so it is difficult to tease apart which behaviors are illegal as opposed to immoral or unethical. The stages of Sinnamon's Adult Sexual Grooming Model are depicted below in Fig. 12.1.

What is clear from Sinnamon's model is that his seven stages directly mirror the five stages of the Sexual Grooming Model (SGM; Winters et al., 2020) for child sexual grooming (see Table 12.1 below) except that in the SGM, the actual perpetration of the abuse (Stage 6: Instigate) is not conceptualized as a separate stage.

Further, Sinnamon's description of the behaviors used in the adult grooming process is almost identical to those identified in the SGM and subsequently assessed using the *Sexual Grooming Scale-Victim Version* (SGS-V; Winters & Jeglic, 2021; see Chap. 13). This suggests that adult sexual grooming may also follow the same (or at least similar) trajectory as child sexual grooming and may be able to be explained using the SGM. It is not clear how Sinnamon derived his stages or behaviors as there were few references in the chapter. If indeed his conceptualization is valid (and this must be determined empirically first), then the SGM framework may also be applicable to adult sexual grooming. As will be discussed in the future research section below, this opens numerous new avenues for further exploration.

12.3 Popular Media Definitions of Adult Sexual Grooming

While there appears to be no consensus on a definition of adult sexual grooming, the existing definitions in the popular media reflect themes of manipulation, dominance, and control (see Table 12.2). Sinnamon (2017) defines adult sexual grooming as:

> ...any situation in which an adult is primed to permit themselves to be abused and/or exploited for sexual gratification of another. (Sinnamon, 2017, p. 462)

The popular cultural definitions of adult sexual grooming suggest that it is a predatory process that is similar to child sexual grooming. There is emphasis on the emotional manipulation that takes place over time and involves various strategies and/or stages including developing a friendship/emotional connection with a potentially vulnerable individual to gain their trust, an effort to separate or isolate them from others, and a gradual onset of abusive behaviors such that the abused adult often does not recognize the abuse before it actually occurs. These popular media definitions of adult sexual grooming appear to overlap significantly with the behaviors, tactics, stages, and themes described in the child sexual grooming literature.

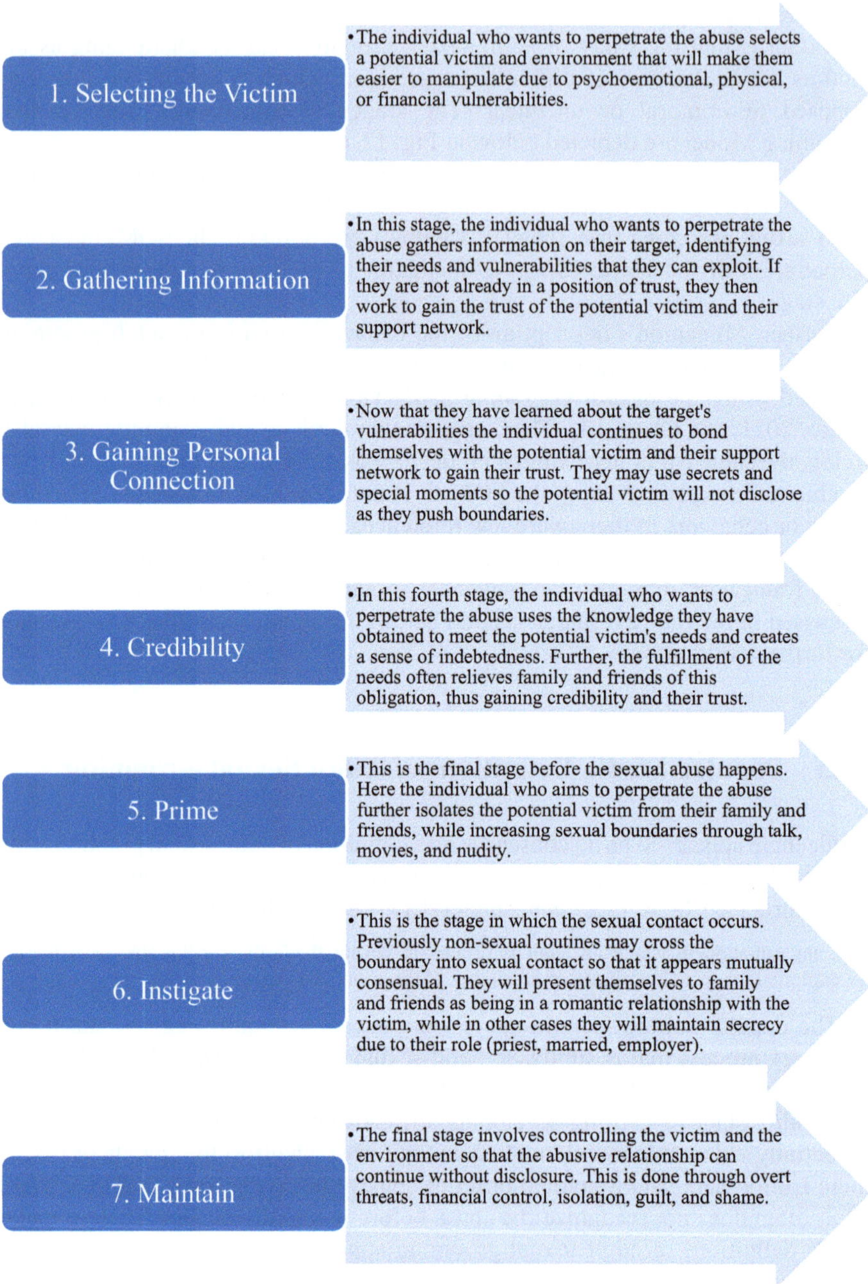

Fig. 12.1 Sinnamon's Seven-Stage Model of Adult Sexual Grooming

Table 12.1 Comparison of SGM and Sinnamon's Seven-Stage Model of Adult Sexual Grooming

SGM stage	Corresponding stage in Sinnamon's Seven-Stage Model of Adult Sexual Grooming
Victim selection	Selecting the victim
Gaining access and isolation	Plan
Trust development	Trust and credibility
Desensitization to sexual content and physical contact	Prime
Post-abuse maintenance behaviors	Maintain

12.4 Related Constructs

There are several constructs that have been discussed in the adult sexual abuse literature that may be related to, or potentially even analogous to, adult sexual grooming, including sexual harassment, sexual coercion, coercive control, and "catfishing," as described below.

12.4.1 Sexual Harassment

The United States (US) Equal Opportunity Commission (EEOC, n.d.) defines sexual harassment as "a form of sex discrimination that violates Title VII of the Civil Rights Act of 1964." According to the EEOC, sexual harassment comprises:

> Unwelcome sexual advances, requests for sexual favors, and other verbal or physical conduct of a sexual nature constitutes sexual harassment when submission to or rejection of this conduct explicitly or implicitly affects an individual's employment, unreasonably interferes with an individual's work performance or creates an intimidating, hostile or offensive work environment.

This definition of sexual harassment describes some behaviors that may overlap with sexual grooming, such as sexual comments, physical touching, and threats/intimidation. Some researchers have developed measures to assess sexual harassment behaviors such as the *Sexual Harassment Inventory* (*SHI*; Murdoch & McGovern, 1998), which was developed and validated by using focus groups, a review of the literature, court cases, and samples of college students, female veterans, and Veterans Affairs Equal Opportunity officers. As is evidenced in the *SHI* (see Table 12.3 for list of items), the items shaded in gray reflect the behaviors in SGM *desensitization to sexual content and physical contact* stage (Winters et al., 2020), such as inappropriate sexual language/jokes, showing pornographic images, exposing their naked body, and increasing sexual touching. As sexual harassment is a manipulative process with the desired goal of gaining sexual relations with a non-consenting adult, there is arguably considerable overlap with the tactics and behaviors used in child sexual grooming.

Table 12.2 Popular media definitions of adult sexual grooming

Popular media definitions	Website
It's a gradual process. The abuser picks their target, build up trust, and the actual abuse, which is usually sexual or financial, doesn't come until much later. It often starts with friendship. The groomer will look for ways to gain their target's trust, often with gifts or promises. Eventually they'll start to ask for something in return, and this eventually leads to abuse. Because groomers work to befriend their victims, some organisations refer to it as "mate crime".	https://www.anncrafttrust.org/signs-of-grooming-in-adults-what-to-watch-out-for/
Similar to child grooming, grooming in adult relationships are all about control and dominance. Grooming is a form of manipulation that is often extremely difficult to spot when a person doesn't know what to look for. Grooming is meant to feel good in the beginning, ensuring the person being groomed has no idea they are being primed for abuse. First, the groomer will attempt to build a friendship or emotional connection with a potential partner that will appear safe and genuine. As time goes on and connection and intimacy builds, the groomer will be slowly and covertly manipulating the victim of grooming to be dependent on them. Maybe the groomer has convinced their partner to open a joint bank account that only the groomer has control over. Perhaps the groomer has been convincing their partner that their support network is actually toxic and that the groomer is the only person who truly cares about them. These tactics may seem obvious, except to someone in the throes of covertly abusive relationship. Once a person realizes they are in a relationship in which they were manipulated, the groomer has likely already done significant damage to their partner's life. If the groomer has been successful with their covertly abusive behaviors, they will have isolated their partner from their support network, instilled a sense of physical, financial, and/or emotional dependence, and manipulated their partner to get what they want, sexually, emotionally, and otherwise.	https://www.modernintimacy.com/understanding-grooming-in-adult-relationships/
Grooming is the predatory act of maneuvering another individual into a position that makes them more isolated, dependent, likely to trust, and more vulnerable to abusive behaviour. The goal is to prepare the other person for abuse (for example, sexual or financial) later. Therefore, the first step the groomer takes is to establish friendship and trust. Adult grooming is correspondent to child grooming and applies to any situation where an adult is primed to allow him or herself to be exploited or abused. It happens online and in real life.	https://www.mobieg.co.za/abuse/adult-grooming/

(continued)

Table 12.2 (continued)

Popular media definitions	Website
Adult grooming is the adult equivalent to child grooming and applies to any behaviour where an adult is prepared so they unwittingly allow abusive behaviour or exploitation to occur later. The abuser typically befriends or builds a relationship with the victim in order to establish a relationship of trust. Well known examples of such abusive behaviours are sexual abuse, elder abuse, financial extortion, human trafficking and sexual slavery. Although it is a common belief that grooming is most relevant to children, the same or similar psychological processes are used to exploit adults. As with child grooming, adult grooming typically involves: Positive reinforcement (gifts, money, praise, superficial charm, flattery, smiling, etc.) Normalization	https://psychology.wikia.org/wiki/Adult_grooming
When an individual (groomer), or group of people ("Grooming gangs"), builds an emotional connection with someone they've targeted to earn trust with the purpose of exploitation for their own motives: sexual abuse, financial, power kicks, even trafficking.	https://caage.org/what-is-adult-grooming/

Table 12.3 Items in the Sexual Harassment Inventory

SHI item
Sexual comments about body (coworkers)
Demeaning comments (coworkers)
Sexual leering
Sexual jokes
Catcalls or sexual remarks
Uncomfortable touching
Sexual comments about body (supervisor)
Unwanted requests for dates (coworkers)
Provocative posters displayed
Unpleasant assignments given because of gender
Threatened to block promotion unless agreed to sex
Threatened to block favorable assignment or transfer prevented because sex refused
Offered favorable assignments in exchange for sex
Unwanted requests for dates (supervisor)
Forced to have sex without consent
Attempted to have sex without consent (coworkers)
Attempted to have sex without consent (supervisor)
Exposed themselves/supervisor

12.4.2 Sexual Coercion

Sexual coercion has been defined as the use of nonphysical strategies and tactics to engage in sexual contact with a nonconsenting individual (DeGue & DiLillo, 2004). Such coercive tactics can include the use of pressure, guilt, shame, badgering, lies, verbal threats, emotional blackmail, ignoring of requests to cease sexual activity, and the use of alcohol and/or drugs to lower inhibitions (DeGue & DiLillo, 2004). It is estimated that between 25% and 33% of all college-aged men have used sexual coercion since age 14 (Abbey et al., 1998, 2001; Koss et al., 1987; Loh et al., 2005). One study of 304 college men found that almost one-third (31.9%) used sexual coercion to obtain sexual contact with a nonconsenting partner. Of those, 86.4% of men reported pretending to care more for the woman than they did, 24.7% reported using verbal threats, 18.5% used continual arguments, and 2.5% threatened to end the relationship. Also, of those who reported using sexual coercion, one-third reported using more than one sexually coercive behavior to obtain sexual contact. While these more aggressive manipulative strategies, such as threats and blackmail, are generally seen post-abuse in child sexual grooming, there is some overlap with the use of feigned affection and the use of substances in the trust development stage of the SGM. Thus, it is possible that sexual coercion may be a facet or manifestation of adult sexual grooming or that it may be that sexual coercion is a separate construct and used in different types of adult sexual abuse.

12.4.3 Coercive Control

The term coercive control was coined by Stark (2006, 2007) to refer to the ongoing tactics and behaviors used by those who perpetrate abuse to restrict a victim's decision-making by preventing their liberty, autonomy, and equality. Consequently, this creates a power imbalance in the relationship that is exploited by the abusive individual. Coercive control was originally conceptualized in the context of intimate partner violence, but subsequently, it has also been applied to any relationship in which one party exploits the vulnerabilities of another in an effort to control them, including sexual violence (Mitchell & Raghavan, 2021). While there is overlap with sexual coercion, these coercive control strategies appear to be more geared toward the maintenance of control in the relationship once the abuse has already happened, whereas sexual coercion is often used to initially instigate the abuse when the individual does not consent.

Recently, Mitchell and Raghavan (2021) conducted a study wherein they examined the relationship between coercive control and sexual coercion, in which an individual is pressured into unwanted sexual activity using nonviolent means such as the absence of consent, resistance, or compliance resulting from threats (Raghavan et al., 2014). Using a sample of 136 men who were attending domestic violence programs for engaging in relationship aggression, they found that those men who used coercive control in their relationships were also likely to use sexually coercive tactics including inducing helplessness, hopelessness, using exploitation, pressure, humiliation and intimidation, relational threats, and bullying. Many of these strategies overlap with those observed in the *post-abuse maintenance* stage of the SGM, and as such, coercive control may be used in sexual grooming to maintain the victim in the abusive situation and prevent escape and detection.

12.4.4 Online Adult Sexual Grooming – Catfishing

There is reference in the popular literature that, similar to child sexual grooming, adult sexual grooming can take place either in person or online. The online sexual grooming of adults has also been referenced as "catfishing," which generally refers to the process of luring someone into a relationship online by using a false persona. In 2013, it was estimated that 5% of all social media accounts were fake and that number is increasing exponentially (D'Onfro, 2013). While there is little empirical research on catfishing, the purpose of the falsely represented relationship appears to have multiple different goals, including financial fraud, playing a hoax on an individual, and in some cases sexual abuse. In cases where sexual abuse is involved, it appears that the goals are the same as the online sexual grooming of children: to get photos, videos, or in-person sexual contact. However, unlike children, adults can consent to these sexual activities. So in adult sexual abuse, the sexual grooming process comes into play as victims are often looking for a consensual relationship with another adult online. However, the person engaging in catfishing manipulates the adult's trust and vulnerability because they are not who they claim to be. As such, due to the nefarious intent of the individual engaging in catfishing, any sexual behaviors are no longer consensual as the victim has been manipulated and deceived (catchthecatfish.com). While the behaviors and tactics of sexually abusive catfishing have not yet been well documented, the goals of manipulating someone into sexual behavior under false pretenses is analogous to the goals of sexual grooming.

12.5 Conclusion

As highlighted in this chapter, there is no empirical research or theoretical literature on adult sexual grooming. However, this chapter also underscores that the majority of sexual abuse against adults is perpetrated by someone known to them and that many sexually abusive relationships exhibit evidence of manipulation and control that gradually escalate over time in order to prevent detection or escape. Many of these strategies and tactics could be understood through the lens of sexual grooming. So while it would be premature to conclude that adult sexual grooming is a valid construct, there are preliminary indicators to suggest that sexual grooming behaviors and tactics are used in at least some sexually abusive behaviors directed toward adults.

There are a few parallel lines of research that are needed. First, since adult sexual abuse has not been examined through the lens of sexual grooming, it would be important to use an inductive approach (i.e., working from the bottom up). Qualitative interviews with survivors of adult sexual abuse about the strategies and tactics that were used can help to yield themes pertaining to the methods and behaviors employed by those who perpetrate adult sexual abuse in the context of a relationship (friend/partner/acquaintance as opposed to stranger rape). Simultaneously, a meta-synthesis of the adult sexual assault literature should be conducted to develop a list of tactics and behaviors that have been described in the research literature. Together, these will form the foundation for the next stage of research wherein these tactics, behaviors, and strategies will be assessed quantitively (i.e., were they present or not) in a large general population sample of adults who have experienced nonstranger sexual abuse as adults and subsequently analyzed to determine which behaviors may fall together. These findings may then be interpreted in light of existing literature on sexual grooming and adult sexual abuse to form a model of adult sexual grooming, which could then be validated empirically.

References

Abbey, A., McAuslan, P., & Ross, L. T. (1998). Sexual assault perpetration by college men: The role of alcohol, misperception of sexual intent, and sexual beliefs and experiences. *Journal of Social and Clinical Psychology, 17*(2), 167–195. https://doi.org/10.1521/jscp.1998.17.2.167

Abbey, A., Zawacki, T., Buck, P. O., Clinton, A. M., & McAuslan, P. (2001). Alcohol and sexual assault. *Alcohol, Research & Health, 25*, 43–51.

Beauregard, E., Proulx, J., Rossmo, K., Leclerc, B., & Allaire, J. F. (2007). Script analysis of the hunting process of serial sex offenders. *Criminal Justice and Behavior, 34*(8), 1069–1084. https://doi.org/10.1177/0093854807300851

Blistein, J. (2021, August 25). Rhye's Michael Milosh hit with suit over alleged abuse, grooming of Alexa Nikolas. *Rolling Stone*. https://www.rollingstone.com/music/music-news/rhye-michael-milosh-complaint-alexa-nikolas-abuse-allegations-1216945/

Creighton, C. D., & Jones, A. C. (2012). Psychological profiles of adult sexual assault victims. *Journal of Forensic and Legal Medicine, 19*(1), 35–39. https://doi.org/10.1016/j.jflm.2011.10.007

DeGue, S., & DiLillo, D. (2004). Understanding perpetrators of nonphysical sexual coercion: Characteristics of those who cross the line. *Violence and Victims, 19*(6), 673–688. https://doi.org/10.1891/vivi.19.6.673.66345

Department of Justice. *National Crime Victimization Survey, 2010–2016 (2017).*

D'Onfro, J. (2013, October 3). *Twitter admits 5% of its "users" are fake*. http://www.businessinsider.com/5-of-twitter-monthly-active-users-are-fake-2013-10

Grow, K., & Newman, J. (2021, November 21). Marilyn Manson: The monster hiding in plain sight. *Rolling Stone*. https://www.rollingstone.com/music/music-features/marilyn-manson-abuse-allegations-1256888/

Jones, J. S., Alexander, C., Wynn, B. N., Rossman, L., & Dunnuck, C. (2009). Why women don't report sexual assault to the police: The influence of psychosocial variables and traumatic injury. *The Journal of emergency medicine, 36*(4), 417–424. https://doi.org/10.1016/j.jemermed.2007.10.077

Kirk-Provencher, K. T., Jeglic, E. L., Calkins, C., & Spillane, N. S. (2021). The use of substances in sexual offending in a United States sample. *Psychiatry, Psychology and Law, 1-15*. https://doi.org/10.1080/13218719.2021.1904445

Koss, M. P., Gidycz, C. A., & Wisniewski, N. (1987). The scope of rape: Incidence and prevalence of sexual aggression and victimization in a national sample of higher education students. *Journal of Consulting and Clinical Psychology, 55*(2), 162–170. https://doi.org/10.1037/0022-006X.55.2.162

Loh, C., Gidycz, C. A., Lobo, T. R., & Luthra, R. (2005). A prospective analysis of sexual assault perpetration: Risk factors related to perpetrator characteristics. *Journal of interpersonal violence, 20*(10), 1325–1348. https://doi.org/10.1177/0886260505278528

McCall-Hosenfeld, J. S., Freund, K. M., & Liebschutz, J. M. (2009). Factors associated with sexual assault and time to presentation. *Preventive Medicine, 48*(6), 593–595. https://doi.org/10.1016/j.ypmed.2009.03.016

Mitchell, J. E., & Raghavan, C. (2021). The impact of coercive control on use of specific sexual coercion tactics. *Violence Against Women, 27*(2), 187–206. https://doi.org/10.1177/1077801219884127

Monroe, L. M., Kinney, L. M., Weist, M. D., Dafeamekpor, D. S., Dantzler, J., & Reynolds, M. W. (2005). The experience of sexual assault: Findings from a statewide victim needs assessment. *Journal of Interpersonal Violence, 20*(7), 767–776. https://doi.org/10.1177/0886260505277100

Morgan, R. E., & Truman, J.L. (2020). Criminal victimization, 2019. *Bureau of Justice Statistics, NCJ 255113*.

Murdoch, M., & McGovern, P. G. (1998). Measuring sexual harassment: development and validation of the Sexual Harassment Inventory. *Violence and Victims, 13*(3), 203–216.

Raghavan, C., Cohen, S., & Tamborra, T. (2014). Development and preliminary validation of the Multidimensional Sexual Coercion Questionnaire (MSCQ). *Journal of Sexual Aggression, 21*, 271–289. https://doi.org/10.1080/13552600.2014.917341

RAINN. (n.d.). *The criminal justice system: Statistics*. https://www.rainn.org/statistics/criminal-justice-system

Rebocho, M. F., & Gonçalves, R. A. (2012). Sexual predators and prey: A comparative study of the hunting behavior of rapists and child molesters. *Journal of Interpersonal Violence, 27*(14), 2770–2789. https://doi.org/10.1177/0886260512438280

Sinnamon, G. (2017). The psychology of adult sexual grooming: Sinnamon's seven-stage model of adult sexual grooming. In *The psychology of criminal and antisocial behavior* (pp. 459–487). Academic Press.

Stark, E. (2006). Commentary on Johnson's "Conflict and control: Gender symmetry and asymmetry in domestic violence". *Violence Against Women, 12*(11), 1019–1025. https://doi.org/10.1177/1077801206293329

Stark, E. (2007). *Coercive control: How men entrap women in personal life*. Oxford University Press.

Stevens, D. J. (1994). Predatory rapists and victim selection techniques. *The Social Science Journal, 31*(4), 421–433. https://doi.org/10.1016/0362-3319(94)90033-7

U.S Bureau of Justice Statistics. National Crime Victimization Survey, [United States], 2017. National Archive of Criminal Justice Data, distributor. March 29, 2020. Available at: https://www.icpsr.umich.edu/icpsrweb/NACJD/studies/36981

U.S. Equal Opportunity Commission. (n.d.). *Facts about sexual harassment*. https://www.eeoc.gov/fact-sheet/facts-about-sexual-harassment

Winters, G. M., & Jeglic, E. L. (2017). Stages of sexual grooming: Recognizing potentially predatory behaviors of child molesters. *Deviant Behavior, 38*(6), 724–733. https://doi.org/10.1080/01639625.2016.1197656

Winters, G. M., & Jeglic, E. L. (2021). The Sexual Grooming Scale–Victim Version: The development and pilot testing of a measure to assess the nature and extent of child sexual grooming. *Victims & Offenders*, 1–22. https://doi.org/10.1080/15564886.2021.1974994

Winters, G. M., Jeglic, E. L., & Kaylor, L. E. (2020). Validation of the sexual grooming model of child sexual abusers. *Journal of Child Sexual Abuse, 29*(7), 855–875. https://doi.org/10.1080/10538712.2020.1801935

Chapter 13
Sexual Grooming Assessment and Treatment

Given the challenges of stopping sexual abuse before it happens, significant attention has been paid to the assessment and treatment of individuals who commit sexual offenses in an effort to prevent future offending (Beech et al., 2009). Understanding sexual grooming may be important to the assessment and treatment of both those who perpetrate the abuse as well as those who have been victimized. Until recently, there has been a dearth of assessment measures that could be used in research or clinical work to assess for sexual grooming. However, within the past several years, researchers have turned their attention to developing measures that can quantitively measure sexual grooming (Winters & Jeglic, 2021; Wolf et al., 2018, 2021). A measure of sexual grooming contributes to a greater understanding and conceptualization of these pre-offense behaviors and could assist in determining the relationship of sexual grooming to treatment outcomes and future risk for sexual violence.

There has been a range of literature regarding the strategies that should be used to treat individuals who committed or were a victim of child sexual abuse (CSA). Many have argued that the incorporation of sexual grooming is an integral part of any treatment given the importance of understanding the sexual offense process for both the victim and person who committed the offense (Leclerc et al., 2009; McAlinden, 2006; Winters et al., 2020), yet there has been little to no research examining the extent to which treatment providers incorporate sexual grooming into their interventions. This chapter will provide an overview of assessment of sexual offenses and sexual grooming, as well as the treatment used for those who perpetrate sexual offenses and those who are victimized, culminating in a discussion of how the construct of sexual grooming can be incorporated into these interventions.

© The Author(s), under exclusive license to Springer Nature Switzerland AG 2022
G. M. Winters, E. L. Jeglic, *Sexual Grooming*,
https://doi.org/10.1007/978-3-031-07222-2_13

13.1 Assessment

The evaluation of individuals who commit sexual offenses may occur for a variety of reasons and at various junctures in the criminal justice process. This includes evaluations to inform sentencing, the intensity and level of supervision needed, treatment needs, sex offender registry or notification, or civil commitment proceedings. Formal assessment instruments have been developed to address areas related to the assessment of sex crimes. Primarily, these measures are intended to inform the individual's risk for reoffending or causes/sources of that potential risk (e.g., deviant sexual interests; ATSA, 2012). Some examples of commonly utilized measures include the *Static-99R* (Phenix et al., 2016), *Minnesota Sex Offender Screening Tool-3* (*MnSOST-3*; Duwe & Freske, 2012), *Sex Offender Risk Appraisal Guide* (*SORAG*; Quinsey et al., 2006), and *Sexual Violence Risk-20* (*SVR-20*; Boer et al., 1997); see Gotch and Hanson (2016) for a comprehensive review of risk assessment measures for individuals who committed a sexual offense.

Scalora and Garbin (2003) investigated factors related to recidivism for a sample of 194 individuals with a history of sexual offenses released from a correctional or an inpatient treatment facility between 1991 and 1995. They found that 79.2% of those who reoffended utilized grooming behaviors against the victim compared to 76.7% of individuals who did not reoffend, although the exact definition used for "grooming" was unclear. Nonetheless, given that nearly three-fifths of individuals who sexually reoffended used sexual grooming, it may be important to incorporate sexual grooming in the assessment of people who have a history of sexual offenses.

Despite sexual grooming being deemed an important component of the offense process and possibly being related to recidivism, these behaviors have been largely neglected in the assessment of those who committed sexual offenses. This may in part be due to the many obstacles of developing and validating a measure for sexual grooming. Bennett and O'Donohue (2014) stressed that while it is possible to assess for whether particular pre-offense behaviors are likely to result in CSA, there are many obstacles to doing so. First, there has historically been a lack of a universal and valid definition of sexual grooming, which makes it difficult to develop a measure to assess for this construct. Second, given sexual grooming behaviors may not differ from normal adult/child interactions, a measure should be able to identify inappropriate behaviors that are used in an effort to increase the likelihood of abuse; that is, a measure should aim to minimize false positives and false negatives. Third, a measure must have established psychometric properties (e.g., interrater reliability, predictive validity) in order to ensure it is a valid and reliable measure of the construct. Despite these obstacles, several researchers have aimed to develop assessment measures intended to address these sexual grooming behaviors utilized in the offense process.

13.1.1 *Perspectives of Individuals Who Committed Sexual Grooming*

The *Modus Operandi Questionnaire* (*MOQ*; Kaufman, 1994) was the first measure to assess for perpetration patterns used by an individual to facilitate a sexual offense against a child or adolescent. This self-report measure contains 339 items used to assess for stages throughout an individual's *modus operandi* (MO); see Table 13.1 for a description of the sections included in the *MOQ*. The items were derived from consultation with both those who have committed or been victimized by CSA and treatment providers for these populations. The measure contains primarily Likert scale responses (0 = never, 3 = almost always), along with several open-ended responses. There is evidence for the measure's internal consistency (0.78–0.93; Kaufman et al., 1997, 1998) and test-retest reliability (Smallbone & Wortley, 2000).

Of note, while the measure intends to assess for MO and not explicitly sexual grooming, the operationalization of MO is actually quite consistent with recent conceptualizations of sexual grooming. That is, many of the sections/items of the *MOQ* mirror those included in the Sexual Grooming Model (SGM; Winters et al., 2020). For example, Section 2 in the *MOQ* appears similar to the SGM *gaining access and isolation* stage, Section 3 addresses the SGM *trust development* stage, and Section 8 describes potential *post-abuse maintenance* strategies.

However, there remains important limitations of this measure. First, while some items may apply to the SGM stages of *victim selection* or *desensitization to sexual content and physical contact,* these sections do not comprehensively assess for these stages/behaviors. For example, the measure does not assess for selecting a victim based on perceived psychological or familial vulnerabilities but rather focuses on physically choosing locations children may frequent. Also, even among the sections that do align with the SGM, the specific items do not necessarily correspond to the behaviors/characteristics that fall under each SGM stage. Second, given that the *MOQ* contains a substantial number of items, both Likert-type and open-ended questions, it is a fairly lengthy and cumbersome measure to administer

Table 13.1 The MOQ sections and description

Section 1	About the children you abused
Section 2	Where you found and had time alone with the children you abused
Section 3	How you gained the trust of the children you abused
Section 4	About the time before the sexual abuse began
Section 5	Questions about the sexual abuse
Section 6	Ways of getting the children you sexually abused involved in sexual activity
Section 7	Threats to get the children you sexually abused involved in sexual activity
Section 8	Keeping the children quiet about sexual abuse

and score; thus, it does not provide a feasible means to assess sexual grooming behaviors given the time and effort required by both the individual who engaged in CSA and the clinician or researcher performing the scoring.

In 2021, Wolf and colleagues proposed the *Sex Offender Grooming Assessment* (*SOGA*). The *SOGA* was developed by the researchers based on "prior research undertaken by the authors on the grooming experiences of adult survivors of CSA, and clinically informed from the researchers' clinical experiences working with convicted sex offenders" (p. 791). The authors further note that many of the questions were adapted from the CSA subscale of the *Computer-Assisted Maltreatment Inventory* (described below). The *SOGA* contains 76 Likert-scale, dichotomous, and open-ended items that fall within the following areas:

1. The individual's crime (number of victims, age of victims, relationship to victim), including time spent grooming the victim
2. Grooming the environment – Defined as the "setting where the offending occurs" (e.g., having a computer in an isolated space, staying up late while the rest of the family sleeps)
3. Online grooming – No definition provided
4. Tricks – No definition provided
5. Mind-altering approaches – No definition provided
6. Coercion – No definition provided
7. Bribes – No definition provided
8. Threats – No definition provided
9. Physical force – No definition provided

The authors administered the measure to a sample of 50 males with a history of a sexual offense (ages 20–72 years old) who were currently in group treatment. The type of offenses included CSA ($n = 42$) and adult sexual assault ($n = 3$), with five participants who declined to provide age of their victim; there were 13 (26%) who did not have a contact offense. The findings showed Cronbach alpha (internal consistency) for the measure was "favorable" (0.91) while the subscales showed more variability (between 0.39 and 0.92). As outlined in Table 13.2, the following results were provided for the endorsement of each subscale, as well as some specific behaviors within the subscale; note, there were missing responses for most of the items, and thus, the total N is not 50 in all cases.

Several limitations should be noted regarding this measure. It is unclear the exact definition of sexual grooming the authors used to create the measure; more specifically, they seemingly assessed for both online and in-person grooming (which are considered conceptually different; see Chap. 5) and included individuals with both adult and child offenses (different tactics may be used on adults versus children; see Chap. 12). Moreover, the subscales were not thoroughly defined in the manuscript; for example, the authors did not explain what was meant by "tricks" or "coercion" and even noted this as a limitation in their paper. Additionally, the authors concluded the subscales were "mostly reliable" although additional types of reliability were not evaluated (e.g., interrater reliability, test-retest reliability) nor was there any mention of validity. Thus, it remains unclear whether this *SOGA* can serve as a

Table 13.2 Results from the SOGA

		N (%) endorsement
Grooming the environment		19 (38)
	Spent time with victim's parents	20 (40)
	Friend to people around the victim	28 (56)
	Took a caretaking role for the victim	26 (52)
	Took a role of being responsible for the victim	28 (56)
	Positive reputation	28 (56)
	Offer help and support to those responsible to the victim	24 (48)
	Career involving children	10 (20)
Online grooming		9 (18)
	Pretended to be a different age	4 (8)
	Mislead victim about who they were	3 (6)
Tricks		12 (24)
	Made victim feel it was a game	5 (10)
	Flattery or attention	30 (60)
Mind-altering approaches		11 (22)
	Give victim alcohol	6 (12)
	Give victim "high" (via drugs)	4 (8)
	Give victim drugs without knowledge	N/A
	Give victim drugs with knowledge	3 (6)
Coercion		18 (36)
	Verbal pressure	8 (16)
	Said, "Everyone is doing it"	5 (10)
	Said, "It's not a big deal"	13 (26)
	Manipulating caretaking	4 (8)
Bribes		21 (42)
	Gifts	19 (38)
	Special privileges	13 (26)
	Special treatment	15 (30)
	Benefits	13 (26)
Threats		3 (6)
	Harm to victim	2 (4)
	Harm to victim's family	0
	Victim's pets	0
	Victim's friends	1 (2)
	Victim's reputation	2 (4)
	Victim's personal possessions	1 (2)
	Tell victim's family	1 (2)
	Punished if they did not go along with the abuse	0

(continued)

Table 13.2 (continued)

		N (%) endorsement
	Intimidation	3 (6)
Physical force		5 (10)
	Use weapon	0
	Use physical restraints	1 (2)

Note: Adapted from Wolf et al. (2021)

Table 13.3 The items of the CAMI grooming subscale

1. Were you promised things like money, gifts, or special treatment?
2. Did he/she threaten to tell your parents or someone else?
3. Were you told that you would be physically hurt?
4. Were you held down or was some other type of physical force used?
5. Were you led to believe there was nothing wrong with these activities or that it was a game?
6. Were you told that the activities would benefit you in some way (e.g., would teach you about sex)?
7. Were you told that you would be punished in some way?
8. Were you continually pestered or pressured verbally?
9. Did you become intoxicated voluntarily and then were unable to resist?
10. Were you was promised alcohol or drugs in exchange for sexual activities?
11. Were you given alcohol or drugs without your knowledge and became unable to resist?
12. Were you threatened that someone/something that you cared about would be hurt?
13. Did someone use his/her status or authority to get you to do these things?
14. Did this person tell you not to tell anyone about these activities?

valid and reliable measure for assessing sexual grooming from the perspective of the individual who committed the offense.

13.1.2 *Perspectives of Victims of Sexual Grooming*

In 2018, Wolf et al. proposed a measure of sexual grooming based on items from the *Computer-Assisted Maltreatment Inventory* (*CAMI*; DiLillo et al., 2010). The *CAMI* measures adults' self-reported experiences related to a range of child maltreatment, including witnessing domestic violence, neglect, and physical, emotional, and sexual abuse. The authors utilized 14 dichotomous items (yes/no) from the CSA subscale of the *CAMI* (which contains 30 total items) to create a Grooming Subscale (see Table 13.3). Using a sample of 295 responses, Wolf et al. (2018) ran an exploratory factor analysis with the first half of the sample, followed by a confirmatory factor analysis with the second half of the sample. They concluded that there were acceptable fit indices and that these findings produced three constructs: *verbal coercion, grooming that used drugs/alcohol,* and *grooming that used threats.*

One of the benefits of the measure is that there are only 14 Grooming Subscale items, which makes the measure quick and easy to administer and score. The major limitation of this measure is that it does not comprehensively examine all possible aspects of the sexual grooming process (such as those delineated by the SGM); rather, the 14 items only represent a subset of potential behaviors that may be used in the process. This may be a product of the use of a preexisting measure assessing child maltreatment rather than a measure specifically developed to assess for sexual grooming based on empirical literature. Additionally, research has shown that two of their subscales (drugs/alcohol and threats) are actually relatively less commonly reported compared to other types of sexual grooming (Winters & Jeglic, 2021). Thus, while this measure provided a first step in assessing sexual grooming, it does not yet provide a comprehensive examination of this process.

In an effort to develop a more comprehensive tool for assessing victims' reports of sexual grooming, we (Winters & Jeglic, 2021) created a measure, the *Sexual Grooming Scale-Victim Version* (*SGS-V*), to assess the extent and nature of sexual grooming used in the offense process as reported by the victim. We developed the *SGS-V* based on the five stages and 42 specific behaviors included in the content-validated SGM (Winters et al., 2020). The *SGS-V* contains a dichotomous (yes/no) item for whether the victim experienced each of the 42 sexual grooming behaviors in the SGM and an additional five "other" options for each of the stages (which allowed respondents to add in other behaviors they may have experienced). Then if a person endorsed a behavior, they are asked to qualitatively describe their experience. See Appendix A for the full *SGS-V*.

Using a sample of 115 adults who experienced CSA, we examined the feasibility and preliminary findings from the measure (Winters & Jeglic, 2021). Regarding implementation, we found that the vast majority (83%) of respondents completed all 47 (42 sexual grooming behaviors plus 5 "other" options) questions of the *SGS-V*, and very few individuals exited out of the survey before completing the *SGS-V*. Moreover, we examined the limited efficacy of the scale by looking at the percent endorsement for each of the *SGS-V* items and the content included in the qualitative analyses. The results showed that the level of endorsement for items varied from 6.1% to 67.7%, and there were no observed ceiling or floor effects (unless an item was expected to have low frequency, e.g., involvement in youth-serving organizations). There was also a range of observed scores within each stage of the SGM and the total scores overall (see Table 13.4). Lastly, when examining qualitative responses, it was evident that respondents were appropriately interpreting the items. This measure has since been used to explore sexual grooming behaviors used by females who committed sexual offenses (Winters et al., in submission), as well as juveniles who engaged in inappropriate sexual behaviors (Chou et al., in submission).

Table 13.4 Preliminary findings for the SGS-V

SGM stage	Valid *N*	Number of *SGS-V* items	Range of observed scores	Mean score	Endorsed at least one item (%)
Victim selection	114	9	0–9	3.2	91.2
Gaining access and isolation	114	5	0–4	1.1	64.9
Trust development	114	10	0–9	4.3	93.9
Desensitization to sexual content and physical contact	114	10	0–10	4.1	93.0
Post-abuse maintenance	115	8	0–8	2.8	82.6
Total	**111**	**42**	**0–37**	**15.3**	**99.1**

Note: Adapted from Winters and Jeglic (2021)

13.2 Treatment

13.2.1 Treatment of Individuals Who Commit Sexual Offenses

It is recommended that individuals who committed a sexual offense engage in treatment in order to reduce the risk for reoffending (ATSA, 2016). Indeed, meta-analytic evidence of 69 studies showed a benefit of treatment for this population (Lösel & Schmucker, 2005). The findings showed that those who were treated had mean rates of sexual recidivism that were 6% lower than the controls, which translates to a reduction of 37% when the low base rate of sexual offending is taking into account. The purpose of treatment for individuals who committed sexual offenses is to prevent future sexually abusive/aggressive behaviors. This includes helping the individual (1) manage the factors that contributed to their offending; (2) address needs by developing strengths and competencies; (3) identifying and modifying thoughts, feelings, and behaviors that contribute to offending; and (4) create and maintain prosocial lives (ATSA, 2016).

Treatment Framework

There are two leading frameworks that inform interventions for sexual offending: (1) the *risk, need, and responsivity (RNR) model* and (2) the *good lives model (GLM)*. The RNR model includes three driving principles that should be considered in treating those with sexual offense histories (see Fig. 13.1). Based on research conducted in the past 30 years, there is evidence to show that when treatment utilizes RNR principles combined with cognitive-behavioral techniques, it can be effective in reducing reoffending rates (ATSA, 2016).

One critique of the RNR model is that the focus on criminogenic needs may not necessarily be sufficient for effective treatment. Thus, a broad strength-based framework for rehabilitation for those with sexual offenses was proposed: the GLM (Ward, 2002; Ward & Stewart, 2003). The GLM views individuals as motivated and goal-seeking; they are driven to actions, behaviors, and experiences that intrinsically benefit them and their well-being (also referred to as *primary human goods*). Criminogenic needs are viewed as obstacles for an individual to attain these goals.

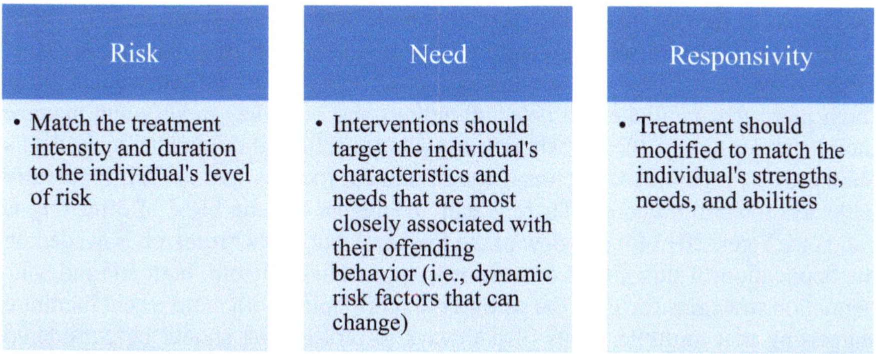

Fig. 13.1 Risk, need, and responsivity model

Thus, GLM-based treatment incorporates an individual's desires and goals in order to most effectively overcome these obstacles while also creating a more prosocial life (Yates, 2003).

Treatment Strategies

Cognitive behavioral therapy (CBT) is the most widely accepted and empirically supported treatment for individuals who committed sexual offenses (e.g., Hanson et al., 2002; Lösel & Schmucker, 2005). In 2008, this was the most frequently used treatment modality for those with sex offenses (McGrath et al., 2010). The treatment targets maladaptive thinking patterns, emotions, and behaviors that contributed to offending by replacing them with more adaptive and prosocial ones. This generally includes targeting the following: modifying offense-supportive attitudes, challenging cognitive distortions, enhancing self-regulation skills, improving social relationships, emotion regulation skills, and reducing deviant sexual arousal (e.g., Barbaree & Marshall, 1998; Marshall et al., 2006; Yates, 2003). Meta-analytic evidence from 2020 showed a significant, moderate effect size for CBT programs in reducing sexual reoffending (Martin & Lösel, 2020); this is consistent with prior research showing its effectiveness (e.g., Hall, 1995; Hanson et al., 2002; Lösel & Schmucker, 2005).

Another approach that is frequently incorporated into CBT interventions for those who committed sexual offenses is relapse prevention (RP; e.g., Laws, 1989; McGrath et al., 2010; Pithers et al., 1988). The goal of RP is to conceptualize and understand the individual's pattern of offending in order to identify, predict, and prevent high-risk situations that are likely to lead to re-offense. When combined with CBT, this approach has been shown to be effective, with recidivism rates being 8% lower than the comparison group (MacKenzie, 2006); however, the findings have been mixed, and other data has not supposed the efficacy of RP (Hanson, 1996, 2000; Laws & Ward, 2006; Yates & Ward, 2007). Notably, use of RP has reduced over the years due to some criticisms, the major one being that RP assumes a single pathway to re-offense and emphasizes avoidance rather than focusing on goals and strengths (Przybylski, n.d.). In more recent years, in an effort to overcome some limitations of RP (i.e., assuming there is a single path to offending), there has been a movement toward a self-regulation model of treatment (SRM; Ward & Hudson, 1998; Ward et al., 1995). The SRM addresses individual's offense-related goals (both those that facilitate and deter offending) and how they modify and manage their behavior to seek these goals. These goals are achieved through an individual's ability to self-regulate their actions; thus, treatment focuses on these self-regulatory pathways toward offending. There is data to suggest that the SRM of offending is valid (see Yates, 2013 for a review of the findings), but further research is needed on the application of this model to treatment approaches. In sum, both RP and self-regulation strategies focus on the pathway to reoffending with more recent literature suggesting that multiple forms of pathways to reoffending should be considered when developing plans for desistance.

Role of Sexual Grooming in Treatment

McAlinden (2013) noted that while it is important to move toward strength- and need-based approaches, there must also be attention to pre-offense behaviors and triggers that contributed to the original offense. This would assist individuals in recognizing patterns of offending and promote self-management of these behaviors in the future. Indeed, there is literature to suggest that individuals plan their offenses and may engage in consistent patterns of offense-related behaviors (Abel et al., 1987; Laws, 1989). Elliott and colleagues (1995) described 91 men with histories of a sexual offense against a child in their study as "creatures of habit" (p. 585). That is, the study findings showed that 84% of the participants in the sample reported that once they developed strategies which were most "successful," they would approach subsequent potential victims in the same manner. Therefore, it has been proposed that sexual grooming is a necessary component of treatment for victims and those who commit these offenses (Craven et al., 2006; Winters et al., 2020).

As noted above, the cognitive behavioral framework addresses distorted thinking and schemas related to sexual offending behaviors. The incorporation of sexual grooming in CBT treatment for individuals with sexual offenses can be beneficial for several reasons (Craven et al., 2006). Identifying and understanding the sexual grooming process may help shed light on an individual's distorted thinking that can be a target of treatment. For example, an individual may justify their offending behaviors given the child was "compliant," yet that compliance was developed using manipulative trust development tactics. As described in Chap. 6, the concept of "self-grooming" refers to the cognitive justification, minimization, or denial of an individual's problematic sexual behavior (van Dam, 2001). Self-grooming is seemingly akin to constructs that facilitate sexual offending, such as neutralization techniques, cognitive distortions, implicit theories of sexual offending, and overcoming internal barriers to offending; these are common constructs targeted during treatment for people with sex offenses. Craven et al. (2006) also suggested that treatment should target motivation for offending, which may vary throughout the pre-offense process. For example, the development of cognitive distortions later in the offense process may reinforce motivation and ultimately facilitate deviant sexual behaviors. Treatment programs can use that information to reduce motivation to offend in the future. Additionally, given sexual grooming is part of the offense process before the abuse occurs, this can aid in managing behaviors of those who have committed an offense. Craven et al. (2006) argued that an individual must understand their sexual grooming behaviors in order to better manage their behaviors in the future. By recognizing and gaining insight into the tactics the individual engaged in to facilitate the offense, they can be better equipped to avoid and reduce problematic sexual behaviors in the future.

The incorporation of sexual grooming into RP or the self-regulation model has also been noted within the research literature (e.g., Leclerc et al., 2009; Winters et al., 2020). That is, understanding and identifying sexual grooming is necessary to fully understand an individual's offense process, which is vital when developing plans for desistance. Indeed, Leclerc et al. (2009) explained that pre-offense behaviors are "important links in the offense chain which leads to reoffending" (p. 9). These tactics should be discussed when treating an individual with a sexual offense to promote insight and awareness of these behavioral patterns and assist the person in recognizing pre-offense tactics in order to prevent reoffending. Ultimately, the goal is to have an individual identify and interrupt the behavioral chain at the earliest possible point when the behaviors are the least dangerous, for example, selecting a victim or attempting to gain access to them. Leclerc et al. (2009) also described the importance of the pre-offense process to identify barriers or obstacles that were present that, at some point, had prevented an individual from committing an offense (i.e., the inability to spend time alone with a child or the presence of someone else who could interfere). By promoting these particular conditions that limit the ability to commit an offense, the RP plan can be further strengthened. Notably, those who commit sexual offenses are heterogenous (Lanning, 2010; Salter, 1995), often having different motivations or tactics used in the pre-offense process; therefore, the identified pathway to offending, and relatedly the plan to remain crime-free, must vary based on the individual.

13.2.2 Treatment of Victims

Victims of CSA may experience a range of negative mental health outcomes, including depression, eating disorders, anxiety, and feelings of shame, guilt, and self-blame (Hall & Hall, 2011; see Chap. 4). An individual may seek treatment for addressing these issues. The primary treatment for individuals who experienced CSA is trauma-informed interventions that are based on CBT principles (Hanson & Wallis, 2018) as these have generally been shown to be effective in treating people who have experienced CSA (McTavish et al., 2021). The goal is to target the maladaptive cognitions related to the sexual abuse and its consequences. Common strategies include (1) psychoeducation about trauma and the impact it may have on victims (e.g., post-traumatic stress symptoms), (2) emotion regulation skills (e.g., breathing, muscle relaxation), (3) exposure to trauma-related memories gradually over time, and (4) cognitive processing to target maladaptive or inaccurate thought patterns (e.g., feeling responsible, feelings of shame or guilt).

Role of Sexual Grooming in Treatment
It has been suggested that the incorporation of grooming into the treatment of victims may be helpful (Leclerc et al., 2009; Winters et al., 2020; Wolf et al., 2018). Leclerc et al. (2009) described the importance of educating victims on the manipulative pre-offense process that may have been used against them. The therapist can also facilitate discussion around the distinction between these behaviors and prosocial relationships, as well as methods to recognize these behaviors in the future. This could assist in dispelling some cognitive distortions the victim may hold surrounding the event or its consequences, such as believing they are responsible for the abuse or that all adults are untrustworthy.

Providing the victim with information regarding sexual grooming may help reduce feelings of shame, guilt, or self-blame. As noted by Hall and Hall (2011), "when the sexual abuse is done by an esteemed trusted adult it may be hard for the child to view the perpetrator in a negative light, thus leaving them incapable of seeing what happened as not their fault" (p. 2). As elaborated on in Chap. 4, victims who experience these negative emotions (e.g., confusion, guilt, shame) may be at increased risk for negative outcomes (e.g., post-traumatic stress disorder, self-harming behaviors); they are also less likely to disclose the CSA, which is notable given nondisclosure is also associated with poorer outcomes (Cunningham, 2020). Therefore, it is possible that garnering insight into the sexual grooming tactics used against them may improve these self-blaming emotions as they can better understand how they were deceptively coerced into this manipulative relationship. Ultimately, the discussion of sexual grooming can potentially help reduce blame and feelings of responsibility for the abuse they experienced.

13.3 Conclusion

In conclusion, the assessment of sexual grooming remains in its early stages. While there have been several proposed measures that have been used for research purposes, these measures have limitations and require further psychometric support (for both validity and reliability) before being widely adopted and used for clinical settings. Future research should seek to validate a measure of sexual grooming, from both the perspective of the victim and person who committed the offense, that is based on empirically supported literature on sexual grooming (such as the SGM; Winters et al., 2020). A measure is only effective if it indeed actually captures the construct of sexual grooming. We are in the process of further validating the *SGS-V*, as well as examining psychometric properties of a version of the measure intended to assess perceptions of sexual grooming from those who committed the offense. Additionally, more research is needed to investigate how sexual grooming is related to important risk assessment constructs. For example, is sexual grooming correlated with risk for sexual recidivism or factors that increase risk (e.g., psychopathic traits, deviant sexual interest)? This information is needed to identify whether sexual grooming has a place in the risk assessment of sexual offenses in the clinical setting, not just within the research context.

Moreover, while there has been significant attention to treatment of those who commit sexual offenses as well as the victims, the incorporation of sexual grooming into interventions has not been widely adopted despite there being overlapping constructs (e.g., self-grooming versus cognitive distortions, understanding the pre-offense process in RP). Research could seek to further investigate whether including psychoeducation and concepts of sexual grooming may indeed result in positive outcomes of those who committed the offenses (e.g., reduced rates of reoffending, improved insight into behaviors, fewer cognitive distortions). Also, research could investigate whether including sexual grooming in the treatment of victims indeed helps reduce feelings of blame, guilt, and responsibility. Overall, there is some preliminary literature to suggest sexual grooming has a place in the assessment and treatment of individuals who commit sexual offenses as well as victims, but additional research is needed.

Appendix A. Sexual Grooming Scale-Victim Version

Victim Selection

There are many reasons that an individual may **select** a victim for their sexually abusive behavior. Please select ***all*** the reasons you believe the individual who abused you may have selected you:

1. I was compliant and/or trusting of adults. (Yes/No)
   - You selected "I was compliant and/or trusting of adults." Please describe.
2. I lacked confidence and/or had low self-esteem. (Yes/No)
   - You selected "I lacked confidence and/or had low self-esteem." Please describe.
3. I was lonely and/or isolated. (Yes/No)
   - You selected "I was lonely and/or isolated." Please describe.
4. I was a troubled child/teen. (Yes/No)
   - You selected "I was a troubled child/teen." Please describe.
5. I was a needy child/teen. (Yes/No)
   - You selected "I was a needy child/teen." Please describe.

6. I felt unwanted or unloved by others. (Yes/No)
   - You selected "I felt unwanted or unloved by others." Please describe.
7. I was not close to my parents and/or they were not resources for me. (Yes/No)
   - You selected "I was not close to my parents and/or they were not resources for me." Please describe.
8. I had a single mother and/or was in need of a "father figure." (Yes/No)
   - You selected "I had a single mother and/or was in need of a 'father figure.'" Please describe.
9. I lacked adult supervision. (Yes/No)
   - You selected "I lacked adult supervision." Please describe.
10. Other reason not listed. (Yes/No)
    - You selected "Other reason not listed." Please describe.

Gaining Access and Isolation

There are many ways that an individual may **gain access to and isolate a victim**. Please select ***all*** the behaviors the individual who abused you may have done to gain access or isolate you:

11. They were involved in youth-serving organizations (e.g., Girl and Boy Scouts, youth sports, church leader, teacher, volunteered with children). (Yes/No)
    - You selected "They were involved in youth-serving organizations (e.g., Girl and Boy Scouts, youth sports, church leader, teacher, volunteered with children)." Please describe.
12. They spent time with my family to gain access to me (e.g., they got close to my family). (Yes/No)
    - You selected "They spent time with my family to gain access to me (e.g., they got close to my family)." Please describe.
13. They did activities alone with me without other adults. (Yes/No)
    - You selected "They did activities alone with me without other adults." Please describe.
14. They took me on overnight stays or outings.
    - You selected "They took me on overnight stays or outings." Please describe.

15. They separated or isolated me from friends, other kids, and/or family. (Yes/No)
    - You selected "They separated or isolated me friends, other kids, and/or family." Please describe.
16. Other reason not listed. (Yes/No)
    - You selected "Other reason not listed." Please describe.

Trust Development

There are many ways that an individual may **develop trust** with the victim or other people around the victim. Please select ***all*** the behaviors the individual who abused you may have done to develop trust with you or those around you:

17. They were charming, nice, and/or likeable. (Yes/No)
    - You selected "They were charming, nice, and/or likeable." Please describe.
18. They had insider status, a good reputation, and/or were considered a "pillar of the community." (Yes/No)
    - You selected "They had insider status, a good reputation, and/or were considered a 'pillar of the community.'" Please describe.
19. They were affectionate and loving toward me. (Yes/No)
    - You selected "They were affectionate and loving toward me." Please describe.
20. They gave me a lot of attention. (Yes/No)
    - You selected "They gave me a lot of attention." Please describe.
21. They showed favoritism toward me and/or formed a special relationship with me. (Yes/No)
    - You selected "They showed favoritism toward me and/or formed a special relationship with me." Please describe.
22. They gave me compliments. (Yes/No)
    - You selected "They gave me compliments." Please describe.
23. They spent a lot of time with me and/or communicated with me often. (Yes/No)
    - You selected "They spent a lot of time with me and/or communicated with me often." Please describe.

24. They engaged in childlike activities with me (e.g., stories, games, sports, music). (Yes/No)
    - You selected "They engaged in childlike activities with me (e.g., stories, games, sports, music). Please describe.
25. They gave me rewards and/or privileges (e.g., gifts, toys, treats, money, trips). (Yes/No)
    - You selected "They gave me rewards and/or privileges (e.g., gifts, toys, treats, money, trips)." Please describe.
26. They provided me with drugs and/or alcohol. (Yes/No)
    - You selected "They provided me with drugs and/or alcohol." Please describe.
27. Other reason not listed. (Yes/No)
    - You selected "Other reason not listed." Please describe.

Desensitization to Sexual Content and Physical Touch

There are many ways that an individual may try to get the victim **used to physical touch or sexual content before the abuse**. Please select ***all*** the behaviors the individual who abused you may have done to get you used to physical touch or sexual content:

28. They asked questions about my sexual experiences and/or relationships. (Yes/No)
    - You selected "They asked questions about my sexual experiences and/or relationships." Please describe.
29. They talked about sexual things they had done. (Yes/No)
    - You selected "They talked about sexual things they had done." Please describe.
30. They used inappropriate sexual language and/or told dirty jokes. (Yes/No)
    - You selected "They used inappropriate sexual language and/or told dirty jokes." Please describe.
31. They educated me about sexual behavior. (Yes/No)
    - You selected "They educated me about sexual behavior." Please describe.
32. They used accidental touching and/or distracted me while touching me. (Yes/No)
    - You selected "They used accidental touching and/or distracted me while touching me." Please describe.

33. They watched me undressing. (Yes/No)
    - You selected "They watched me undressing." Please describe.
34. They exposed their naked body to me. (Yes/No)
    - You selected "They exposed their naked body to me." Please describe.
35. They showed me pornography photographs or videos. (Yes/No)
    - You selected "They showed me pornography photographs or videos." Please describe.
36. They used seemingly innocent and/or nonsexual touching (e.g., hugs/tickling). (Yes/No)
    - You selected "They used seemingly innocent and/or nonsexual touching (e.g., hugs/tickling)." Please describe.
37. They gradually increased the amount of sexual touching over time. (Yes/No)
    - You selected "They gradually increased the amount of sexual touching over time." Please describe.
38. Other reason not listed. (Yes/No)
    - You selected "Other reason not listed." Please describe.

Post-abuse Maintenance

There are many ways that an individual may try to **prevent the victim from disclosing the abuse or to continue the abuse over time.** Please select ***all*** the behaviors you believe the individual who abused you may used to try to prevent disclosure or continue the abuse:

39. They told me not to tell anyone what happened. (Yes/No)
    - You selected "They told me not to tell anyone what happened." Please describe.
40. They encouraged secrets. (Yes/No)
    - You selected "They encouraged secrets." Please describe.
41. They told me they loved me and/or that I was special. (Yes/No)
    - You selected "They told me they loved me and/or that I was special." Please describe.
42. They gave me rewards and bribes or allowed me to avoid punishment. (Yes/No)
    - You selected "They gave me rewards and bribes or allowed me to avoid punishment." Please describe.

43. They convinced me it was acceptable and/or normal behavior. (Yes/No)
    - You selected "They convinced me it was acceptable and/or normal behavior." Please describe.
44. They misstated the moral standards regarding touch (e.g., they told me touching was okay or normal). (Yes/No)
    - You selected "They misstated the moral standards regarding touch (e.g., they told me touching was okay or normal)." Please describe.
45. They made me feel responsible for the abuse. (Yes/No)
    - You selected "They made me feel responsible for the abuse." Please describe.
46. They threatened abandonment, rejection, or my family breaking up. (Yes/No)
    - You selected "They threatened abandonment, rejection, or my family breaking up." Please describe.
47. Other reason not listed. (Yes/No)
    - You selected "Other reason not listed." Please describe.

References

Abel, G. G., Becker, J. V., Mittelman, M., Cunningham-Rathner, J., Rouleau, J. L., & Murphy, W. D. (1987). Self-reported sex crimes of nonincarcerated paraphiliacs. *Journal of Interpersonal Violence, 2*(1), 3–25. https://doi.org/10.1177/088626087002001001

Association for Treatment of Sexual Abusers. (2012). *Sex offender risk assessment.* https://www.atsa.com/pdfs/SexOffenderRiskAssessmentBriefWithBibliography2012.pdf

Association for Treatment of Sexual Abusers. (2016). *Sex offender treatment for adult males.* https://www.atsa.com/pdfs/Policy/SexOffenderTreatmentAugust2016.pdf

Barbaree, H. E., & Marshall, W. L. (1998). Treatment of the sexual offender. In R. M. Wettstein (Ed.), *Treatment of offenders with mental disorders* (pp. 265–328) Guilford.

Beech, A. R., Craig, L. A., & Browne, K. D. (Eds.). (2009). Assessment and treatment of sex offenders: A handbook. *The Howard Journal of Crime and Justice, 49*, 312–312.

Bennett, N., & O'Donohue, W. (2014). The construct of grooming in child sexual abuse: Conceptual and measurement issues. *Journal of Child Sexual Abuse, 23*(8), 957–957. https://doi.org/10.1080/10538712.2014.960632

Boer, D. P., Hart, S. D., Kropp, P. R., & Webster, C. D. (1997). Manual for the sexual violence risk- 20: Professional guidelines for assessing risk of sexual violence. *Mental Health, Law, & Policy Institute.*

Chou, C., Neumann, N., Smith, K., & Winters, G. (In submission). *Sexual grooming behaviors of juvenile offenders in child sexual abuse.* Submitted for poster presentation at the American Psychological Association Conference.

Craven, S., Brown, S., & Gilchrist, E. (2006). Sexual grooming of children: Review of literature and theoretical considerations. *Journal of Sexual Aggression, 12*(3), 287–299. https://doi.org/10.1080/13552600601069414

Cunningham, K. C. (2020). Shame and guilt in PTSD. In *Emotion in posttraumatic stress disorder* (pp. 145–171). Academic. https://doi.org/10.1016/B978-0-12-816022-0.00006-5

DiLillo, D., Hayes-Skelton, S. A., Fortier, M. A., Perry, A. R., Evans, S. E., Moore, T. L. M., Walsh, K., Nash, C., & Fauchier, A. (2010). Development and initial psychometric properties of the computer assisted maltreatment inventory (CAMI): A comprehensive self-report measure of child maltreatment history. *Child Abuse & Neglect, 34*(5), 305–317. https://doi.org/10.1016/j.chiabu.2009.09.015

Duwe, G., & Freske, P. (2012). Using logistic regression modeling to predict sexual recidivism: The Minnesota sex offender screening tool-3 (MnSOST-3). *Sexual Abuse: A Journal of Research and Treatment, 24*, 350–377. https://doi.org/10.1177/1079063211429470

Elliott, M., Browne, K., & Kilcoyne, J. (1995). Child sexual abuse prevention: What offenders tell us. *Child Abuse & Neglect, 19*(5), 579. https://doi.org/10.1016/0145-2134(95)00017-3

Gotch, K., & Hanson, R. K. (2016). *Risk assessment for males who have engaged in harmful or illegal sexual behavior.* Association for the Treatment of Sexual Abusers. https://www.atsa.com/pdfs/ATSA_Risk_Assessment_for_Males_(2016).pdf

Hall, G. C. N. (1995). The preliminary development of a theory-based community treatment for sexual offenders. *Professional Psychology: Research and Practice, 26*(5), 478–483. https://doi.org/10.1037/0735-7028.26.5.478

Hall, M., & Hall, J. (2011). The long-term effects of childhood sexual abuse: Counseling implications. http://counselingoutfitters.com/vistas/vistas11/Article_19.pdf

Hanson, R. K. (1996). Evaluating the contribution of relapse prevention theory to the treatment of sexual offenders. *Sexual Abuse: A Journal of Research and Treatment, 8*, 201–208. https://doi.org/10.1007/BF02256635

Hanson, R. K. (2000). What is so special about relapse prevention? In D. R. Laws (Ed.), *Relapse prevention with sex offenders* (pp. 1–31). Guilford.

Hanson, R. F., & Wallis, E. (2018). Treating victims of child sexual abuse. *Treatment in Psychiatry, 175*(11), 1064–1070. https://doi.org/10.1176/appi.ajp.2018.18050578

Hanson, R. K., Gordon, A., Harris, A. J. R., Marques, J. K., Murphy, W. D., Quinsey, V. L., & Seto, M. C. (2002). First report of the collaborative outcome data project on the effectiveness of psychological treatment for sex offenders. *Sexual Abuse: A Journal of Research and Treatment, 14*, 169–194. https://doi.org/10.1177/107906320201400207

Kaufman, K. L. (1994). *Modus operandi questionnaire. Revised version.* Author (Children's hospital).

Kaufman, K. L., McCrady, F. E., Holmberg, J. K., Rotzien, A. L., Orts, K. A., … Hilliker, D. R. (1997). *Factor structure of the behaviors of sexual offenders as measured by the modus operandi questionnaire.* Paper presented at the 16th Annual Conference of the Association for the Treatment of Sexual Abusers.

Kaufman, K. L., Holmberg, J. K., Orts, K. A., McCrady, F. E., Rotzien, A. L., Daleiden, E. L., & Hilliker, D. R. (1998). Factors influencing sexual offenders' modus operandi: An examination of victim–offender relatedness and age. *Child Maltreatment, 3*(4), 349–361. https://doi.org/10.1177/1077559598003004007

Lanning, K. V. (2010). *Child molesters: A behavioral analysis* (5th ed.). National Center for Missing & Exploited Children.

Laws, D. R. (1989). *Relapse prevention with sex offenders.* Guilford.

Laws, D. R., & Ward, T. (2006). When one size doesn't fit all: The reformulation of relapse prevention. In W. L. Marshall, Y. M. Fernandez, L. E. Marshall, & G. A. Serran (Eds.), *Sexual offender treatment: Controversial issues* (pp. 241–254). Wiley.

Leclerc, B., Proulx, J., & Beauregard, E. (2009). Examining the modus operandi of sexual offenders against children and its practical implications. *Aggression and Violent Behavior, 14*(1), 5–12. https://doi.org/10.1016/j.avb.2008.08.001

Lösel, F., & Schmucker, M. (2005). The effectiveness of treatment for sexual offenders: A comprehensive meta-analysis. *Journal of Experimental Criminology, 1*, 117–146. https://doi.org/10.1007/s11292-004-6466-7

MacKenzie, D. L. (2006). *What works in corrections: Reducing the criminal activities of offenders and delinquents.* Cambridge University Press.

Marshall, W. L., Marshall, L. E., Serran, G., & Fernandez, Y. M. (2006). *Treating sexual offenders: An integrated approach*. Routledge.
Martin, S., & Lösel, F. (2020). Sexual offender treatment for reducing recidivism among convicted sex offenders: A systematic review and meta-analysis. *Campbell Systematic Reviews, 13*(1), 1–75. https://doi.org/10.4073/csr.2017.8
McAlinden, A. M. (2006). Setting 'em up': Personal, familial and institutional grooming in the sexual abuse of children. *Social & Legal Studies, 15*(3), 339–362. https://doi.org/10.1177/0964663906066613
McAlinden, A. (2013). 'Grooming' and the sexual abuse of children: Implications for sex offender assessment, treatment and management. *Sexual Offender Treatment, 8*(1) http://www.sexual-offender-treatment.org/118.html
McGrath, R. J., Cumming, G. F., Burchard, B. L., Zeoli, S., & Ellerby, L. (2010). *Current practices and emerging trends in sexual abuser management: The Safer Society 2009 North American survey*. Safer Society Press.
McTavish, J. R., Santesso, N., Amin, A., Reijnders, M., Ali, M. U., Fitzpatrick-Lewis, D., & MacMillan, H. L. (2021). Psychosocial interventions for responding to child sexual abuse: A systematic review. *Child Abuse & Neglect, 116*, 104203–104203. https://doi.org/10.1016/j.chiabu.2019.104203
Phenix, A., Helmus, L. M., & Hanson, R. K. (2016). Static-99R & Static-2002R evaluators' workbook.
Pithers, W. D., Kashima, K. M., Cumming, G. F., & Beal, L. S. (1988). Relapse prevention: A method of enhancing maintenance of change in sex offenders. In A. C. Salter (Ed.), *Treating child sex offenders and victims: A practical guide* (pp. 131–170). Sage.
Przybylski, R. (n.d.). Chapter 7: Effectiveness of treatment for adult sex offenders. https://smart.ojp.gov/somapi/chapter-7-effectiveness-treatment-adult-sex-offenders
Quinsey, V. L., Harris, G. T., Rice, M. E., & Cormier, C. A. (2006). *Violent offenders: Appraising and managing risk* (2nd ed.). American Psychological Association.
Salter, A. C. (1995). *Transforming trauma: A guide to understanding and treating adult survivors of child sexual abuse*. Sage Publications, Inc.
Scalora, M. J., & Garbin, C. (2003). A multivariate analysis of sex offender recidivism. *International Journal of Offender Therapy and Comparative Criminology, 47*(3), 309–323. https://doi.org/10.1177/0306624X03047003005
Smallbone, S., & Wortley, R. (2000). *Child sexual abuse in Queensland: Offender characteristics and modus operandi (full report)*. Queensland Crime Commission.
van Dam, C. (2001). *Identifying child molesters: Preventing child sexual abuse by recognizing the patterns of the offenders*. Haworth Maltreatment and Trauma Press/The Haworth Press.
Ward, T. (2002). The management of risk and the design of good lives. *Australian Psychologist, 37*(3), 172–179. https://doi.org/10.1080/00050060210001706846
Ward, T., & Hudson, S. M. (1998). The construction and development of theory in the sexual offending area: A metatheoretical framework. *Sexual Abuse: A Journal of Research and Treatment, 10*, 47–63. https://doi.org/10.1023/A:1022106731724
Ward, T., & Stewart, C. (2003). Criminogenic needs and human needs: A theoretical model. *Psychology, Crime & Law, 9*, 125–143. https://doi.org/10.1080/1068316031000116247
Ward, T., Louden, K., Hudson, S. M., & Marshall, W. L. (1995). Descriptive model of the offence chain for child molesters. *Journal of Interpersonal Violence, 10*, 452–472. https://www.ojp.gov/ncjrs/virtual-library/abstracts/descriptive-model-offense-chain-child-molesters
Winters, G. M., & Jeglic, E. L. (2021). The sexual grooming scale – Victim version: The development and pilot testing of a measure to assess the nature and extent of child sexual grooming. *Victims & Offenders, 1-22*, 1–22. https://doi.org/10.1080/15564886.2021.1974994
Winters, G. M., Jeglic, E. L., & Kaylor, L. E. (2020). Validation of the sexual grooming model of child sexual abusers. *Journal of Child Sexual Abuse, 29*(7), 855–875. https://doi.org/10.1080/10538712.2020.1801935

Winters, G., Jeglic, E., & Kaylor, L. (In submission). Victims' perspectives of sexual grooming behaviors of females who commit child sexual abuse.

Wolf, M. R., Linn, B. K., & Pruitt, D. K. (2018). Grooming child victims into sexual abuse: A psychometric analysis of survivors' experiences. *Journal of Sexual Aggression, 24*(2), 215–224. https://doi.org/10.1080/13552600.2018.1504555

Wolf, M. R., Pruitt, D. K., & Leet, T. (2021). Lessons learned: Creation and testing of a new instrument (sex offenders grooming assessment) for measuring sex offenders' perceptions of their grooming behaviors. *Journal of Child Sexual Abuse, 30*(7), 785–805. https://doi.org/10.1080/10538712.2021.1970681

Yates, P. M. (2003). Treatment of adult sexual offenders: A therapeutic cognitive-behavioral model of intervention. *Journal of Child Sexual Abuse, 12*, 195–232. https://doi.org/10.1300/J070v12n03_08

Yates, P. M. (2013). Treatment of sexual offenders: Research, best practices, and emerging models. *International Journal of Behavioral Consultation and Therapy, 8*(3–4), 89–95. https://doi.org/10.1037/h0100989

Yates, P. M., & Ward, T. (2007). Treatment of sexual offenders: Relapse prevention and beyond. In K. Witkiewitz & G. A. Marlatt (Eds.), *Therapists' guide to evidence-based relapse prevention* (pp. 215–234). Elsevier.

Chapter 14
Sexual Grooming Prevention

Child sexual abuse (CSA) is a serious problem globally and has severe long-lasting consequences, yet it is a problem that is "100% preventable" (Letourneau, 2017, p. 1). Given that sexual grooming encompasses many *pre*-offense behaviors, understanding sexual grooming tactics and identifying sexual grooming behaviors are areas that are ripe for consideration in sexual violence prevention efforts. As such, this chapter will begin with a review of the history and current state of CSA prevention. We will then review what efforts have been made to specifically address in-person and online sexual grooming. The chapter will conclude with a discussion of future directions for the prevention of CSA and how child sexual grooming behaviors should be integrated into prevention initiatives.

14.1 History of Child Sexual Abuse Prevention

The first legal protections for children from abuse only began 150 years ago (Eide, 1990). This arose following the high-profile case of 10-year-old Mary Ellen Wilson, who in 1874 was physically and emotionally abused by her adoptive parents. However, at the time, there was no legal recourse for intervention in a child's home. The case came to the attention of a social worker named Marietta "Etta" Wheeler, who was shocked by the state of the child. After many failed efforts to intervene, Wheeler sought out Henry Bergh, the founder of the American Society for the Prevention of Cruelty to Animals (ASPCA), in hopes that he could help her legally find a way to remove Mary Ellen from the home. Together with Bergh's lawyer, they were able to remove Mary Ellen from her home, and her adoptive mother faced legal charges. Later that same year, Bergh, along with Elbridge Gerry and James Wright, founded the New York Society for the Prevention of Cruelty to Children (SPCC) to help with the legal protection of children from abuse (Eide, 1990). While this case did not pertain to CSA specifically, it brought the issue of child maltreatment to

© The Author(s), under exclusive license to Springer Nature Switzerland AG 2022

G. M. Winters, E. L. Jeglic, *Sexual Grooming*,
https://doi.org/10.1007/978-3-031-07222-2_14

public attention and resulted in legal reform and protections for children from all types of abuse, including CSA.

The next pivotal moment in CSA prevention did not happen until almost 100 years later when in 1962, pediatrician Henry Kempe and his colleagues wrote an article entitled "battered child syndrome," which was published in the *Journal of the American Medical Association* (a publication that targeted medical professionals). In their article, Kempe and his colleagues described the battered child syndrome as "a clinical condition in young children who have received serious physical abuse, generally from a parent or foster parent. The condition has also been described as 'unrecognized trauma' by radiologists, orthopedists, pediatricians and social service workers" (p. 17). The authors indicated that the syndrome often goes unrecognized, and if it is recognized, it is generally poorly handled by physicians as they are hesitant to bring it to the attention of the authorities (Kempe et al., 1962). While this article pertained almost exclusively to physical abuse, it was seminal for two reasons. First, it acknowledged that there are long-term psychological consequences to child abuse. Second, it provided physicians with concrete strategies and examples to identify and report cases of suspected child abuse to authorities. Most importantly, Kempe's work led state and federal governments to develop a formal system of reporting cases of suspected child abuse and enact legislation about formal reporting of suspected cases of child abuse (Child Welfare Information Gateway, 2017).

The next major step in protecting children from abuse came in 1974 when the United States (US) Congress enacted the Child Abuse Prevention and Treatment Act (CAPTA P.L. 93–247). CAPTA requires that as a condition of receiving funding, states are required to have policies and procedures in place to deal with allegations of child abuse and neglect. Further, CAPTA requires states to have definitions of child abuse and neglect that are consistent with what is described in CAPTA, which reads, "At a minimum, any recent act or failure to act on the part of a parent or caretaker, which results in death, serious physical or emotional harm, sexual abuse or exploitation, or an act or failure to act which presents an imminent risk of serious harm." (CAPTA P.L. 93–247). There have been many amendments and reauthorizations of CAPTA over the years to enhance the prevention, assessment, investigation, prosecution, and treatment of child abuse, as well as to provide grants to public agencies and nonprofit organizations and fund research endeavors to prevent child abuse. CAPTA was most recently amended on January 7, 2019, by the Victims of Child Abuse Act Reauthorization Act of 2018 (P.L. 115–424).

Since the institution of CAPTA, there has been increased recognition of the scope of the problem of CSA and society's role in protecting vulnerable children. As described below, the Centers for Disease Control (CDC) developed prevention guidelines though in recent years, several other legislative efforts have been put forth in the US to address CSA prevention (see Chap. 16 for a more in-depth review), such as the Family First Prevention Services Act (FFPSA), the Protecting Young Victims from Sexual Abuse and Safe Sport Authorization Act of 2017, and the Child Protection Improvements Act of 2017.

14.2 Prevention of Child Sexual Abuse

Given the breadth and scope of the problem of CSA, the public health approach for prevention has been adopted. The public health approach is rooted in scientific principles and is data driven, seeking to target the population as opposed to the individual in order to impact the largest number of people possible. According to the CDC (n.d.), there are four main steps to the public health approach, which include: (1) defining and monitoring the problem, (2) identifying risk and protective factors, (3) developing and testing prevention strategies, and (4) assuring widespread adoption. There are two models of prevention rooted in the public health approach that are used in the prevention of sexual violence as described below:

(1) *The public health model of prevention.*
(2) *The socioecological model of prevention.*

14.2.1 The Public Health Model

The *public health model* of sexual violence prevention addresses *when* the intervention takes place (CDC, 2004). Ideally, we would be able to prevent all acts of sexual violence before they occur; however, at present, this is not possible. As such, efforts to minimize the short- and long-term negative impacts of sexual violence must also be included in prevention strategies. As shown in Fig. 14.1, the model includes three levels of intervention: primary, secondary, and tertiary.

Primary prevention of sexual abuse involves targeting large groups of people before the sexual violence occurs, and it targets both the general population and those who may be at increased risk of victimization (e.g., women and children) and perpetration (O'Donohue et al., 2013; Townsend, 2008). This encompasses teaching youth about healthy relationships, developing policies and procedures to minimize known risks for perpetration, and changing societal norms (Saul & Audage, 2007). There is debate about whether targeting at-risk populations falls under primary (CDC, 2004) or secondary prevention (McCartan et al., 2018). Regardless of whether labeled primary or secondary prevention, these interventions aim to identify and target individuals who may be at increased risk for perpetration. For example, over a 6-year period between 2005 and 2011, Project Dunkelfeld in Germany targeted undetected individuals who had pedophilic and hebephilic sexual interests and provided anonymous and confidential cognitive behavioral treatment. Compared to a wait-list control group, Beier et al. (2015) found that dynamic risk factors (e.g., emotional deficits and offensive supportive cognitions) decreased post treatment, while sexual self-management increased for those in the treatment.

As noted above, while some identify *secondary prevention* as targeting individuals who are at a high risk for victimization or perpetration (see McCartan et al., 2018), according to the CDC (2004), the goals of secondary prevention are to inform

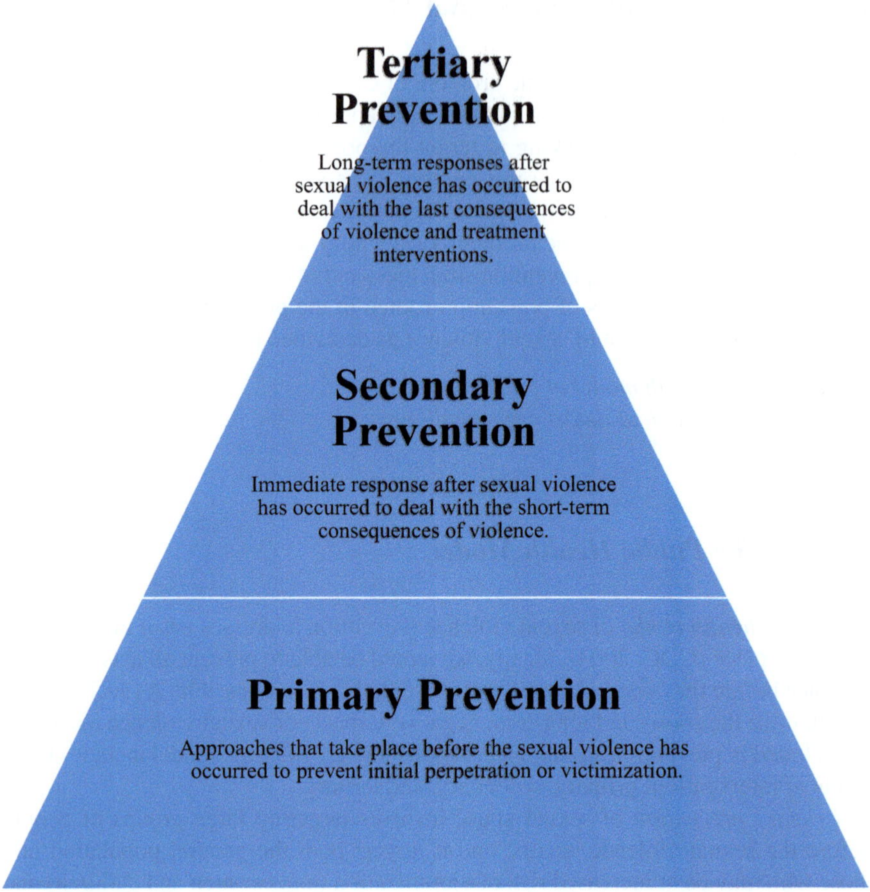

Fig. 14.1 Public health approach to sexual violence prevention. (*Note:* Adapted from the CDC, 2004)

responses after the sexual abuse has occurred. This includes addressing how organizations and services respond to survivors of sexual violence immediately after the abuse happens or is disclosed in order to minimize the short-term consequences. This might include advocacy, legal interventions, psychological support, and access to health care.

Finally, *tertiary prevention* takes place after the abuse has been perpetrated and focuses on addressing the long-term consequences of sexual abuse and making sure that it does not happen again (Becker & Reilley, 1999; CDC, 2004). This can involve working with those who committed sexual violence to provide evidence-based interventions to decrease risk for recidivism (Jeglic & Calkins, 2016) or working with survivors of sexual violence to prevent and minimize the long-term impacts of sexual abuse.

14.2.2 The Socioecological Model of Prevention

While the *public health model* of prevention addresses *when* prevention takes place, the *socioecological model* describes *what* the focus of the prevention program should be. According to the *socioecological model*, there are many determinants of behavior, and individuals do not engage in behavior within a vacuum, but rather, they interact with others and the systems within their environment. This model is rooted in the work of Kelly (1966, 1968, 1971) and Bronfenbrenner (1979, 1986, 1995), who emphasized the systems (e.g., the family, community, and society) that intertwine to result in violence (as discussed in Chap. 7 on familial grooming). Kelly's *ecological model* highlights persons, constructs, events, and environments, while Bronfenbrenner's *ecological model* consists of microsystems, mesosystems, exosystems, macrosystems, and chronosystems, all of which contribute to the behavior of the individual. Similarly, as seen in Fig. 14.2, the socioecological model encompasses four levels of influence: individual, relationship, community, and societal.

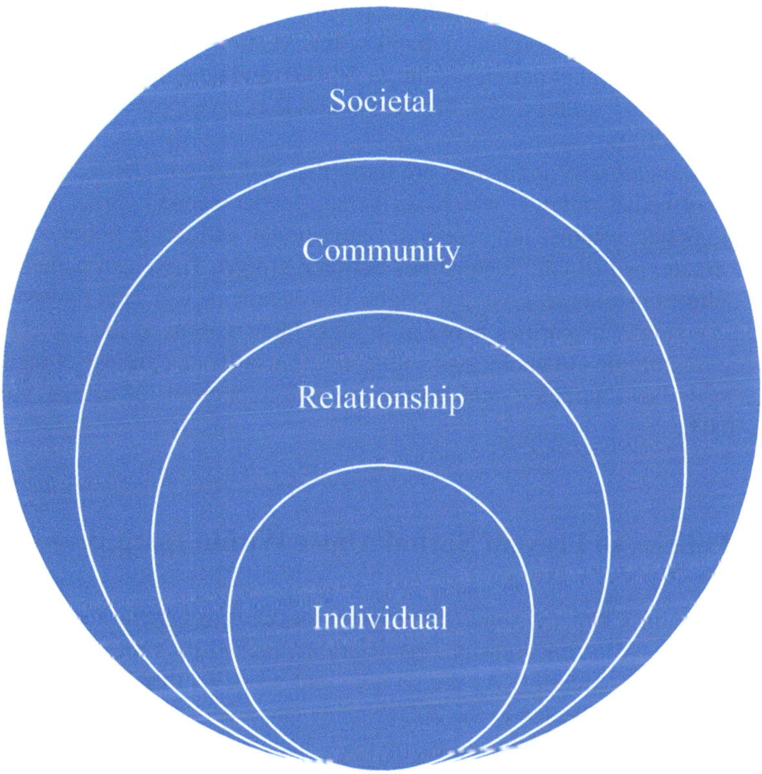

Fig. 14.2 The socioecological model of sexual violence prevention

At the *individual level*, prevention efforts can target characteristics, biological factors, behaviors, and experiences that can put an individual at increased risk for sexual violence victimization and perpetration. Risk factors at the individual level can include attitudes and beliefs that are supportive of sexual violence, a personal history of child abuse, witnessing violence in the home, antisocial behaviors, and substance abuse. Prevention programs can target these risk factors through individual or group counseling, therapy, or other educational programs (CDC, 2004; Krug et al., 2002).

At the next level, sexual violence prevention should also focus on *relationship* influences. Prevention programming can involve addressing relationships that either increase risk, such as negative or abusive relationships with peers, intimate partners, and family members, or decrease risk, such as social support. Specific risk factors of this level can include family strife, marital instability, poor parenting and/or a lack of supervision of minors, and delinquent peer relationships. Relationship-level prevention programs can involve bystander interventions, family therapy, and educational interventions at schools or colleges (CDC, 2004).

Community level interventions focus on community environments that may increase the risk for perpetration or victimization, such as youth-serving organizations, workplaces, and neighborhoods. Risk factors can include neighborhood disorganization, lack of social connectedness, poverty, limited economic or recreational opportunity, and toxic workplace dynamics. Interventions can involve community building, anti-harassment policies in the workplace, and other interventions that are designed to address policies, systems, or climates that are supportive of sexual violence (CDC, 2004).

Finally, *societal level* influences are those that address societal factors that are supportive of sexual violence, which can include gender inequality, societal/cultural norms and belief systems, and economic, educational, and health policies that create, exacerbate, or maintain inequalities between groups. These can include countries or cultures that oppress women's rights or systemic racism and oppression that maintain economic disparities between groups. Interventions at the societal level may require multiple collaborations with commitment from a variety of leaders to change such laws, policies, and norms that are supportive of sexual violence (CDC, 2004).

14.3 Policies to Prevent Sexual Abuse Within Institutions

As described in Chap. 8, some perpetrators of CSA sought access to minors through their work in child-serving organizations, such as the Catholic Church and the Boy Scouts of America. As the breadth and scope of this institutional child abuse was publicly revealed in the 2000s, many countries commissioned inquiries and reviews to examine how cases of CSA happened within the institutional context. McAlinden (2012) summarized the common themes that emerged from these investigations including:

1. The abuse was undetected over many years.
2. There were often multiple perpetrators and multiple victims.
3. The institutional culture prevented employees from reporting inappropriate behaviors or suspicions of CSA.
4. Victims were afraid to report the abuse, and as such, many complaints were not formally reported.
5. When cases of CSA were reported, often nothing was done because the institution either wanted to cover up the abuse or the perpetrator was believed over the victim.
6. There were poor internal management and external governance frameworks in place to oversee the preventing and reporting of CSA.

These findings, among others, spurred youth-serving institutions to develop new policies and guidance for preventing CSA. While many organizations developed their own policies, in 2007, the CDC published a report entitled *Preventing CSA Within Youth-Serving Organizations: Getting Started on Policies and Procedures* (Saul & Audage, 2007), which contained a list of six components to be addressed as part of comprehensive sexual abuse prevention policies and procedures within youth-serving organizations (see Table 14.1). As such, all youth-serving organizations should have policies in place addressing the following six components.

1. Screening and Selecting Employees and Volunteers In addition to general job-related skills, youth-serving organizations need to consider child abuse prevention when screening potential candidates for any positions in which they will have contact with minors (both paid and unpaid). This should include both adolescents and adults as one-third of all minors are abused by another minor (Jeglic & Calkins, 2018). Further, this should apply to all candidates, including individuals that are well known to the employers or employees that have worked with the organization in the past. With criminal records checks, red flags would be any charges or convictions involving endangering a minor or a sexually related crime, including noncontact offenses such as possession of child sexual exploitation material. It should be noted that an absence of a criminal record does not mean that the person is safe as many sex crimes go unreported or undetected and not all criminal record checks show information pertaining to arrests and charges that did not result in a conviction. Also, if there is a gap on the resume, this should be followed up to make sure that no positions were omitted. In addition, personal interviews using open-ended questions should be conducted, specifically when asking about the potential employee/volunteer's desire to work with youth.

2. Guidelines for Interactions Between Individuals Youth-serving organizations should seek to encourage positive interactions between adults and youth and minimize harmful ones. Institutions should have a clearly spelled out code of conduct for

Table 14.1 CDC's (2007) six key components and corresponding strategy recommendations

Component	Strategy recommendations
Screening and selecting employees and volunteers	• A review of the organizational code of conduct and ethics. • A thorough background check including criminal records (should encompass arrests, charges, and convictions). • A search of the internet, including social media. • Calling all previous employers and verifying dates of employment, which should correspond to those listed on the resume and reasons for leaving.
Guidelines for interactions between individuals	• Having at least two adults present at all times when working with youth (i.e., no one-on-one interactions). • Guidelines for physical contact (i.e., no hugs; physical contact only as required for safety, such as spotting in gymnastics or to correct form [body placement]). • A zero-tolerance policy for sexual comments or jokes. • Prohibiting contact with minors outside of institutional-related events (i.e., do not drive minors home in personal vehicles, take minors out for meals, or non-organization-related excursions). • Recognizing that youth can abuse other youth, so having policies for certain high-risk activities or areas, such as changing rooms having two adults present during times when youth are changing.
Monitoring behavior	• Establish behavioral policies and make a list of behaviors that are and are not permitted. • Develop policies on how to handle boundary violations. • Document all instances of boundary violations. • Determine which boundary violations will result in immediate terminations and which ones can be remediated. • Establish clear reporting and accountability chains. • Yearly evaluations where issues related to sexual violence prevention are evaluated and discussed. • Regular unscheduled observation of employees/volunteers working with youth.
Ensuring safe environments	• Clear lines of sight. • Bright lights. • Video cameras or security in areas that may be hidden from view. • Locked closets and storerooms. • Windows in all doors. • Open-door policies. • The use and monitoring of video cameras.

(continued)

Table 14.1 (continued)

Component	Strategy recommendations
Responding to inappropriate behavior, breaches in policy, and allegations and suspicions of child sexual abuse	• Collaborating with a lawyer regarding reporting policies. • Identifying who within the organization is a mandated child abuse reporter. • Defining the continuum of appropriate, inappropriate, and harmful behaviors. • Defining which violations will be handled internally and which ones require contacting the authorities. • Developing confidentiality and community/press notification policies when an accusation of CSA is made and/or confirmed. • Having a policy about what to do regarding the employment of staff/volunteers who are accused of sexual abuse while the accusation is being investigated. • Having clear documentation of all reports and investigation proceedings and results.
Training about child sexual abuse prevention	• General information about CSA, including a discussion of sexual grooming and its warning signs. • Organizational policies and procedures for CSA prevention. • How to handle disclosures of sexual abuse and reporting. • Definitions of appropriate and inappropriate conduct and behaviors.

employees/volunteers as it pertains to preventing sexual violence. There should be regular training on this code of conduct, and employees should sign off on having read and understood them on, at minimum, a yearly basis.

3. Monitoring Behavior Once staff and volunteer behavior policies have been established, then violations of these policies must be monitored, enforced, and documented. Inappropriate behaviors may include showing favoritism to certain youth, giving gifts, and spending time alone with youth. Each violation or boundary violation should be examined by a team including human resources and legal representatives. While some boundary violations may warrant a warning and behavior plan, other violations, such as those involving potential serious grooming behaviors and sexual content, should result in immediate termination and the potential involvement of authorities (if sexual contact or behavior was involved). While ultimately supervisors are responsible for those who work under them, to prevent sexual violence, all employees and volunteers are responsible for monitoring behavior within the organization, and there should be a clear reporting chain. All employees and volunteers should also have regular (at least annual) training on sexual abuse prevention policies, as well as regular supervision and evaluations where these issues are evaluated and discussed. Supervisors should also regularly conduct unscheduled observations (in-person or via video) of employees and volunteers as they are engaging with youth.

4. Ensuring Safe Environments Youth-serving organizations must also create environments that can help prevent sexual abuse. Policies and guidelines should also be created to address safety when on the toilet, showering, and changing clothes. Further protocols must be established for transportation to and from institution-sanctioned events as well as policies regarding youth traveling in employee/volunteers' cars.

5. Responding to Inappropriate Behavior, Breaches in Policy, and Allegations and Suspicions of Child Sexual Abuse It is the responsibility of the youth-serving organization to develop policies and procedures to protect against sexual abuse; however, if sexual abuse is suspected, then it is the authorities, such as police and child protection services, who should be notified to investigate the allegations or suspicions. The CDC report (2007) notes that conducting internal investigations can harm the youth and/or the legal investigative process.

6. Training About Child Sexual Abuse Prevention The final component of a comprehensive child abuse prevention policy is training. Training should be done yearly, be documented, and consist of separate training for employees/volunteers, caregivers, and the youth themselves. Caregivers and youth should receive training on CSA information, including the stages of grooming and what may constitute grooming behaviors. They should also be trained on organizational policies and procedures and what to do if abuse is suspected.

While none of these policies are in and of themselves foolproof, having the aforementioned policies and procedures in place, as well as having all employees and volunteers within the organization trained about the signs of sexual grooming and CSA and how to respond, will make it less likely that a perpetrator can use their institutional affiliation to gain access to youth for the purposes of sexual abuse.

14.4 Sexual Grooming-Specific Prevention

14.4.1 In-Person Sexual Grooming Prevention

Many of the aforementioned child abuse prevention strategies target behaviors, tactics, and risk factors that are associated with sexual grooming. For example, institutional guidelines regarding touching between adult staff and youth are designed to prevent the behaviors involved in the *desensitization to sexual content and physical contact* stage identified in the Sexual Grooming Model (SGM; Winters et al., 2020). Organizational policies that require two adults to be present around minors prevent the isolation of minors as delineated in the *gaining access and isolation* stage of the SGM. Further, many educational interventions now mention sexual grooming as a strategy used by some individuals to perpetrate CSA, but to our knowledge, there is no data evaluating whether such interventions are effective at increasing adults' abilities to detect sexual grooming behaviors. While we hope that education about the SGM and its associated behaviors and tactics can aid in prevention efforts, we know that without targeted educational interventions, individuals are poor at identifying sexual grooming behaviors before the abuse occurs (see Winters & Jeglic, 2017). Further, research suggests that individuals are better able to identify sexual grooming behaviors related to sexual content and touch as possibly indicative of future sexual abuse but struggle to recognize other types of sexual grooming behaviors (see Winters & Jeglic, 2016).

Based upon our current understanding of child sexual grooming, Craven et al. (2007) recommended five points at which prevention and intervention strategies could be used, as detailed in Table 14.2 below.

From a tertiary prevention perspective, grooming knowledge and education has an important role in the treatment of those who perpetrate sexual crimes, especially among those who abuse children and adolescents. A central component of treatment is the understanding of the events and risk factors that contribute to perpetration. Identifying the grooming behaviors and tactics employed by the perpetrator can be incorporated into sexual management plans in order to detect high-risk behaviors and develop strategies that can prevent future abuse (see Chap. 13; Moster et al., 2008; Schaffer et al., 2010).

It should be noted that many of these prevention strategies are dependent upon the further empirical study of sexual grooming behaviors and tactics. As such, none have been studied sufficiently to deem them effective at preventing sexual abuse. However, given the current state of knowledge of sexual grooming and the degree to which such behaviors and strategies appear to be embedded in the sexual abuse of children, adolescents, and potentially adults as well (see Winters & Jeglic, 2021 and Chap. 12), we recommend that at present, sexual abuse prevention efforts explicitly address sexual grooming behaviors and tactics as delineated in the SGM.

Table 14.2 Strategies for prevention/intervention of child sexual grooming

Point of prevention/intervention	Strategy
Identifying potential offenders at the onset of their sexual interest in children	• Prevention programs with those who have pedophilic interest but have not acted on them like stop it now or stopitnow.org (in the United States).
Identification of potential offenders as they initiate self-grooming behaviors	• Better understanding of how motivations to sexually abuse develop so that potential offenders can seek help.
Identification of potential offenders as they groom the environment and significant others	• Training youth-serving institutions about sexual grooming strategies and behaviors. • Implementation of policies and procedures to limit access to minors.
Identification of potential offenders once they start grooming the child	• Increasing public awareness about sexual grooming behaviors and tactics.
Work with identified offenders to prevent future offending	• Cognitive behavioral sex offender treatment. • Circles of support and accountability to support released individuals in the community.

14.4.2 Online Sexual Grooming Prevention

As detailed in Chap. 5, the behaviors and tactics used in online sexual grooming differ somewhat from those used in in-person sexual grooming, and the online process may take place more rapidly than sexual grooming that happens in-person (Black et al., 2015; Marcum et al., 2007; Winters et al., 2017). In addition, the online nature of the grooming makes it more pervasive as those who want to engage in online sexual abuse have easy access to minors around the world. As online sexual grooming has proliferated over the last decade due to the increase in number of minors who have access to electronic devices, so too have the calls for prevention. As described in Chap. 5, the majority of prevention initiatives have been legislative, with many countries introducing legislation to make the luring of children via electronic means a crime (Ezioni, 2020). However, such crimes are hard to prosecute, and often, the abuse has already occurred. Prevention efforts to date have largely focused on education for youth and parents as well as digital protection applications that can be installed on devices. For example, Wurtele and Kenny (2016) discussed five types of prevention efforts:

1. **Cybersafety websites**. Some websites are designed to provide minors with information about the dangers of online solicitation and sexting although Wurtele and Kenny (2016) caution that much of the information is based upon "stranger danger," and they fail to address risky teen online behaviors.
2. **Online sexual grooming software**. Microsoft has developed software that can scan chats to detect child sexual grooming. Project Artemis scans chats to detect words and speech patterns that may be indicative of sexual grooming, and if detected, they are flagged for review by a human moderator (Lyons, 2020).
3. **Parenting education.** Parental education focuses on teaching parents about the risks online and helps to facilitate parent-child dialogues about Internet safety. Whittle et al. (2013) found that parents who oversaw their teen's online activity were less likely to experience a negative online event, such as solicitation. Other parental education can include the use of protective software and situational prevention (e.g., use of devices in public areas).
4. **School-based safety education**. Schools have been identified as a likely place for online safety education as not all parents/guardians may feel comfortable/capable of having such conversations with their children. Standardized Internet safety programs have been designed to be administered in educational settings, which enable youth to practice skills such as what to do if they are contacted online by a stranger (Jones et al., 2014).
5. **Guidelines for youth-serving organizations.** As detailed above in the guidelines for sexual abuse prevention in youth-serving organization, policies and procedures regarding the acceptable and unacceptable use of Internet-enabled communications should be established. While personal devices are increasingly being used for educational purposes, personal communications between staff and youth should always be public and not via text messaging or social media.

Similar to many CSA prevention initiatives, these guidelines and practices are intuitive and are likely helpful in preventing online sexual grooming; however, few have been tested empirically.

14.5 Conclusion

While the past few decades have witnessed an increase in sexual violence prevention programs and strategies, many of these programs are still lacking data to demonstrate their effectiveness. In part, this is due to measurement challenges. For example, when implementing educational interventions, environmental approaches, or general policies and procedures, it is hard to determine how much sexual violence these approaches prevent. It is not clear how outcomes should be measured (i.e., change in attitudes or the number of cases of sexual abuse prevented). While there are many strategies that appear intuitive to prevent sexual violence (such as parental education), the CDC highlights that, at present, evidence-based primary prevention strategies are limited. The CDC has detailed key gaps that require more research including:

- Improving surveillance systems and data collection for monitoring CSA.
- Increasing our understanding of risk and protective factors for CSA perpetration and victimization.
- Strengthening existing and developing new evidence-based policies, programs, and practices for the primary prevention of CSA.
- Increasing dissemination and implementation of evidence-based strategies for CSA prevention (CDC, n.d.)

Furthermore, many current strategies fail to adequately address the role of child sexual grooming in CSA. The CDC guidelines for youth-serving organizations take into consideration that many nonfamilial individuals who want to abuse children seek out roles in youth-serving organizations, and as such, the CDC has recommended that youth-serving organizations have policies and environmental protections in place to minimize access to vulnerable youth. However, many training programs still only gloss over sexual grooming. They either have an incomplete understanding of sexual grooming (i.e., does not include the fact that minors or women may engage in sexual grooming, does not include all stages of sexual grooming, or fails to address online sexual grooming), or they do not address sexual grooming at all. Further, if sexual grooming is included in trainings, its applicability to teens and possibly adults as well is rarely addressed. Ultimately, much work remains in developing and empirically validating prevention strategies.

References

Becker, J. V., & Reilly, D. W. (1999). Preventing sexual abuse and assault. *Sexual Abuse, 11*(4), 267–278. https://doi.org/10.1177/107906329901100403

Beier, K. M., Grundmann, D., Kuhle, L. F., Scherner, G., Konrad, A., & Amelung, T. (2015). The German Dunkelfeld project: A pilot study to prevent child sexual abuse and the use of child abusive images. *The Journal of Sexual Medicine, 12*(2), 529–542. https://doi.org/10.1111/jsm.12785

Black, P. J., Wollis, M., Woodworth, M., & Hancock, J. T. (2015). A linguistic analysis of grooming strategies of online child sex offenders: Implications for our understanding of predatory sexual behavior in an increasingly computer-mediated world. *Child Abuse & Neglect, 44*, 140–149. https://doi.org/10.1016/j.chiabu.2014.12.004

Bronfenbrenner, U. (1979). *The ecology of human development*. Harvard University Press.

Bronfenbrenner, U. (1986). Ecology of the family as a context for human development: Research perspectives. *Developmental Psychology, 22*, 723–742. https://doi.org/10.1037//0012-1649.22.6.723

Bronfenbrenner, U. (1995). Developmental ecology through space and time: A future perspective. In P. Moen, G. H. Elder Jr., & K. Luscher (Eds.), *Examining lives in context: Perspectives on the ecology of human development* (pp. 619–647). APA Books.

Centers for Disease Control. (2004). *Sexual violence prevention: Beginning the dialogue*. Centers for Disease Control and Prevention.

Centers for Disease Control (n.d.) *Preventing child sexual abuse*. https://www.cdc.gov/violenceprevention/childsexualabuse/fastfact.html

Child Abuse Prevention and Treatment Act of 1974. 42 USC §§5101–5106.

Child Abuse Prevention and Treatment Amendment Act of 2018. USC §§115–424.

Child Welfare Information Gateway. (2017). *Child maltreatment prevention: Past, present, and future*. U.S. Department of Health and Human Services, Children's Bureau.

Craven, A., Brown, S., & Gilchrist, E. (2007). Current responses to sexual grooming: Implications for prevention. *The Howard Journal, 46*(1), 60–71. https://doi.org/10.1111/j.1468-2311.2007.00454.x

Eide, M. (1990). The first chapter of children's rights. *American Heritage, 41*(5) https://www.americanheritage.com/first-chapter-childrens-rights

Ezioni, L. (2020). The crime of grooming. *Child & Family Law Journal, 8*(1) https://lawpublications.barry.edu/cflj/vol8/iss1/1

Jeglic, E. L., & Calkins, C. (Eds.). (2016). *Sexual violence: Evidence based policy and prevention*. Springer.

Jeglic, E. L., & Calkins, C. (2018). *Protecting your child from sexual abuse: What you need to know to keep your kids safe*. Skyhorse Publishing.

Jones, L. M., Mitchell, K. J., & Walsh, W. A. (2014). *A content analysis of youth internet safety programs: Are effective prevention strategies being used?* Crimes Against Children Research Center, University of New Hampshire.

Kelly, J. G. (1966). Ecological constraints on mental health services. *American Psychologist, 21*, 535–539. https://doi.org/10.1037/h0023598

Kelly, J. G. (1968). Towards an ecological conception of preventive interventions. In J. W. Carter Jr. (Ed.), *Research contributions from psychology to community mental health* (pp. 75–99). Behavioral Publications.

Kelly, J. G. (1971). Qualities for the community psychologist. *American Psychologist, 26*, 897–903. https://doi.org/10.1037/h0032231

Kempe, C. H., Silverman, F. N., Steele, B. F., Droegemueller, W., & Silver, H. K. (1962). The battered-child syndrome. *JAMA, 181*, 17–24. https://doi.org/10.1001/jama.1962.03050270019004

Krug, E. G., Mercy, J. A., Dahlberg, L. L., & Zwi, A. B. (2002). The world report on violence and health. *The Lancet, 360*(9339), 1083–1088. https://doi.org/10.1016/S0140-6736(02)11133-0

Letourneau, E. (2017, September 14). Watch my TEDMED talk on child sexual abuse prevention: Prevention is the only way to end victimization. *Psychology Today*. https://www.psychologytoday.com/intl/blog/prevention-now/201709/watch-my-tedmed-talk-childsexual-abuse-prevention

Lyons, K., (2020, January 14). Microsoft tries to improve child abuse detection by opening its Xbox chat tool to other companies. *The Verge*. https://www.theverge.com/2020/1/14/21063491/microsoft-tool-artemis-abuse-chat-xbox

Marcum, C. D. (2007). Interpreting the intentions of internet predators: An examination of online predatory behavior. *Journal of Child Sexual Abuse: Research, Treatment, & Program Innovations For Victims, Survivors, & Offenders, 16*(4), 99–114. https://doi.org/10.1300/J070v16n04_06

McAlinden, A. M. (2012). *'Grooming'and the Sexual Abuse of Children: Institutional, Internet and Familial Dimensions*. Oxford University Press.

McCartan, K. F., Merdian, H. L., Perkins, D. E., & Kettleborough, D. (2018). Ethics and issues of secondary prevention efforts in child sexual abuse. *International Journal of Offender Therapy and Comparative Criminology, 62*(9), 2548–2566. https://doi.org/10.1177/0306624X17723951

Moster, A., Wnuk, D. W., & Jeglic, E. L. (2008). Cognitive behavioral therapy interventions with sex offenders. *Journal of Correctional Health Care, 14*(2), 109–121. https://doi.org/10.1177/1078345807313874

O'Donohue, W., Geer, J. H., & Elliott, A. (2013). The primary prevention of child sexual abuse. In *The sexual abuse of children* (pp. 485–526). Routledge.

Saul, J., & Audage, N. C. (2007). *Preventing child sexual abuse within youth-serving organizations: Getting started on policies and procedures*. US Department of Health and Human Services, Centers for Disease Control and Prevention, National Center for Injury Prevention and Control, Division of Violence Prevention.

Schaffer, M., Jeglic, E. L., Moster, A., & Wnuk, D. (2010). Cognitive-behavioral therapy in the treatment and management of sex offenders. *Journal of Cognitive Psychotherapy, 24*(2), 92–103. https://doi.org/10.1891/0889-8391.24.2.92

Townsend, S. M. (2008). Primary prevention of sexual violence: A technical assistance guide for planning and evaluation.. Pennsylvania Coalition Against Rape.

Whittle, H., Hamilton-Giachritsis, C., Beech, A., & Collings, G. (2013). A review of young people's vulnerabilities to online grooming. *Aggression and Violent Behavior, 18*(1), 135–146. https://doi.org/10.1016/j.avb.2012.11.008

Winters, G. M., & Jeglic, E. L. (2016). I knew it all along: The sexual grooming behaviors of child molesters and the hindsight bias. *Journal of Child Sexual Abuse, 25*(1), 20–36. https://doi.org/10.1080/10538712.2015.1108945

Winters, G. M., & Jeglic, E. L. (2017). Stages of sexual grooming: Recognizing potentially predatory behaviors of child molesters. *Deviant Behavior, 38*(6), 724–733. https://doi.org/10.1080/01639625.2016.1197656

Winters, G. M., & Jeglic, E. L. (2021). The sexual grooming scale–victim version: The development and pilot testing of a measure to assess the nature and extent of child sexual grooming. *Victims & Offenders*, 1–22. https://doi.org/10.1080/15564886.2021.1974994

Winters, G. M., Kaylor, L. E., & Jeglic, E. L. (2017). Sexual offenders contacting children online: An examination of transcripts of sexual grooming. *Journal of Sexual Aggression, 23*(1), 62–76. https://doi.org/10.1080/13552600.2016.1271146

Winters, G. M., Jeglic, E. L., & Kaylor, L. E. (2020). Validation of the sexual grooming model of child sexual abusers. *Journal of Child Sexual Abuse, 29*(7), 855–875. https://doi.org/10.1080/10538712.2020.1801935

Wurtele, S. K., & Kenny, M. C. (2016). Technology-related sexual solicitation of adolescents: A review of prevention efforts. *Child Abuse Review, 25*(5), 332–344. https://doi.org/10.1002/car.2445

Chapter 15
Law Enforcement and the Courts and Sexual Grooming

Instances of sexual abuse often go unreported, but there are some cases of child sexual abuse (CSA) that are formally reported to law enforcement and subsequently processed through the courts. There is a so-called "funnel" effect from reporting, formal investigation, prosecution, and conviction for sexual offenses; that is, the number of cases at each step in the process reduces (Block & Williams, 2019; Manson, 1984). As a result, there are few cases of CSA being reported to law enforcement and even fewer that are processed through the courts and ultimately convicted. Nonetheless, law enforcement personnel must be prepared to investigate the CSA cases that are being brought to the attention of the authorities. The construct of sexual grooming may be helpful in informing those working these cases on what information to seek during investigation, as well as how to guide the questioning of those involved (e.g., victims, suspects, witnesses) about the instances that occurred before, during, and after the offense. Also, for the cases that are eventually prosecuted, court personnel must be informed about the characteristics of these offenses in the decision-making process (e.g., decisions regarding plea bargains, adjudication, sentencing, etc.). While sexual grooming has yet to be researched in the context of the court system and sentencing, it may be useful in informing the determination of guilt and sentencing phases of the process. In this chapter, we will explore ways in which sexual offense cases are processed through law enforcement and the courts as well as describe how sexual grooming should be incorporated during these steps in the criminal justice system.

© The Author(s), under exclusive license to Springer Nature Switzerland AG 2022
G. M. Winters, E. L. Jeglic, *Sexual Grooming*,
https://doi.org/10.1007/978-3-031-07222-2_15

15.1 Overview of Sexual Offenses in the Criminal Justice System

In general, there is a step-by-step process for how criminal cases, including sex crimes, are processed through law enforcement and the court (American Bar Association [ABA], 2020). See Fig. 15.1 for an overview of the criminal justice procedure.

As noted previously, there is a funnel effect that occurs with sexual offenses through the criminal justice system (see Fig. 15.2). That is, there are fewer cases at each stage of the process, from reports to authorities, arrest, prosecution, and ultimately conviction (Manson, 1984).

Regarding initial disclosure, there is recent research to suggest that fewer than half of victims of CSA disclose the abuse informally to a social support (Winters et al., 2020), with prior estimates suggesting this number may be as low as 16–25% (Jonzon & Lindblatt, 2004; London et al., 2005, 2008; Lyon & Ahern, 2010; National Children's Advocacy Center, 2014). More so, even fewer of these cases will become known to law enforcement. For example, one retrospective review of 13 studies showed a range between 5% and 13% of alleged cases of CSA were reported to authorities (London et al., 2008). Based on data from the National Incident-Based Reporting System (NIBRS; i.e., a system that gathers information from criminal offenses and arrests reported to 8,500 law enforcement agencies across 20 states in the United States [US]), there were 65,728 reported rape incidents that were ultimately reported to law enforcement in 2020, which includes 26,736 cases committed against victims ages 10–19 (Federal Bureau of Investigation [FBI], 2021). Although this data is limited by the number of states/agencies that participate, as well as the lack of inclusion of victims under the age of 10, the

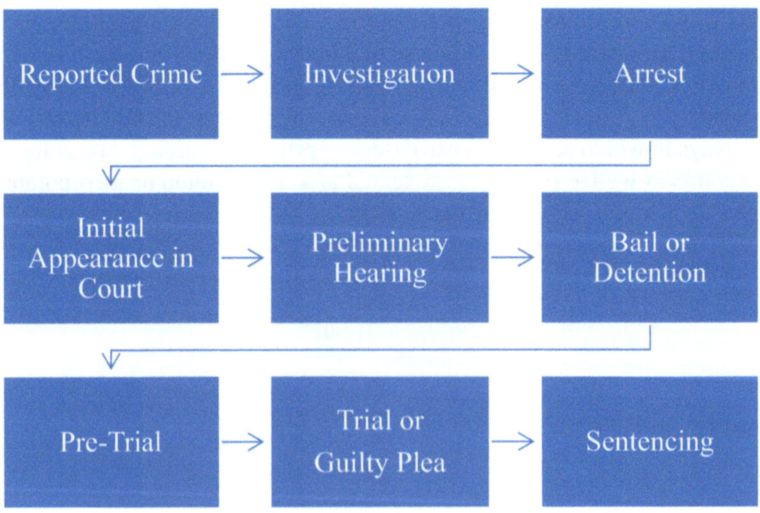

Fig. 15.1 Overview of the criminal court process

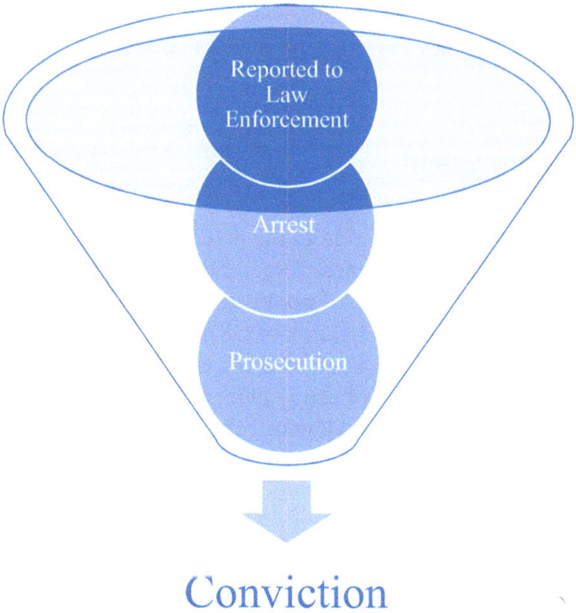

Fig. 15.2 The funnel effect of sex offense cases

numbers reflect that around one-third of the cases being reported to law enforcement are against minors.

The next critical step in the criminal justice process is whether there is enough evidence to formally charge an individual accused of a sexual offense following the report to law enforcement. Compared to the 65,728 rape incidents that were reported to law enforcement, only 16,895 (~25%) of these resulted in an arrest (FBI, 2021). This is consistent with data from prior decades (1991–1996), showing that 27% of sexual assault victimizations reported in NIBRS resulted in an arrest (Snyder, 2000). When looking specifically at the percentage of arrests in child victimization cases from 1991 to 1996, the results showed arrests in only 19% of cases when the victim was under age six, which is lower than the percentages for victims ages six to 11 (33%) or 12 to 17 (32%). This is consistent with another study on CSA cases that found approximately one in five cases out of 500 examined were prosecuted, and half of those resulted in a conviction or guilty plea (Block & Williams, 2019).

Lastly, if an individual is found guilty, there is a sentencing phase in the court. According to the US Sentencing Commission, there were 1,067 defendants of sexual abuse sentenced in 2018 (this includes the following crimes: rape, statutory rape, criminal sexual abuse of a ward, abusive sexual contact, promoting a commercial sex act, travel to engage in prohibited sexual conduct with a minor, production of child pornography, or child exploitation enterprises). Nearly all (98.8%) were sentenced to prison time, with the average sentence being 191 months. Taken together, when examining cases from the disclosure through sentencing process, there are fewer and fewer cases; nonetheless, there is still a significant number of cases that are received by law enforcement and the courts each year.

15.2 Law Enforcement

Law enforcement serves a critical role in the detection, investigation, and arrest of those who perpetrate sexual offenses. Recommendations for law enforcement departments include the importance of establishing and enforcing specific policies, procedures, and trainings for investigation of CSA cases (US Department of Justice [DOJ], 2001). The important aspects of the CSA investigation process can be broadly described in terms of 1) collecting evidence (e.g., through search warrants or medical examination) and 2) interviewing relevant sources (e.g., the child victim, caregivers, other family or friends, the suspect; US DOJ, 1997).

15.2.1 Investigations

Generally speaking, law enforcement follows a set of guidelines during CSA investigations. Table 15.1 presents the recommended steps for law enforcement throughout the investigation process (US DOJ, 2001).

15.2.2 Interviews

Forensic interviews often serve as the first, and an incredibly important, aspect of a CSA investigation (Newlin et al., 2015), given there may not be physical evidence to substantiate a CSA allegation (e.g., in cases where there was delayed disclosure). Law enforcement investigating these cases should consider interviewing the child involved, as well as the suspect, non-offending caregivers, or other individuals who might have knowledge of the abuse (e.g., siblings, other relatives, friends; US DOJ, 1997).

A forensic interview of a child is "a developmentally sensitive and legally sound method of gathering factual information regarding allegations of abuse or exposure to violence. This interview is conducted by a competently trained, neutral professional utilizing research and practice-informed techniques as part of a larger investigative process" (Newlin et al., 2015, p. 3). It has been recommended that these types of child forensic interviews occur in three phases (see Table 15.2). These steps are used to ensure the emotional well-being of the child while gathering as much substantive information regarding the allegations in order to facilitate evidence collection and eventual prosecution. In sum, the investigation and interviewing

Table 15.1 Steps in law enforcement investigations of CSA

Once a referral is received
• Identify personal biases in order to maintain objectivity • Know the state statutes and department guidelines • Know what community resources are available for the family and victim • Introductions that explain the officer's role and focus of the investigation • Interview the child alone, focusing on evidence that may help corroborate the accusation • Assure that the child will receive the best treatment to protect them
Getting information for the preliminary report
• Ask about the history of the abuse (especially dates) and any other elements that are necessary for the report • Provide supportive facts in the report and refrain from forming an opinion until the end of the report
Preserving the crime scene
• Treat the scene as a crime scene (even if the abuse occurred previously) • Secure any instruments of abuse or corroborative evidence that the child identified in their report • Photograph the scene and injuries of the child if applicable
Follow-up investigation
• Be supportive of the child and family • Arrange for a medical examination and transportation, and collect clothing items for evidence if applicable • Use applicable investigative techniques • Refer the child and family to community resources/therapy • Provide the child and family with information on how to contact the detective
During the court phase
• Visit the court with the child to familiarize them with the setting, or coordinate this with the prosecution • Prepare the courtroom exhibits • File all evidence in accordance to policy • Update the family about the progress of the investigation and court process • Follow up with probation department for preparation of a presentence report

processes conducted by law enforcement are vital in gathering evidence toward convicting an individual who committed a sexual offense.

15.2.3 *Sexual Grooming in Law Enforcement Investigations*

The construct of sexual grooming and related terms (e.g., seduction, modus operandi) have been referenced in relation to law enforcement investigations since the 1970s and 1980s (Lanning, 2018). In Lanning's (2010) guide for professionals investigating cases of child exploitation, he emphasized that some individuals may utilize sexual grooming techniques during the offense process, and thus, sexual grooming strategies and tactics must be considered when investigating CSA cases. Table 15.3 presents some examples of how sexual grooming has been incorporated

Table 15.2 The phases of a child forensic interview

Rapport building phase
• Introductions • Provision of an age- and context-consistent explanation of the interview process (e.g., documentation, content of interview) • Discussion about the importance of telling the truth and practice providing narratives/episodic memory training
Substantive phase
• Inquire about the narrative description of the events using open-ended and objective questions • Includes seeking details, clarifying content, and exploring alternative hypotheses
Closure phase
• Attention to the child's emotional needs • Transition discussion to non-substantive topics • Allowing the child to ask questions • Discuss safety planning or provide psychoeducation

Table 15.3 Investigation guidelines referencing sexual grooming

Victim selection	Regarding the victim's family situation: 1. "Extreme over-protectiveness and/or parental dominance; 2. Social isolation; 3. Conflict or alienation between parents; 4. Substance abuse; 5. Lack of supervision, controls, communication"[a]
Gaining access and isolation	"Whether access to the victim by the suspect was possible and if he or she had the opportunity to commit the offense"[a]
Trust development	"Lures: The suspect may have used toys, games, or stuffed animals to entice the child into the situation or to try to maintain the child's interest in the perpetrator"[b] "Playful, lures with toys, games," and "gifts"[a] "Special attention"[a] "Interacts with child at child level of emotional development"[a]
Desensitization to sexual content and physical contact	"Unobtrusive touch leading to overt sexual assault"[a] "Show pornography"[a] "Gradually lowers inhibitions"[a]
Post-abuse maintenance	"Child victims are often sworn to keep the sexual behavior a secret"[b] "Secrecy associated with the sexual activity, or threats of personal harm to the child or to the child's family"[c]

[a]California Commission on Peace Officer Standards and Training (CCPOST) (1998)
[b]United States Department of Justice (1997)
[c]Office of the Attorney General (1998)

into existing guidelines for law enforcement investigations (i.e., what information they should be seeking to obtain during the investigation). However, from our review, there appears to be limited attention to the importance of sexual grooming in training and in guidelines for law enforcement investigating CSA cases in general.

Investigations

We argue that given the high number of cases that involve at least some aspects of sexual grooming (e.g., Canter et al., 1998; Winters & Jeglic, 2021), it would be beneficial for law enforcement to consider sexual grooming when collecting evidence and during interview procedures. If law enforcement personnel conducting the CSA investigation have a thorough understanding of the sexual grooming process, they can potentially use that information in guiding their gathering of evidence. For example, the investigators can seek evidence to suggest that the individual took the child on overnight stays, provided the child with gifts or drugs/alcohol, or used sexualized behaviors before the alleged abuse (e.g., showing the child their naked body, showing the child pornography). Looking for these types of sexual grooming behaviors in the suspect-child interactions can help shed light on the presence, extent, severity, and frequency of the alleged sexual abuse.

Moreover, if an allegation of CSA is brought to the attention of law enforcement but no suspect has been identified (e.g., if the child is reluctant to disclose out of fear, concern for the individual, etc.), law enforcement can gather information regarding the child's interactions with adults or juveniles in their life to see if any of these pre-offense tactics may be present. Of course, these behaviors in and of themselves are not necessarily definitive signs of abuse, but they could lead law enforcement to potential suspects or witnesses that may have helpful information. Relatedly, it is possible that an individual is offending against more than one child. Therefore, in cases where a suspect is identified, law enforcement may want to search for the presence of sexual grooming behaviors with other potential victims, such as whether the adult had access to or spent time alone with other children, as it may be beneficial to interview these individuals. There is evidence that once someone who abuses children has developed tactics that have led to abuse, they will then repeat these "successful" behaviors and tactics when they abuse other children (Elliott et al., 1995). Ultimately, having an established modus operandi across crimes can help in conviction if the case is taken to court, although a caveat with all sexual grooming behaviors is that many sexual grooming behaviors and tactics are also consistent with normal adult-child interactions and are not always deviant in nature. As such, law enforcement should look for clusters of grooming behaviors or evidence of those grooming behaviors that are frequent or more severe (e.g., those that include touch and sexual content).

Interviewing

Next, in regard to interviewing, having an interviewer in CSA investigations who is familiar with sexual grooming may help facilitate the questions during the substantive phase. The interviewer could be attentive to aspects of the sexual grooming process (such as the stages and behaviors in the Sexual Grooming Model [SGM] in Winters et al., 2020) as these may provide credence to the allegations of abuse if they are observed in a high frequency or severity. For example, an interviewer could utilize the *Sexual Grooming Scale-Victim Version* (*SGS-V*; Winters et al., 2021) to guide questions about the offense process. This could include using particular items/questions to gather specific information or to administer the entire measure in certain cases (e.g., with older victims, given the *SGS-V* has not yet been validated with youth). The stages of sexual grooming may be helpful in guiding the child through the temporal sequence of the offense process, from the earlier behaviors (e.g., selecting a vulnerable victim, gaining access and isolating the child) through the increasing concerning sexual acts (e.g., gradual increase in physical touch and sexual conversations). Also, evidence of the use of post-abuse maintenance tactics by the individual accused of the offense may shed light on how the victim responded to abuse (e.g., if their disclosure was delayed, it may be in part due to the use of these post-abuse sexual grooming strategies). It has also been suggested that during interviews with caregivers or witnesses, it may be beneficial to educate them about sexual grooming so they can potentially identify any behaviors or statements that could corroborate the child's allegations (The Institute for Human Services, 2010). For example, a caregiver might be asked about whether the suspect spent time alone with the child without other adults present and whether there were any sexual conversations or behaviors observed between the victim and the suspect.

15.3 Courts

As outlined in Fig. 15.1, there is a step-by-step process for how criminal cases, including sex crimes, are processed through court (ABA, 2020). Following the arrest and formal charges, the defendant proceeds through an initial court appearance, preliminary hearing, and pretrial. Subsequently, they either enter a guilty plea (i.e., plea bargain) or go to trial. If the case goes to trial and the defendant is found guilty, they undergo a sentencing process through the courts.

Consistent with other crimes in the criminal justice system, prosecuted sexual offense cases are more likely to result in a guilty plea via a plea bargain than to go to trial (Block & Williams, 2019). Block and Williams (2019) found that in a sample of 89 cases of CSA that were prosecuted, 14 (15.7%) went to trial compared to 32 (36.0%) that resulted in a plea bargain, with the remaining cases including those where guilt was admitted but adjudication was deferred ($n = 15$; 16.8%), the charges were dismissed ($n = 24$; 27%), or the charges were pending ($n = 4$; 4.5%). The study also found that of the 14 cases that went to trial, 10 (71.4%) were found guilty, and 4 (28.6%) were found not guilty. It is recommended that those involved in the court process for child CSA cases (e.g., attorneys, judges) should understand sexual crimes (ABA, 2015; United Nations Office of Drugs and Crime, 2017), including the unique characteristics (e.g., reasons for nondisclosure) and processes (e.g., use of sexual grooming tactics) that may be involved. This information may be helpful in the decision-making steps for processing a sexual offense in the court system—from decisions regarding whether the case should be pleaded out or go to trial, all the way through the adjudication and sentencing phases—as it can help shed light on duration, intensity, and validity of the CSA allegations.

15.3.1 *Using Sexual Grooming as Evidence for Adjudication*

According to the ABA (2015), evidence of sexual grooming may be helpful to convict defendants in jurisdictions that have laws that sexual grooming alone is a crime (this topic is addressed in Chap. 16) as well as to substantiate allegations of CSA through presenting evidence of sexual grooming and/or having expert testimony on the subject. The ABA even includes an information page on their website to inform attorneys regarding the definition of sexual grooming, behaviors that may be involved in the process, and the contexts in which these behaviors are likely to occur in (e.g., in-person, online, or institutions; ABA, 2015).

According to Manero (2012), sexual grooming evidence must be considered admissible under the Federal Rules of Evidence 404(b), which states:

> Evidence of other crimes, wrongs, or acts is not admissible to prove the character of a person in order to show action in conformity therewith. It may, however, be admissible for other purposes, such as proof of motive, opportunity, intent, preparation, plan, knowledge, identity, or absence of mistake or accident, provided that upon request by the accused, the prosecution in a criminal case shall provide reasonable notice in advance of trial, or during trial if the court excuses pretrial notice on good cause shown, of the general nature of any such evidence it intends to introduce at trial.

Thus, it has been suggested that sexual grooming evidence can help shed light on a defendant's preparation, planning, and opportunity leading up to the offense, as well as the individual's intent and motivation (Manero, 2012). Interestingly, however, the use of expert testimony and evidence on sexual grooming has been the subject of numerous court appeals, primarily as it relates to the admissibility of this type of evidence. Arguments are typically related to whether such evidence is relevant and probative of the crime for which the defendant is charged and not "unduly prejudicial" (i.e., the evidence detracts from the material issues and is likely to result in improper decisions by the trier of fact; Manero, 2012). Table 15.4 provides examples of cases (not an exhaustive list) across the US that have addressed the issue of whether sexual grooming testimony should be admitted in court or not.

Most recently, the issue of sexual grooming testimony in court was brought up during the federal trial of Ghislaine Maxwell (see Chap. 9 for a description of this case; United States v. Ghislaine Maxwell, 2021). A clinical psychologist was permitted by the federal judge to testify in the case about the process of "grooming" in CSA cases. Per court documentation, the expert would testify to the following:

1. First, that perpetrators of sexual abuse of minors frequently use manipulation or coercion short of physical force as part of a strategic pattern, often referred to as grooming, to make the minor vulnerable to abuse.
2. Second, that manipulation and grooming can prevent the minor from understanding their experience as abuse and so prevent disclosure.
3. Third, that abuse can cause long-term traumatic and psychological consequences.
4. Fourth, that the presence of another individual can facilitate sexual abuse of minors.
5. And fifth, that nondisclosure, incremental disclosure, and secrecy are common among victims of sexual abuse and that memory can be affected by a variety of factors, including the effects of trauma.

Table 15.4 Example cases of admissibility of sexual grooming testimony

Cases that sexual grooming testimony was upheld
Krause v. State of Texas (2019) • The appellate argued that the trial court abused its discretion by permitting expert testimony on the defendant having "groom[ed]" the complainant. • Expert testimony from Young, an investigative law enforcement officer, included: "In this case, the suspect would have to obviously be very, very close to his victim, would have to gain the trust, have to gain the love of the victim or it doesn't work in their advantage. I mean, they can't do this type of stuff if they don't have the love and trust, you know, of the children they do this to." • The court concluded that sexual grooming is a "legitimate subject of expert testimony," and Young "possessed sufficient qualifications" (i.e., 19 years in law enforcement) to testify on the matter. They also noted that the testimony did not "increase the depth of understanding of the jurors" as sexual grooming is "not a complex topic.".
Morris v. State of Texas (2011) • The appellate argued that "grooming" was not a legitimate subject of expert testimony given the lack of scientific research on the subject and questioned the expert's qualifications for this testimony. • Testimony on sexual grooming was provided by former Texas Ranger Hullum, who described the term as "an attempt by the offender to get the victim compliant with what he wants to happen." Hullum noted this might include giving the child alcohol or pornography, engaging in sexual banter, giving or withholding gifts, or telling the child about the adult's own prior sexual experiences. • The court recognized the experience-based study of "grooming" to be a legitimate "subject of expert testimony has been established sufficiently to be judicially noticed."
Bryant v. State of Texas (2010) • Appellate argued that the trial court erred by permitting testimony regarding "grooming" given the expert was not qualified to offer this testimony due to the lack of sufficient experience and training. • The expert, a law enforcement officer for two years investigating crimes against children, testified about grooming, including: "Grooming is a common technique used. There's plenty of research on it, and it's common." • The court determined the trial court did not err in including the expert testimony as the required field of the expert's expertise was not "complex" and the testimony about grooming was "not conclusive about anything," nor was it central to determine guilt or innocence.
Cases that sexual grooming testimony was deemed inadmissible
State of Oregon v. Henley (2018) • Appellate argued the court erred in allowing testimony about "grooming" as "scientific" evidence as it does not meet the standard of scientific validity and reliability under the evidentiary standard. • An expert, Palfreman, a forensic interviewer, testified that the defendant used sexual grooming behaviors based on her interview with the victim. Specifically, she stated, "Um, when she just talked about the massaging where she wanted it on her neck but he would go lower into her chest area." • The court concluded the trial court erred in admitting the evidence of sexual grooming without a proper foundation, but the court declined to form an opinion regarding whether the evidence had requisite reliability and validity of scientific evidence. They reversed the decision and remanded the case for further proceedings in circuit court.

(continued)

Table 15.4 (continued)

State of Louisiana v. Vidrine (2009) • The appellate argued the trial court erred in allowing the expert to testify on the issue regarding the defendant's behaviors being consistent with sexual grooming. • The expert, Benitez, a social worker, testified that the victim's testimony about the defendant pulling down his pants and touching his penis were consistent with "grooming" when the individual tests the boundaries of his victim. • The court determined that the statements were beyond providing a scientific perspective to help the jury evaluate the victim's testimony, and the opinion regarding grooming was "unduly prejudicial" given it suggested the behaviors were consistent with a person who committed a sexual offense.
State of Washington v. Braham (1992) • The appellate contended the court erred in permitting expert testimony about "grooming" given it is a type of "profile" evidence that would be unfairly prejudicial. • The expert, Berliner, a director of a research center and assistant professor, testified that sexual grooming is a "clinical term . . . has been applied to what we would call a process of victimization . . . [W]hat is basically meant by that is that in most cases where sexual abuse happens, it isn't something that just happens suddenly out of the blue. Generally there is a period of time where the person who intends to abuse the child gradually gets the child to feel more comfortable and may gradually sexualize the relationship or form a bond with the child so that the child will either not understand that what's happening to them is wrong or the child will not tell anyone about it after it happens." • The court held that the testimony served "virtually no probative value," and thus, the trial court erred in admitting the evidence as it was unfairly prejudicial. However, the court refrained from holding that this type of evidence would always be inadmissible.

The judge also determined that the defense could not call another expert witness to counter the testimony presented. In favor of the defense, the judge did determine that the expert could not provide testimony on one particular topic, grooming-by-proxy (i.e., sexual grooming in the present of a third-party; item 4, above) as "this phenomenon is not identified in the relevant literature regarding CSA and has not been subjected to peer review." Ultimately, there remains inconsistency across courts regarding whether sexual grooming should or should not be permitted as evidence in the court.

15.3.2 Using Sexual Grooming as Evidence for Sentencing

If an individual pleads guilty or is found guilty at trial, there is a subsequent phase in the court process during which the person is sentenced. There is typically a sentencing hearing for the judge to determine the appropriate sentence based on mitigating (e.g., factors suggesting a lower sentence may be appropriate) and aggravating (e.g., factors suggesting a longer sentence is appropriate) factors (Officers of the United States Attorneys, n.d.). While there are guidelines provided by the US Sentencing Commissions containing suggestive ranges for sentences for particular types of crimes (Officers of the United States Attorneys, n.d.), these additional motivating and aggravating factors can also be considered. The judge considers the content in a presentence report, as well as any statements from victims, defendant, or attorneys, in determining the sentence.

Butrus (2018) examined 37 cases of violent and sexual offenders to determine what types of factors were considered aggravating or mitigating in sentencing for these defendants. Based on the analysis of 12 sexual offenses cases, Butrus presented the most common aggravating and mitigating factors (see Table 15.5).

While the sample size in the Butrus (2018) study is small, the findings are relevant for consideration when discussing the role of sexual grooming in sentencing. First, *victim vulnerability* is considered an aggravating factor; per the SGM (Winters et al., 2020), those who sexually groomed their victim may seek out children with emotional/psychological or familial vulnerabilities, meaning that victim selection process may be relevant in considering victim vulnerability as an aggravating factor. Second, presence of a *breach of trust* is certainly related to the construct of sexual grooming as one of the stages involved in the process encompasses the development, and eventual betrayal, of trust with the victim. Third, there is evidence that sexual grooming may result in more *negative consequences for the victim* (Cunningham, 2020; see Chap. 5 for a full review); thus, sexual grooming utilized in the offense may speak to the issue of prolonged negative effects on a victim, especially if a *victim impact statement* is present describing these types of pre-offense behaviors. Fourth, the judge may consider the defendant's *denial, lack of remorse, or declining to accept responsibility* as aggravating factors (or lack thereof as a mitigating factor). As outlined in Chap. 6, some individuals may use "self-grooming" to promote and justify the offending behavior, which may be relevant when considering how these factors relate to the defendant's cognitive responses to

Table 15.5 Butrus (2018) findings for aggravating and mitigating factors for sexual offense cases

Aggravating factors	Mitigating factors
1. Age/vulnerability of victim(s)	1. Pled guilty
2. Prolonged negative effects on victim	2. Mental health problems
3. Breach of trust	3. Substance use problems
4. Victim impact statement	4. Childhood adversity
5. Prior offenses 6. History of substance use problems	5. Accepted responsibility for offending/showed remorse
7. Denial/lack of remorse/refusal to accept responsibility	6. Motivated for treatment 7. Defendant age
	8. No relevant past criminal record
	9. Less serious type of offense
	10. Was intoxicated at time of offending
	11. Cooperated with law enforcement
	12. Reduced risk of recidivism
	13. Good candidate for rehabilitation

the allegations. Fifth, while empirical research is needed on the association between use of sexual grooming and risk, it is possible that the prolonged, frequent, and intense use of these behaviors could result in more victims, longer periods of abuse, or more severe abuse—all factors that are relevant for consideration in the construct of *risk for future offending*.

15.3.3 Probation and Parole Stipulations

In addition to sexual grooming being potentially helpful to inform the factors considered in sentencing, the court may also benefit from considering sexual grooming in the context of parole/probation. After being released from incarceration, individuals with a history of sexual offenses will typically be supervised in the community under parole or probation conditions. The number of sexual offenders under community supervision has increased substantially over the past two decades (Lobanov-Rostovsky, 2015), with there being 800,000 registered sex offenders in the US in 2017 (NCMEC, 2017). The supervision of these individuals may include a range of conditions, such as polygraph testing, electronic monitoring (e.g., GPS), sex offender registration and community notification, residence restrictions, and mandatory treatment. When determining these conditions, it may be beneficial to consider the individual offense processes before, during, and after offending to inform applicable restrictions, recommended services, and areas of inquiry during probation/parole check-ins. For example, an individual who sexually groomed their victim through youth-serving organization (e.g., school) may be an appropriate candidate for residency restrictions so they are unable to reside near youth-serving institutions. During probation or parole meetings and polygraph tests, the professional overseeing the case could inquire about behaviors or tactics known to the individual's sexual grooming patterns to ensure these behaviors are not being enacted again.

15.4 Conclusion

In all, sexual grooming may serve an important role in the investigation and court proceedings for cases involving CSA. For investigations, law enforcement can utilize information on sexual grooming in the gathering of evidence, as well as interview of relevant persons (e.g., victim, suspect, witnesses). While law enforcement personnel are typically trained broadly on CSA, it appears there is little attention to the pre-offense tactics that might be used and how these can inform their investigations. Guidelines and trainings for those investigating CSA cases could include information about the overarching process of sexual grooming, as well as specific and observable behaviors that might have been present in order to collect valuable evidence to substantiate abuse claims. It may also be that the stages of sexual grooming could help guide victims or witnesses in their account of the abuse to ensure that information is gathered from before, during, and after the abuse. It would be helpful to have additional empirical research on whether law enforcement uses the construct of sexual grooming during investigations and if so, whether including sexual grooming behaviors and tactics in evidence gathering or interviews proves to be effective in substantiating (or refuting) cases of alleged CSA.

Additionally, court personnel may want to use this information in the adjudication or sentencing process. As was described above, there remains controversy within the courts regarding whether sexual grooming can be used as evidence or expert testimony at trial. We recommend that if this type of evidence does enter the courtroom, it must be based on empirical research and avoid conclusions based on personal experiences—as sexual grooming is a complex and nuanced topic. Also, consistent with recommendations from Manero (2012), we feel it is important that experts testifying on these issues are indeed experts in this area. That is, the individual should have *substantial* experience working in the field (research, clinical work, investigation) but must also rely upon reliable and valid empirical data on the subject. Lastly, we recommend improved quality and quantity of sexual grooming research in general. The more empirical and valid research that law enforcement, court personnel, expert witnesses, treatment providers, and probation/parole officers have on the subject, the more effective and accurate the processing of these cases in the criminal justice system will be.

References

American Bar Association. (2015). *Understanding sexual grooming in child cases*. https://www.americanbar.org/groups/public_interest/child_law/resources/child_law_practiceonline/child_law_practice/vol-34/november-2015/understanding-sexual-grooming-in-child-abuse-cases/

American Bar Association. (2020). *Steps in a trial*. https://www.americanbar.org/groups/public_education/resources/law_related_education_network/how_courts_work/casediagram/

Block, S. D., & Williams, L. M. (2019). *The prosecution of child sexual abuse: A partnership to improve outcomes: Final summary overview*. University of Massachusetts.

Bryant v. State of Texas, No. 01-09-00200-CR. (2010). https://caselaw.findlaw.com/tx-court-of-appeals/1535126.html

Butrus, N. (2018). Judicial sentencing considerations in cases of violent offenders versus sexual offenders. *Psychiatry, Psychology and Law, 25*(5), 653–674. https://doi.org/10.1080/13219719.2018.1473175

California Commission on Peace Officer Standards and Training. (1998). *Guidelines for the investigation of child physical abuse and neglect, child sexual abuse and exploitation*. file:///E:/FDU/Research/Grooming%20Book/Articles/Law%20Enforcement/Child_Abuse_Investigation%20-%20notes%20grooming.pdf

Canter, D., Hughes, D., & Kirby, S. (1998). Paedophilia: Pathology, criminality, or both? The development of a multivariate model of offence behaviour in child sexual abuse. *Journal of Forensic Psychiatry, 9*(3), 532–555. https://doi.org/10.1080/09585189808405372

Cunningham, K. C. (2020). Shame and guilt in PTSD. In *Emotion in posttraumatic stress disorder* (pp. 145–171). Academic Press. https://doi.org/10.1016/B978-0-12-816022-0.00006-5
Elliott, M., Browne, K., & Kilcoyne, J. (1995). Child sexual abuse prevention: What offenders tell us. *Child Abuse & Neglect, 19*(5), 579–579. https://doi.org/10.1016/0145-2134(95)00017-3
Federal Bureau of Investigation [FBI]. (2021). *Crime data explorer.* https://crime-data-explorer.fr.cloud.gov/
Jonzon, E., & Lindblad, F. (2004). Disclosure, reactions, and social support: Findings from a sample of adult victims of child sexual abuse. *Child Maltreatment, 9*, 190–200. https://doi.org/10.1177/1077559504264263
Krause v. State of Texas, No. 14–11–00884–CR. (2012). https://caselaw.findlaw.com/tx-court-of-appeals/1601524.html
Lanning, K. V. (2010). *Child molesters: A behavioral analysis* (5th ed.). National center for missing & exploited children.
Lanning, K. (2018). The evolution of grooming: Concept and term. *Journal of Interpersonal Violence, 33*(1), 5–16. https://doi.org/10.1177/0886260517742046
Lobanov-Rostovsky, C. (2015). *Adult sex offender management.* U.S. Department of Justice. https://smart.ojp.gov/sites/g/files/xyckuh231/files/media/document/adultsexoffendermanagement.pdf
London, K., Bruck, M., Ceci, S. J., & Shuman, D. W. (2005). Disclosure of child sexual abuse: What does the research tell us about ways that children tell? *Psychology, Public Policy, and Law, 11*, 194–226. https://doi.org/10.1037/1076-8971.11.1.194
London, K., Bruck, M., Wright, D. B., & Ceci, S. J. (2008). Review of the contemporary literature on how children report sexual abuse to others: Findings, methodological issues, and implications for forensic interviewers. *Memory, 16*, 29–47. https://doi.org/10.1080/09658219791725732
Lyon, T. D., & Ahern, E. C. (2010). Disclosure of child sexual abuse. In J. E. B. Myers (Ed.), *APSAC handbook on child maltreatment* (3rd ed., pp. 233–252). Sage Publications.
Manero, G. D. (2012). Introducing grooming as 'other acts' evidence. *National Center for Prosecution of Child Abuse, 23*(7), 1–4. http://www.ncdsv.org/images/NCPCA_IntroducingGroomingAsOtherActsEvidence_2012.pdf
Manson, D. A. (1984). *Tracking offenders – The child victim.* Bureau of Justice Statistics. https://www.bjs.gov/index.cfm/content/data/index.cfm?ty=pbdetail&iid=3521
Morris v. State of Texas, No. PD–0796–10. (2011). https://caselaw.findlaw.com/tx-court-of-criminal-appeals/1587579.html
National Center for Missing and Exploited Children [NCMEC]. (2017). *Map of registered sex offenders in the United States.* https://web.archive.org/web/20170717203105/; http://www.missingkids.com/en_US/documents/Sex_Offenders_Map.pdf
National Children's Advocacy Center. (2014). *Sexual abuse: Perpetrators, grooming, and prevention.* http://www.nationalcac.org/images/pdfs/LocalServices/Prevention/ForParents/PerpetratorInformation.pdf
Newlin, C., Steel, L. C., Chamberlin, A., Anderson, J., Kenniston, J., Russell, A., Stewart, H., & Vaughan-Eden, V. (2015). *Child forensic interviewing: Best practices.* Office of Juvenile Justice and Delinquency Prevention. file:///E:/FDU/Research/Grooming%20Book/Articles/Law%20Enforcement/Child%20Forensic%20Interviewing.pdf\
Office of the Attorney General. (1998). *Texas evidence collection protocol.* https://www.texasattorneygeneral.gov/sites/default/files/files/divisions/crime-victims/evidence_collection.pdf
Officers of the United States Attorneys. (n.d.). *Sentencing.* United States Department of Justice. https://www.justice.gov/usao/justice 101/sentencing
Snyder, H. N. (2000). *Sexual assault of young children as reported to law enforcement: Victim, incident, and offender characteristics.* A NIBRS Statistical Report. https://files.eric.ed.gov/fulltext/ED446834.pdf
State of Louisiana v. Vidrine, 9 So.3d 1095. (2009).
State of Oregon v. Henley, 422 P.3d 217, 363 Or. 284. (2018).
State of Washington v. Braham, 67 Wn. App. 930. (1992).

The Institute for Human Services. (2010). *Investigative interviewing in child sexual abuse cases.* http://www.pacwrc.pitt.edu/curriculum/203%20InvIntInCSA/Content/Final%20Content_2-10.pdf

U.S. Department of Justice. (2001). *Law enforcement response to child abuse.* file:///E:/FDU/Research/Grooming%20Book/Articles/Law%20Enforcement/zResponse%20to%20CA.pdf

United Nations Office of Drugs and Crime. (2017). *Trainers guide: Prosecuting & adjudicating cases of sexual exploitation of children.* https://www.unodc.org/documents/southeastasiaand-pacific/download/2017/PJ_SEC_Modules_1-4_3_August_2017_FINAL-03.pdf

United States Department of Justice. (1997). *Criminal investigation of child sexual abuse.* https://www.ojp.gov/pdffiles1/Digitization/162426NCJRS.pdf

United States v. Ghislaine Maxwell, 20-CR-330. (2021). https://s3.documentcloud.org/documents/21103204/maxwell-lisa-rocchio-111221.pdf

United States Sentencing Commission (2018). *Quick Facts - Sexual Abuse Offenders.* https://www.ussc.gov/sites/default/files/pdf/research-and-publications/quick-facts/Sexual_Abuse_FY18.pdf

Winters, G. M., & Jeglic, E. L. (2021). The Sexual Grooming Scale–Victim Version: The development and pilot testing of a measure to assess the nature and extent of child sexual grooming. *Victims & Offenders*, 1–22. https://doi.org/10.1080/15564886.2021.1974994

Winters, G. M., Colombino, N., Schaaf, S., Laake, A., Jeglic, E. L., & Calkins, C. (2020a). Why do child sexual abuse victims not tell anyone about their abuse? An exploration of factors that prevent and promote disclosure. *Behavioral Sciences & the Law, 38*(6), 586–611. https://doi.org/10.1002/bsl.2492

Winters, G. M., Jeglic, E. L., & Kaylor, L. E. (2020b). *Validation of the sexual grooming model of child sexual abusers.* Research, Treatment, & Program Innovations for Victims, Survivors, & Offenders. https://doi.org/10.1080/10538712.2020.1801935

Chapter 16
Sexual Grooming Legislation and Policy

To adequately protect individuals from sexual abuse, especially children, it is integral that we have the legal means in which to intervene before the sexual abuse begins. All states and the federal government have laws in place making the act of sexual abuse illegal. However, many of these laws pertain only to the sexual abuse once it has already occurred. While these types of laws are obviously needed to apprehend perpetrators and prevent further abuse, they do little to prevent sexual abuse before it occurs. Thus, individuals who are victimized are likely to experience the negative short- and long-term effects of abuse unless policies and legislation are put in place to prevent the abuse. Legislation targeting pre-abuse behaviors is starting to be developed and applied to cases involving sexual grooming, especially online sexual grooming. Given the role that sexual grooming plays in many cases of child sexual abuse (CSA; Canter et al., 1998; Winters & Jeglic, 2021) and potentially adult sexual abuse (see Chap. 12), this chapter will begin by discussing some of the challenges faced when developing sexual grooming legislation, followed by a review of current United States (US) Federal and State Enticement statutes, as well as international sexual grooming legislation. We will also review how sexual grooming may be applied in civil cases of sexual abuse. Then we will propose additional laws that can be used to prevent sexual grooming and conclude with a discussion of the development of future legislation and policies to prevent sexual grooming.

16.1 Challenges in Developing Sexual Grooming Legislation

Efforts to create anti-grooming legislation have been hampered by a number of issues. First and foremost, while there has been a general consensus in the clinical and research community that child sexual grooming is used in many cases of CSA, there has not been a consensus as to how child sexual grooming is defined and which behaviors and tactics comprise it (Bennett & O'Donohue, 2014). As described

© The Author(s), under exclusive license to Springer Nature Switzerland AG 2022

G. M. Winters, E. L. Jeglic, *Sexual Grooming*,
https://doi.org/10.1007/978-3-031-07222-2_16

in Chap. 3, there have been no fewer than one dozen definitions of sexual grooming put forth in the literature. Further, the characteristics of sexual grooming can differ based upon the age of the victim, the relationship between the victim and the perpetrator, and the context in which the abuse takes place (see Winters et al., 2021). Without a clear understanding of the construct of child sexual grooming, including specific observable behaviors and tactics, it has not been possible to develop legislation grounded in scientific principles. It has been our hope that with the development of the content-validated SGM (Winters et al., 2020) and the ensuing child sexual grooming definition (Winters et al., 2021), its stages, behaviors, and tactics can form the basis of future sexual grooming legislation.

Child sexual grooming behaviors differ by the setting and, thus, may be exhibited somewhat differently when they happen online versus in-person. As highlighted in Chap. 5, online sexual grooming follows many of the same patterns or stages as in-person sexual grooming; however, it tends to take place over a shorter period of time (Black et al., 2015: Marcum et al., 2007; Winters et al., 2017). Further, while some individuals seek to meet minors offline for sexual contact, others are seeking child sexual exploitation material (CSEM) or sexualized talk. As such, typologies of online offenders tend to reflect the goal of the sexual contact, such as obtaining or transmitting CSEM or engaging in sexual fantasy (i.e., sexual talk without the intention to meet; see Chap. 5; Briggs et al., 2011; DeHart et al., 2017; McLaughlin, 1998). Therefore, sexual grooming legislation must be broad enough to be able to capture behaviors exhibited both in online and in in-person cases of sexual grooming. Existing sexual grooming legislation primarily focuses on the online sexual solicitation of minors and does not encompass in-person sexual grooming (International Centre for Missing and Exploited Children [ICMEC], 2017). Some state enticement laws even stipulate that the Internet or electronic devices *must* be involved in the sexual grooming (e.g., Alaska, Minnesota).

One of the biggest issues with legislating pre-abuse behaviors is determining intent. To find someone guilty of sexual grooming before the abuse has occurred, it is necessary to prove to the courts that the individual had mens rea (translated from Latin to "guilty mind"), which means the individual intended to commit a crime, and actus reus (translated from Latin to "guilty act"), which means the wrongful behaviors that encompass the physical elements of the crime (Ezioni, 2020; Goodman-Delahunty & Martschuk, 2020; Kool, 2011). Many of the sexual grooming behaviors mimic normal and healthy adult-child interactions (Knoll, 2010; McAlinden, 2013). For example, an uncle playing childish games and tickling a young child can be a seen as a loving bonding moment between family members. However, when those same behaviors are exhibited with the desire to prepare the child for sexual abuse, then the once loving behaviors are now potentially criminal. However, it is often not until the abuse is perpetrated that we are able to see in hindsight that the behaviors were indicative of sexual grooming (Winters & Jeglic, 2016), and intent is nearly impossible to prove with some sexual grooming behaviors before the abuse has taken place (e.g., the individual is charming, nice, and likeable). However, as noted by Winters et al. (2020), intent is likely when these sexual grooming behaviors are seen in clusters, when there is a high frequency of the behaviors (e.g., constant tickling, sitting on lap, saying "I love you"), or the most severe behaviors (e.g., exposing their naked body to the child or the gradual increase of sexual touching) are observed. For instance, cases which have successfully prosecuted sexually grooming as a stand-alone crime have used the sexual touch and content behaviors from stage four of the SGM as the actus rea (*United States v. Chambers*, 2011).

16.2 Federal Enticement Statute

In the US, sex crimes can be prosecuted at the federal or state level. At the federal level, sexual grooming behaviors may be able to be prosecuted under the Federal Enticement Statute, which is section §2422 of the US Criminal Code. The US Federal Enticement Statue reads:

(a) Whoever knowingly persuades, induces, entices, or coerces any individual to travel in interstate or foreign commerce, or in any Territory or Possession of the United States, to engage in prostitution, or in any sexual activity for which any person can be charged with a criminal offense, or attempts to do so, shall be fined under this title or imprisoned not more than 20 years, or both.
(b) Whoever, using the mail or any facility or means of interstate or foreign commerce, or within the special maritime and territorial jurisdiction of the United States knowingly persuades, induces, entices, or coerces any individual who has not attained the age of 18 years, to engage in prostitution or any sexual activity for which any person can be charged with a criminal offense, or attempts to do so, shall be fined under this title and imprisoned not less than 10 years or for life.

On the surface, the Federal Enticement Statute appears to focus on individuals engaging in sex trafficking as it includes reference to interstate travel and prostitution. However, case law pertaining to section B determined that travel is *not* required if the minor is induced, enticed, or coerced into prostitution or sexual activity (*United States v. Nitschke*, 2011). The use of the words "induce," "entice," and "coerce" suggests that the minor is manipulated, lured, or pressured against their will to engage in the sexual behavior. These constructs are analogous to the manipulation seen in sexual grooming and, as such, could apply to cases of both in-person and online sexual grooming.

16.3 State Level Anti-grooming Legislation

In addition to the Federal Enticement Statute, approximately 42 US states have also developed their own anti-grooming legislation (Chetosky, 2019, Kaylor et al. 2022). Numerous states such as Alabama, Alaska, Connecticut, Florida, Idaho,

Illinois, Louisiana, Minnesota, Missouri, Nebraska, New Hampshire, New Mexico, North Carolina, Texas, Utah, and West Virginia all specify that the enticement, solicitation, or luring must involve the use of an electronic device, computer, Internet, or text messaging, meaning that the law may not encompass in-person sexual grooming. However, other states are vaguer in their language and use words such as "entice," "coerce," or even "groom" the child to engage in sexual activity (see Arkansas below). Further, some states use the word "attempt" when describing the sexual behavior, suggesting that the abuse does not yet have to occur for a crime to be committed (e.g., see Iowa). Below in Table 16.1 are several examples of state anti-grooming legislation that may apply both to online and in-person sexual grooming (see Kaylor et al. 2022 for a list of state grooming legislation).

What is clear after reviewing state legislation is that it is varied and there is little consistency across states. Further, some states, such as Washington, do not have legislation to address pre-offense behaviors at all, and thus, unless sexual abuse has occurred, the perpetrator cannot be charged (Sadler, 2018). Given that historically individuals who have used sexual grooming tactics to abuse minors and avoid detection have been known to move from one institution to another, often across state lines, it is important that there is consistency in the language of state anti-grooming legislation in order for it to be effective at preventing CSA and sexual grooming-based CSA in particular.

Table 16.1 Examples of state level grooming legislation

Arkansas Protection of Children Against Exploitation Act of 1979 § 5-27-307 – Sexually grooming a child.
(b) A person commits sexually grooming a child if he or she knowingly disseminates to a child thirteen (13) years of age or younger … visual or print medium depicting sexually explicit conduct with the purpose to entice, induce, or groom the child … to engage in the following with a person: (1) sexual intercourse; (2) sexually explicit conduct; or (3) deviate sexual activity.
Iowa Code § 728.12
1. It shall be unlawful to employ, use, persuade, induce, entice, coerce, solicit, knowingly permit, or otherwise cause or attempt to cause a minor to engage in a prohibited sexual act or in the simulation of a prohibited sexual act.
New York Consolidated Laws, Penal Law – PEN § 100.08 Criminal solicitation in the third degree
A person is guilty of criminal solicitation in the third degree when, being over eighteen years of age, with intent that another person under sixteen years of age … he solicits, … attempts to cause such other person to engage in such conduct.
Oregon ORS 167.057 – Luring a minor.
(1) If the person … uses with, a minor, a police officer posing as a minor or an agent of a police officer posing as a minor, a visual representation or explicit verbal description or narrative account of sexual conduct for the purpose of inducing the minor … to engage in sexual conduct.

16.4 International Sexual Grooming Legislation

Given the global reach of the Internet, the focus of international sexual grooming legislation has been on online sexual grooming and the transmission of CSEM. In 2017, the ICMEC published the findings of their study in which they examined national level legislation in 196 countries to determine whether it contained the following five characteristics of what model online sexual grooming legislation should encompass:

1. Exists with regard to the online grooming of children for sexual purposes;
2. Provides a definition of (or describes) grooming, including online grooming, and utilizes computer- and Internet-specific terminology;
3. Criminalizes online grooming, with the intent to meet the child offline;
4. Criminalizes online grooming, regardless of the intent to meet the child offline; and.
5. Criminalizes showing pornography to a child (p. 6; ICMEC, 2017).

Overall, they found that 63 countries had some sexual grooming legislation, and of those, 24 countries (including Argentina, Australia, Brazil, Colombia, Canada, France, Germany Ireland, Italy, Malaysia, Philippines, United Kingdom, and the US, among others) met all the aforementioned criteria. Of greater concern was that 133 countries had no legislation for online sexual grooming, with 82 other countries meeting none of the five criteria. While it is encouraging that countries from all areas of the globe are recognizing online sexual grooming, much work has yet to be done, and to our knowledge, there is no comprehensive review of international in-person sexual grooming legislation at this time.

16.5 Civil Litigation and Sexual Grooming

Civil litigation may also be pursued in cases involving sexual grooming under three conditions:

1. There were no criminal charges.
2. There were criminal charges, but the charges were dismissed, or the perpetrator was found not guilty.
3. There were criminal charges, and the individual was found guilty (Goguen, 2021).

Civil litigation differs from criminal prosecution in that the standard of proof is "preponderance of evidence" as opposed to "beyond a reasonable doubt" in criminal cases, and as such, plaintiffs are often more successful obtaining justice in civil court due to the lower standard of proof (Bublick, 2006). In civil litigation, plaintiffs can seek compensation for personal injury resulting from the CSA.

Civil courts may be particularly relevant for those experiencing sexual grooming on two fronts. First, it is possible to sue for damages inflicted by the sexual grooming behaviors themselves even if contact sexual abuse did not occur. Sexual grooming is defined as a manipulative, deceptive, and coercive process used to prepare the victim for sexual abuse (Craven et al., 2006; Winters et al., 2020). According to Wolf and Pruitt (2019, p. 347):

> As the perpetrator 'grooms' toward the goal of desensitizing victims and normalizing increasingly severe physical and psychological boundary violations (Bennett & O'Donohue, 2014), it is difficult for those being groomed to recognize the escalation and identify it as unhealthy. Similarly, for victims who once thrived on the affirming strategies, a shift in the process (i.e., withholding of gifts or attention, more vulgar sexual 'jokes,' 'accidental' touch or exposure, past consumption of drugs or alcohol now being used against them) may result in a sense of shame or guilt, which may lead them to question their own integrity, moral character, or responsibility in the offense. (Bennett & O'Donohue, 2014; McAlinden, 2006)

As described in Chap. 4 on the consequences of sexual grooming, such behaviors can constitute psychological abuse and maltreatment which the research literature links to depression, anxiety, suicidal ideation, and post-traumatic stress disorder among youth (Arslan, 2016). Second, some cases of sexual abuse involve sexual grooming that takes place within the context of child-serving organizations (i.e., schools, athletic clubs, religious organizations). In some of these cases, the perpetrator was able to take advantage of institutional failure to have adequate policies and procedures in place to protect the minor from CSA, and thus, the institution can be held liable for the damages incurred to the minor (Bublick, 2014; Moran, 2019).

16.6 Legislation That Can Help Prevent Grooming

Following the revelations of the breath and scope of institutional CSA (see Chap. 8), many organizations and state governments passed laws to mandate the reporting of cases of suspected CSA as well as to better screen for those at risk of engaging in CSA, which will be reviewed in further depth below.

16.6.1 Mandatory Reporting of Child Sexual Abuse

As the problem of CSA was beginning to be recognized in the 1960s, the US was the first country to begin passing Mandatory Child Abuse Reporting Laws for designated individuals between 1963 and 1967 (Mathews & Kenny, 2008). In 2007, the International Society for Prevention of Child Abuse and Neglect surveyed 161 countries globally about child abuse reporting legislation, and at that time, of the 72 countries that responded, 29 had mandatory policies in place while 12 indicated they had voluntary reporting by professionals (Daro, 2007). In the US, the mandated reporters vary by state, but educators, psychologists, and medical doctors are all mandated reporters. While these policies are not specific to sexual grooming, they do enable individuals to report people who may be engaging in sexual grooming behaviors before the abuse has occurred without fear of reprisal. As with every other policy, there are failings and loopholes such as teen sexual activity; however, at minimum, such a report can trigger an investigation that can alert guardians and institutions of potential risks that this individual may pose to minors (Mathews & Kenny, 2008).

16.6.2 Mandatory Background Checks

Many of these laws have been applied to educational settings as they fall under the authority of the states. In 1993, then President Bill Clinton passed the National Child Protection Act (NCPA), which permitted states to enact legislation to facilitate criminal background checks, which could include mandatory or voluntary fingerprinting for those that work with minors (NCPA, 1993). Subsequently, most states established laws requiring public school teachers to be fingerprinted and undergo background checks for employment and certification (Buschmann, 2002). The goal of fingerprinting was so that educators who had allegations or charges of misconduct could not alter their identities and obtain employment in another district or state. However, some states enacted legislation only requiring the fingerprinting for certification or first-time employment (Buschmann, 2002), while others left the background checks to the districts, unintentionally creating a loophole as district level background checks can be incomplete, inconsistent, or absent altogether (Kelly, 2017). Regarding sexual grooming, mandatory background checks and fingerprinting can help to identify those who were previously charged or convicted of CSA or CSA-related behaviors and, in many cases, were using their access to child-serving organizations, such as schools, to gain access to minors.

16.6.3 "Pass the Trash" Legislation

A limitation of background checks and fingerprinting is that they only identify individuals that have already been charged with and/or convicted of a crime. However, sexual abuse is the most underreported crime, and 95% of all new sex offenses are committed by someone who is not on the sex offender registry (Sandler et al., 2008). In investigating many historical cases of sexual misconduct within educational settings, it was found that when allegations of boundary violations or CSA came to the attention of the administration, educators were often permitted to resign instead of being investigated. Thus, when new potential employers called for references, they were only told the dates that the individual was employed there—a practice that has been dubbed "pass the trash" (Grant et al., 2019). This enabled individuals who were engaging in sexual grooming to move to a new district and begin anew with a clean slate, their history of misconduct unbeknownst to their new employers. To overcome this significant problem, in 2015, then President Barack Obama signed the Every Student Succeeds Act, which contained the "prohibition on aiding and abetting sexual abuse." This law mandates educational institutions to report allegations of educational misconduct to the appropriate authorities (ESSA, 2015). The law further encourages schools not to enter into confidential agreements with teachers who have allegations of misconduct (Grant et al., 2019). This led state legislators in Pennsylvania, New Jersey, Connecticut, Nevada, Washington, Oregon, and Maryland to enact "pass the trash" legislation, which makes it illegal for school districts to engage in such practices (Grant et al., 2019; sesamenet.org, n.d.). In addition, given that schools are governed by the states, a national database of educator misconduct was created by the National Association of State Directors of Teacher Education and Certification (NASDTEC) where districts could report cases of educator misconduct that would be available to schools across the country. However, Kelly (2017) found that since the database is voluntary, it is not complete (Grant et al., 2019).

16.7 Development of Future Legislation and Policies to Prevent Sexual Grooming

As described in this chapter, while there is some legislation both in the US and internationally to address sexual grooming, much work is left to be done. Existing legislation is primarily focused on online sexual grooming or sex trafficking, and there is little clear legislation that can be applied to in-person sexual grooming before the contact sexual abuse takes place. While there may be some recourse for victims in civil court, the goal is to have policies and laws in place to prevent the sexual abuse before it occurs, and this is precisely where properly formed anti-sexual grooming legislation can be helpful.

ICMEC (2017) proposes several components of model online grooming legislation that can also be applied to laws addressing in-person sexual grooming that broadly focuses on (1) definition, (2) offenses, and (3) sanctions and sentencing:

1. Define what is meant by child/minor: As was evidenced in the state legislation, the definition of a minor and age of consent varies from state to state, and there is even more variability between countries. ICMEC proposes that for online legislation, a child should be defined as "any person under the age of 18" (p. 9).
2. Define the act of grooming, including online grooming: As was noted at the onset of this chapter, you can only prosecute a known construct, meaning that it has to be defined. However, all aspects of the legislation must be explicit and based upon observable characteristics, tactics, and behaviors of sexual grooming. We believe that the SGM and its ensuing definition can be used as the basis with which to craft more clearly defined sexual grooming legislation.
3. Incorporate grooming and online grooming into the penal code: As was observed with the US state laws, grooming is rarely explicitly legislated; instead, it is

either criminal based upon case law or requires "reading between the lines" to make the sexual grooming behaviors fit the written legislation instead of the other way around.

4. Criminalize the process of online grooming (and in-person grooming): ICMEC highlights that until recently, sexual grooming is considered to be part of the process of CSA instead of a stand-alone entity. As such, they advocate for making the sexual grooming behaviors themselves a crime regardless of whether contact sexual abuse or the transmission of CSEM takes place. They further specify that online grooming should be grooming regardless of whether the intent was to meet the child and that showing pornography to a child should also be illegal.
5. They also propose several guidelines for punishment and sentencing including:
   (a) Punishing parents or legal guardians who participate in the grooming of a child under their care.
   (b) Punishing online sexual grooming as a stand-alone offense.
   (c) Providing extraterritorial jurisdiction for sexual abuse committed against children.
   (d) Not holding the child criminally liable for their involvement with online grooming offenders.
   (e) Establish minimum sentence for those who engage in grooming.
   (f) Enhance penalties for repeat offenders and aggravating factors.

In addition to these guidelines, policies and laws for individuals and institutions who interact with minors must be strengthened in line with the current research and knowledge on CSA perpetration generally and sexual grooming specifically. Further, these policies and laws need to be standardized and have a shared understanding of the behaviors and tactics that those who offend against children use to groom them so that this information can be easily disseminated to employees, guardians, and those who investigate allegations of CSA.

16.8 Conclusion

As described in this chapter, legislation currently exists that may be applied to sexual grooming such as Federal and State Enticement statutes and international online grooming laws. However, these laws are limited as they lack a consistent and research based definition of sexual grooming, and they do not clearly apply to in-person sexual grooming considering that many laws reference travel or the use of electronic devices/computers. Further, at present, it would be difficult to prove intent without contact CSA, and thus, these laws are limited in their ability to prevent abuse. While there may be some recourse for individuals in civil court as there is a different burden of proof, we know little about how sexual grooming is being applied. As the body of knowledge about sexual grooming continues to expand, this knowledge needs to be integrated into legislation to create evidence-based anti-grooming laws that can be used to prevent sexual abuse and prosecute perpetrators.

References

Arkansas Protection of Children Against Exploitation Act of 1979, AR Code § 5-27-307. (2017). https://law.justia.com/codes/arkansas/2017/title-5/subtitle-3/chapter-27/subchapter-3/section-5-27-307/

Arslan, G. (2016). Psychological maltreatment, emotional and behavioral problems in adolescents: The mediating role of resilience and self-esteem. *Child Abuse & Neglect, 52*, 200–209. https://doi.org/10.1016/j.chiabu.2015.09.010

Bennett, N., & O'Donohue, W. (2014). The construct of grooming in child sexual abuse: Conceptual and measurement issues. *Journal of Child Sexual Abuse, 23*(8), 957–976. https://doi.org/10.1080/10538712.2014.960632

Black, P. J., Wollis, M., Woodworth, M., & Hancock, J. T. (2015). A linguistic analysis of grooming strategies of online child sex offenders: Implications for our understanding of predatory sexual behavior in an increasingly computer-mediated world. *Child Abuse & Neglect, 44*, 140–149. https://doi.org/10.1016/j.chiabu.2014.12.004

Briggs, P., Simon, W. T., & Simonsen, S. (2011). An exploratory study of internet-initiated sexual offenses and the chat room sex offender: Has the internet enabled a new typology of sex offender? *Sexual Abuse: Journal of Research and Treatment, 23*(1), 72–91. https://doi.org/10.1177/1079063210384275

Bublick, E. M. (2006). Tort suits filed by rape and sexual assault victims in civil courts: Lessons for courts, classrooms and constituencies. *SMU Law Review, 59*(1), 55. https://scholar.smu.edu/smulr/vol59/iss1/3

Bublick, E. M. (2014). Who is responsible for child sexual abuse – A view from the Penn State scandal. *Journal of Gender Race & Justice, 17*(2), 297–312.

Buschman, C. (2002). Mandatory fingerprinting of public school teachers: Facilitating background checks or infringing on individuals' constitutional rights. *William & Mary Bill of Rights Journal, 11*(3), 1273. https://scholarship.law.wm.edu/cgi/viewcontent.cgi?referer=https://www.google.com/&httpsredir=1&article=1298&context=wmborj

Canter, D., Hughes, D., & Kirby, S. (1998). Paedophilia: Pathology, criminality, or both? The development of a multivariate model of offence behaviour in child sexual abuse. *The Journal of Forensic Psychiatry, 9*(3), 532–555. https://doi.org/10.1080/09585189808405372

Chetosky, K. K. (2019). Minnesota v. Muccio: The Constitutionality of Minnesota's Sexual Grooming Law. *Northwestern University Law Review. Online, 114*, 1.

Craven, S., Brown, S., & Gilchrist, E. (2006). Sexual grooming of children: Review of literature and theoretical considerations. *Journal of Sexual Aggression, 12*(3), 287–299. https://doi.org/10.1080/13552600601069414

Daro, D. (Ed.). (2007). *World perspectives on child abuse* (7th ed.). International Society for Prevention of Child Abuse and Neglect.

DeHart, D., Dwyer, G., Seto, M. C., Moran, R., Letourneau, E., & Schwarz-Watts, D. (2017). Internet sexual solicitation of children: A proposed typology of offenders based on their chats, e-mails, and social network posts. *Journal of Sexual Aggression, 23*(1), 77–89. https://doi.org/10.1080/13552600.2016.1241309

Every Student Succeeds Act of. (2015). Pub. L. No. 114-95 § 114 Stat. 1177 (2015–2016), 114th Congress: Every Student Succeeds Act.

Ezioni, L. (2020). The crime of grooming. *Child & Family Law Journal, 8*(1). https://lawpublications.barry.edu/cflj/vol8/iss1/1

Federal Enticement Statute, 18 U.S.C. § 2422. https://www.law.cornell.edu/uscode/text/18/2422#:~:text=Whoever%20knowingly%20persuades%2C%20induces%2C%20entices,to%20do%20so%2C%20shall%20be

Goguen, D. (2021). *Filing a civil lawsuit for child sexual abuse.* https://www.alllaw.com/articles/nolo/personal-injury/filing-civil-lawsuit-child-sexual-abuse.html

Goodman-Delahunty, J., & Martschuk, N. (2020). Mock jury and juror responses to uncharged acts of sexual misconduct. *Zeitschrift für Psychologie, 228*(3), 199–209. https://doi.org/10.1027/2151-2604/a000410

Grant, B. J., Wilkerson, S., & Henschel, M. (2019). Passing the trash: Absence of state laws allows for continued sexual abuse of K–12 students by school employees. *Journal of Child Sexual Abuse, 28*(1), 84–104. https://doi.org/10.1080/10538712.2018.1483460

International Centre for Missing and Exploited Children [ICMEC] (2017). *Online grooming of children for sexual purposes: Model legislation & global review.* https://www.icmec.org/wp-content/uploads/2017/09/Online-Grooming-of-Children_FINAL_9-18-17.pdf

Kaylor, L. E., Winters, G. M., Jeglic, E. L., & Cilli, J. (2022). An analysis of child sexual grooming legislation in the United States. *Psychology, Crime & Law*, 1–19.

Kelly, J. (2017, October, 23). How USA TODAY graded the states on teacher background checks. *USA Today.* https://www.usatoday.com/story/news/2016/02/14/how-we-graded-states-teacher-background-checks/80214540/

Knoll, J. (2010). Teacher sexual misconduct: Grooming patterns and female offenders. *Journal of Child Sexual Abuse, 19*(4), 371–386. https://doi.org/10.1080/10538712.2010.495047

Kool, R. (2011). Prevention by all means – A legal comparison of the criminalization of online grooming and its enforcement. *Utrecht Law Review, 7*(3), 46–69. https://doi.org/10.18352/ulr.171

Luring a Minor, OR Rev Stat § 167.057. (2011). https://law.justia.com/codes/oregon/2011/vol4/167/167-057/#:~:text=(1)%20A%20person%20commits%20the,to%20engage%20in%20sexual%20conduct

Marcum, C. D. (2007). Interpreting the intentions of internet predators: An examination of online predatory behavior. *Journal of Child Sexual Abuse: Research, Treatment, & Program Innovations For Victims, Survivors, & Offenders, 16*(4), 99–114. https://doi.org/10.1300/J070v16n04_06

Mathews, B., & Kenny, M. C. (2008). Mandatory reporting legislation in the United States, Canada, and Australia: A cross-jurisdictional review of key features, differences, and issues. *Child Maltreatment, 13*(1), 50–63. https://doi.org/10.1177/1077559507310613

McAlinden, A. M. (2006). Setting 'Em up': Personal, familial and institutional grooming in the sexual abuse of children. *Social & Legal Studies, 15*(3), 339–362. https://doi.org/10.1177/0964663906066613

McAlinden, A. M. (2013). 'Grooming' and the sexual abuse of children: Implications for sex offender assessment, treatment and management. *Sexual Offender Treatment, 8*(1) http://www.sexual-offender-treatment.org/118.html

McLaughlin, J. (1998). Technophilia: A modern day paraphilia. *Knight stick, 51*(Spring/Summer 98), 47–51. https://www.iletsbeiforumjournal.com/images/Issues/FreeIssues/ILEEF%202002-2.3.pdf

Moran, M. (2019). Cardinal sins: How the Catholic Church sexual abuse crisis changed private Law. *Georgetown Journal of Gender & the Law, 21*, 95. https://www.law.georgetown.edu/gender-journal/wp-content/uploads/sites/20/2020/01/Article-4.pdf

National Child Protection Act of 1993, Pub. L. No. 103–209, § 3, 107 Stat. 2490,2491.

New York Consolidated Laws, Penal Law, PEN § 100.08. https://codes.findlaw.com/ny/penal-law/pen-sect-100-08.html

Sadler, S. R. (2018). *"Communication with a minor for immoral purposes" what Washington state law is not talking about.* Master's thesis, University of Washington Bothell.

Sandler, J. C., Freeman, N. J., & Socia, K. M. (2008). Does a watched pot boil? A time series analysis of New York State's sex offender registration and notification law. *Psychology, Public Policy, and Law, 14*(4), 284. https://doi.org/10.1037/a0013881

Sesamenet.org. (n.d.). *S.E.S.A.M.E stop educator sexual abuse misconduct and exploitation.* https://www.sesamenet.org/legislation

Sexual Exploitation of a Minor, Iowa Code § 728.12. https://www.legis.iowa.gov/docs/ico/section/728.12.pdf

United States v. Chambers, 642 F.3d 588, 592 (7th Cir. 2011).

United States v. Nitschke, 843 F. Supp. 2d 4 (D.D.C. 2011).

Winters, G. M., & Jeglic, E. L. (2016). I knew it all along: The sexual grooming behaviors of child molesters and the hindsight bias. *Journal of Child Sexual Abuse, 25*(1), 20–36. https://doi.org/10.1080/10538712.2015.1108945

Winters, G. M., & Jeglic, E. L. (2021). The sexual grooming scale–victim version: The development and pilot testing of a measure to assess the nature and extent of child sexual grooming. *Victims & Offenders*, 1–22. https://doi.org/10.1080/15564886.2021.1974994

Winters, G. M., Kaylor, L. E., & Jeglic, E. L. (2017). Sexual offenders contacting children online: An examination of transcripts of sexual grooming. *Journal of Sexual Aggression, 23*(1), 62–76. https://doi.org/10.1080/13552600.2016.1271146

Winters, G. M., Jeglic, E. L., & Kaylor, L. E. (2020). Validation of the sexual grooming model of child sexual abusers. *Journal of Child Sexual Abuse: Research, Treatment, & Program Innovations for Victims, Survivors, & Offenders*. https://doi.org/10.1080/10538712.2020.1801935

Winters, G. M., Kaylor, L. E., & Jeglic, E. L. (2021). Toward a universal definition of child sexual grooming. *Deviant Behavior*, 1–13. https://doi.org/10.1080/01639625.2021.1941427

Wolf, M. R., & Pruitt, D. K. (2019). Grooming hurts too: The effects of types of perpetrator grooming on trauma symptoms in adult survivors of child sexual abuse. *Journal of Child Sexual Abuse, 28*(3), 345–359. https://doi.org/10.1080/10538712.2019.1579292

Chapter 17
Conclusion

Sexual grooming has been deemed "a ubiquitous feature of the sexual abuse of children" (Thornton, 2003, p. 144). We have argued throughout this book that given that these observable behaviors largely occur *before* the sexual abuse occurs, they can serve as an integral factor in the prevention, investigation, prosecution, assessment, and treatment of sexual offenses. If we can better understand the pre-offense tactics that might be used during the offense process, preventative efforts (e.g., educational materials, organizational policies, legislation) can incorporate this construct in order to identify "red flags" before the abuse happens. Moreover, if a case of child sexual abuse (CSA) is identified and reported, we feel it is important to have law enforcement and court personnel who thoroughly understand the offense process (including before and after the actual abuse) to investigate and prosecute these cases most effectively. We must also have clinical assessment and treatment strategies that are informed by the research on sexual grooming, especially if these behaviors are indeed integral to the sexual abuse process. All of these aforementioned implications highlight why we believe it is vitally important to understand the sexual grooming behaviors of those who commit child sexual offenses. Ultimately, these reasons led us to write this book.

What we find to be troubling is that despite the importance of understanding sexual grooming, there has been a significant lack of empirical research and literature on the subject—both in quality and quantity. We suggest this may be a product of various factors, including the lack of agreement regarding a proper definition and model of the construct, inconsistent methods of operationalizing and measuring sexual grooming, and difficulty differentiating these behaviors from normative adult/child interactions. With these obstacles in mind, in this book, we sought to synthesize the literature on sexual grooming while also drawing upon related constructs to provide a broad yet comprehensive examination of sexual grooming.

Chapters 1, 2, 3 and 4 included an overview of what is known about sexual grooming more generally, such as the proposed definitions and models of the construct as well as the consequences of victimization. In Chaps. 2 and 3, we argued

© The Author(s), under exclusive license to Springer Nature Switzerland AG 2022

G. M. Winters, E. L. Jeglic, *Sexual Grooming*,
https://doi.org/10.1007/978-3-031-07222-2_17

that numerous definitions and models of a single construct can cause confusion and disagreement across various fields—which led us to develop a content-validated model of sexual grooming (Sexual Grooming Model [SGM], Winters et al., 2020) along with a definition based on this model (Winters et al., 2021). We hope that this parsimonious, yet comprehensive, model and definition can serve as a basis for future research and practice related to sexual grooming. Subsequently, in Chap. 4, we described the potential consequences of sexual grooming for the child (e.g., less likely to disclose; trauma symptoms; increased shame, guilt, and fear), family (e.g., feeling of guilt, emotional distress, familial discord), and institutions/community (e.g., community distrust or anger, lawsuits), which supports the need to better understand sexual grooming in order to prevent such outcomes.

In Chaps. 5, 6, 7 and 8, we addressed different types of sexual grooming, including online, self, familial and community, and institutional grooming. Chapter 5 outlines various models of the online sexual grooming process, many of which mirror the stages in the SGM; we suggest that developing a more parsimonious and easily understood model of online sexual grooming might help bring cohesiveness to that line of research. We then described in Chap. 6 how the construct of self-grooming is seemingly analogous to terms previously proposed in the literature (e.g., neutralization techniques, cognitive distortions, implicit theories of sexual offending, overcoming internal barriers to offending), which broadly suggests a person seeking to commit CSA may progress through self-grooming stages including (1) preparation, (2) justification, and (3) maintenance. Subsequently, Chaps. 7 and 8 identified how the person seeking to commit the offense may sexually groom not only the child but also the child's family, community, and institutions (e.g., religious and education settings, sporting organizations, and youth-serving organizations).

Chapters 9, 10, 11 and 12 examined how sexual grooming may be utilized by specific populations (i.e., women, sex traffickers, juveniles, adults seeking to offend against other adults). While very little is known about how sexual grooming patterns may be unique to these different groups, the literature nonetheless suggests that pre-offense behaviors may indeed be observed by a range of people seeking to commit sexual offenses. However, we stress that additional research is needed to better understand the nuances of sexual grooming utilized by these different populations.

Finally, Chaps. 13, 14, 15 and 16 evaluated how sexual grooming can be used in different contexts—such as assessment and treatment, preventative efforts, law enforcement and courts, and legislation. In Chap. 13, we address the proposed measures to assess for sexual grooming, including our recently published measure the *Sexual Grooming Scale-Victim Version* (*SGS-V*; Winters et al., 2021) based upon the SGM; we also stressed the importance of incorporating sexual grooming into the treatment of both those who committed CSA as well as those who were victimized. Chapter 14 included our analysis of how prevention of CSA can be informed by sexual grooming, including in institutional and online settings. Lastly, in Chaps. 15 and 16, we argued that law enforcement and the courts can benefit from sexual grooming-informed practices and that the criminalization of sexual grooming behaviors is vital to stopping CSA before it occurs.

17.1 The Next Steps Forward

While significant progress has been made in the past five years to describe, quantify, and measure sexual grooming, writing this book has highlighted how much we still do not know. As such, there are logical next steps in terms of research, education, treatment, detection, prosecution, and policy that we hope will be spurred from this book.

17.1.1 Research

As this project developed, we often found ourselves with more questions than answers, and we have developed a long list of research questions that we need to address. Some are currently underway, and some are planned for the future as described below:

1. *Further Validation of the Sexual Grooming Model (SGM;* Winters et al., 2020*) and the SGS-V (*Winters & Jeglic, 2021*)*. While both the SGM and *SGS-V* have been a big step forward in terms of our ability to identify specific stages and behaviors related to child sexual grooming, both the model and the measure require further validation. We are currently in the process of testing the validity of the model in a large sample of adults who have experienced CSA. We are also testing additional psychometric properties (including validity and reliability) of the *SGS-V*.
2. *The Identification of Sexual Grooming Behaviors That Are Most Indicative of Sexual Abuse*. As noted throughout this book, one of the difficulties in identifying child sexual grooming before it happens is that on the surface, many of the child sexual grooming behaviors appear to be the same as normal and healthy adult/child interactions, but their underlying intent is nefarious (Knoll, 2010; McAlinden, 2013). It is the ambiguity of the intent of these behaviors that aides the perpetrator in avoiding detection as the behaviors are either not identified or, if they do arouse suspicion, they are often explained away or minimized. So to prevent both CSA and false allegations against someone who is simply behaving in a caring manner, we must identify which specific grooming behaviors differentiate caring adults from perpetrators. We are currently attempting to do so by comparing the endorsement of sexual grooming behaviors as listed in the *SGS-V* between adults who have experienced CSA and adults who have not. We are asking those who did not experience CSA to complete the *SGS-V* describing their interactions with the closest adult male in their lives who is not their father. We hope that in doing so, we will be able to identify which sexual grooming behaviors may be uniquely predictive of CSA.
3. *Investigate Adult Sexual Grooming*. As described in Chap. 12, the term sexual grooming has been used in popular culture to describe the behaviors and tactics of those who perpetrate adult sexual abuse. While there are some constructs that

are similar to sexual grooming, such as sexual coercion, coercive control, and sexual harassment, that have been studied as they pertain to adult sexual abuse, to the best of our knowledge, there is no qualitative or quantitative research examining sexual grooming behaviors as they pertain to adult sexual abuse. As such, we are about to embark on a mixed methods study examining the presence of sexual grooming behaviors among a large sample of adults who have experienced unwanted sexual contact as adults. The results of this study will help to form the basis of future inquiries into sexual grooming or grooming-like behaviors exhibited by those who abuse adults.
4. *Investigate Female and Juvenile Sexual Grooming*. There is increasing evidence and awareness that women and juveniles can perpetrate sexual abuse and that it may be more prevalent than previously believed. In Chaps. 9 and 11, we discussed what is known about female- and juvenile-perpetrated sexual abuse and the sexual grooming behaviors that may be exhibited by these populations. However, the extant research remains largely theoretical, and thus, we aim to explore females' and juveniles' sexual grooming behaviors and the contexts within which they are used.
5. *Study Characteristics of Sexual Grooming for Unique Populations and Contexts*. As the characteristics of sexual grooming may differ based upon the traits of the victim, perpetrator, and situation, it is important to study sexual grooming across a number of different contexts and groups. For example, as described in Chap. 8, there is evidence that priests within the Catholic Church employed reverential fear and religious duress as grooming tactics that would be unique to their position and the religious setting (see Spraitz and Bowen, 2019). Further, as described in Chap. 10, sexual grooming within the context of sex trafficking may have some unique features. Thus, our goal is to examine the SGM and its related behaviors and tactics across different contexts, such as those who have been abused by clergy, victims of sex trafficking, those who have been abused within the context of sport, and children abused in the Boy Scouts of America. We also seek to examine how these behaviors may differ depending upon the age and gender of the victim and their relationship to the perpetrator.

This is not a comprehensive list of all the research needed going forward but rather a road map as we anticipate that as each project is completed, it will provide some answers and likely many more questions for further exploration.

17.1.2 Education

Most youth-serving organizations now require child abuse prevention training for staff, and states require mandated reporter training for licensed professionals that work with minors. While training staff is an integral component of comprehensive sexual abuse prevention policies, the content of the training is crucial. In a review of state-based mandated reporter training, Baker et al. (2021) concluded that in general, the existing state-based trainings are not presenting comprehensive definitions, examples, and indicators of the major types of child maltreatment, including sexual abuse. Further, there was almost no mention of sexual grooming behaviors or tactics, (only 11% of the trainings mentioned grooming) and the focus of the training materials was on identifying indications of abusive behaviors perpetrated by the minor's parent or guardian and not on identifying abusive behaviors that may be exhibited by staff who work with minors. Understanding and identifying sexual grooming tactics and behaviors are crucial to preventing CSA before it happens as almost all cases of CSA involve at least some elements of sexual grooming (Winters & Jeglic, 2021). As such, all state-based and organizational child maltreatment and sexual abuse prevention trainings must contain research-based information on the stages and behaviors involved in the sexual grooming process and how these may be manifested by employees within child-serving organizations.

While trainings take place in the context of work settings, parents and children are often left out. Arguably, since parents/guardians are the gatekeepers to their children, they should be prioritized when it comes to teaching about sexual abuse prevention (Steedman et al., in submission). While it is incumbent upon parents to protect their children, parents can also be groomed, as described in Chap. 7 on familial grooming. Thus, it is important to teach children what to do if an adult behaves in a way that makes them uncomfortable. Given that all children must attend school, the school is the most logical setting through which these trainings should occur, and they can be incorporated in back-to-school nights or educational outreach.

17.1.3 Treatment

Chapter 13 highlights the role of sexual grooming in treatment. It is vital that clinicians who provide services to both those who engage in sexual abuse and those who have experienced sexual abuse are knowledgeable about sexual grooming behaviors and tactics and how to incorporate this knowledge into their work. As discussed in Chap. 6, it remains unclear whether sexual grooming is a conscious process or not, and thus, it is important to help the individual recognize the sexual grooming behaviors they have used as part of their offense chain and work with them to integrate these high-risk grooming behaviors into their self-management plan.

For those who work with individuals who have experienced CSA, as discussed in Chap. 4, it is important to understand how sexual grooming may impact their clients. There is some evidence to suggest that sexual grooming may negatively exacerbate the long-term impact of CSA (Wolf & Pruitt, 2019), which highlights the need for providers to recognize the role that sexual grooming may play in the early detection and reporting of CSA as well as how the manipulation involved in sexual grooming can create long-lasting feelings of guilt and shame. Working with the client to understand that they were sexually groomed helps the client to recognize that the abuse was not their fault; that is, they and those around them were sexually groomed, and the only fault lies with the perpetrator.

17.1.4 Investigation and Prosecution

Equipping law enforcement and legal professionals with up-to-date information about sexual grooming is essential for the detection and prosecution of sexual grooming-based sexual abuse. Understanding the sexual grooming behaviors and tactics employed by those who sexually offend can help in the investigation and prosecution of sexual abuse. Checklists for law enforcement to use as part of their interrogations can help to form the basis of the cases. Access to expert witnesses who can explain sexual grooming behaviors to juries can help lawyers successfully build and prosecute perpetrators (see Kaylor et al., 2022).

17.1.5 Policy

Preventing CSA is incumbent upon legislation and policy. Legislation targeting pre-abuse behaviors such as sexual grooming can prevent CSA before it occurs. However, in order for grooming legislation to be effective, ICMEC (2017) recommends that a clear definition is needed. Chapter 16 highlights the challenges and inconsistencies of existing legislation as it pertains to sexual grooming. Going forth, sexual grooming, both in person and online, regardless of whether it results in a contact offense or the transmission of child sexual abuse material, needs to be made into a crime onto itself. To achieve this, legislation needs to be clear and consistent across jurisdictions and based upon the current research literature.

17.2 Concluding Remarks

The writing of this book involves both a culmination and a beginning. On one hand, it represents the culmination of years of work and is the most current comprehensive resource on sexual grooming. On the other hand, this book is really a beginning since, as we highlighted throughout the text, there is very little empirical evidence about sexual grooming. We have also identified areas in which other constructs may be related and intertwined with the sexual grooming literature, which may help shed light on the construct of sexual grooming. Ultimately, this book sets the foundation for the future empirical study of sexual grooming. The interest and research on sexual grooming have been proliferating rapidly, and we hope that in a few short years, many of the gaping holes we have identified will have answers. Most importantly, we hope that this book provides the information about sexual grooming needed for individuals, families, communities, practitioners, administrators, institutions, and policy-makers to better detect, prosecute, and most importantly prevent sexual abuse.

References

Baker, A. J., LeBlanc, S., Adebayo, T., & Mathews, B. (2021). Training for mandated reporters of child abuse and neglect: Content analysis of state-sponsored curricula. *Child Abuse & Neglect, 113*(104932). https://doi.org/10.1016/j.chiabu.2021.104932

International Centre for Missing and Exploited Children [ICMEC]. (2017). *Online grooming of children for sexual purposes: Model legislation & global review*. https://www.icmec.org/wp-content/uploads/2017/09/Online-Grooming-of-Children_FINAL_9-18-17.pdf

Kaylor, L. E., Winters, G. M., Jeglic, E. L., & Cilli, J. (2022). An analysis of child sexual grooming legislation in the United States. *Psychology, Crime & Law,* 1–19. https://doi.org/10.1080/1068316X.2022.2043313

Knoll, J. (2010). Teacher sexual misconduct: Grooming patterns and female offenders. *Journal of Child Sexual Abuse, 19*(4), 371–386. https://doi.org/10.1080/10538712.2010.495047

McAlinden, A. M. (2013). 'Grooming' and the sexual abuse of children: Implications for sex offender assessment, treatment and management. *Sexual Offender Treatment, 8*(1) http://www.sexual-offender-treatment.org/118.html

Spraitz, J. D., & Bowen, K. N. (2019). Examination of a nascent taxonomy of priest sexual grooming. *Sexual Abuse, 31*(6), 707–728. https://doi.org/10.1177/1079063218809095

Steedman, L., Jeglic, E., & Winters, G. (in submission). Examining parental abilities to recognize sexual grooming behaviors of child sexual abusers.

Thornton, D. (2003). The Machiavellian sex offender. In A. Matravers (Ed.), *Sex offenders in the community: Managing and reducing the risks* (Cambridge Criminal Justice Series). Willan Publishing.

Winters, G. M., & Jeglic, E. L. (2021). The Sexual Grooming Scale–Victim Version: The development and pilot testing of a measure to assess the nature and extent of child sexual grooming. *Victims & Offenders*, 1–22. https://doi.org/10.1080/15564886.2021.1974994

Winters, G. M., Jeglic, E. L., & Kaylor, L. E. (2020). Validation of the sexual grooming model of child sexual abusers. *Journal of Child Sexual Abuse, 29*(7), 855–875. https://doi.org/10.1080/10538712.2020.1801935

Winters, G., Schaaf, S., Grydehoj, R., Allan, C., Lin, A., & Jeglic, E. (2021). The sexual grooming model of child sex trafficking. *Victims & Offenders*. https://doi.org/10.1080/15564886.2021.1926031

Wolf, M. R., & Pruitt, D. K. (2019). Grooming hurts too: the effects of types of perpetrator grooming on trauma symptoms in adult survivors of child sexual abuse. *Journal of Child Sexual Abuse, 28*(3), 345–359. https://doi.org/10.1080/10538712.2019.1579292

Index

© The Editor(s) (if applicable) and The Author(s), under exclusive license to Springer Nature Switzerland AG 2022
G. Winters, E. L. Jeglic, *Sexual Grooming*,
https://doi.org/10.1007/978-3-031-07222-2

I

J

L

M

N

O

P